Novel Antibacterial Biomaterials for Medical Applications and Modeling of Drug Release Process

This book provides a comprehensive review of synthesis and physicochemical and biological characterization of novel antibacterial biomaterials produced according to original procedures and aimed at medical applications such as wound dressing, soft and hard tissue implants, drug delivery devices, and carriers for cell cultivation. It is intended for all researchers working in the fields of biomaterials and biomedical engineering, as well as medical professionals, science and engineering graduate students, academics, and industrial researchers.

- Includes in-depth discussions on synthesis and physicochemical characterization of novel polyvinyl alcohol-based hydrogels aimed at wound dressings and soft tissue implants.
- Explores synthesis and physicochemical characterization of novel bioceramic hydroxyapatite-based coatings on metal surface aimed for hard tissue implants.
- Reviews cytotoxicity and antibacterial activity of novel polyvinyl alcohol-based hydrogels aimed for wound dressing and soft tissue implants.
- Discusses cytotoxicity and antibacterial activity of bioceramic hydroxyapatite-based coatings on metal surface aimed for hard tissue implants.
- Provides original fractional derivative models of drug release process from hydrogels and bioceramic coatings on metal surface and explores diffusion mechanism.

Vesna Mišković-Stanković is Professor at the Faculty of Ecology and Environmental Protection, University Union-Nikola Tesla, Belgrade, Serbia. She obtained her BSc, MSc, and PhD degrees in chemical engineering from the School of Technology and Metallurgy, University of Belgrade, Serbia, and postdoc fellowship from the University of Trento, Italy. She was Professor at the Faculty of Technology and Metallurgy, University of Belgrade. She was also Visiting Professor at the University of Trento, Italy; Ohio University, USA; Laval University, Canada; Shandong University, Jiangsu Normal University, and Fudan University, China; and Kyung Hee University, Seoul, South Korea. Her research activities include biomaterials, biomedicine, and electrochemistry. She is a member of the Academy of Engineering Sciences of Serbia and was listed among the top 2% of scientists in the world by Stanford University.

Teodor Atanackovic is Professor Emeritus at the Department of Mechanics, Faculty of Technical Sciences, University of Novi Sad, Serbia, and a member of the Serbian Academy of Arts and Sciences. He works in theoretical mechanics and the application of fractional kinetics in pharmacology and dentistry. He was listed among the top 2% of scientists in the world by Stanford University.

Novel Antibacterial Biomaterials for Medical Applications and Modeling of Drug Release Process

Vesna Mišković-Stanković
and Teodor Atanackovic

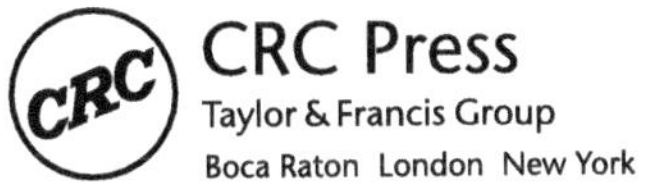

CRC Press
Taylor & Francis Group
Boca Raton London New York

CRC Press is an imprint of the
Taylor & Francis Group, an **informa** business

Designed cover image: Shutterstock

First edition published 2024
by CRC Press
2385 NW Executive Center Drive, Suite 320, Boca Raton FL 33431

and by CRC Press
4 Park Square, Milton Park, Abingdon, Oxon, OX14 4RN

CRC Press is an imprint of Taylor & Francis Group, LLC

ISBN: 978-1-032-66886-4 (hbk)
ISBN: 978-1-032-66887-1 (pbk)
ISBN: 978-1-032-66889-5 (ebk)

DOI: 10.1201/9781032668895

Typeset in Times
by Deanta Global Publishing Services, Chennai, India

Contents

Preface

This book provides a comprehensive overview of synthesis, physico-chemical, and biological characterization of novel antibacterial biomaterials produced according to original procedures for wound dressings, soft and hard tissue implants, drug delivery devices, and cell cultivation carriers. It focuses on recent advancements in alginate-based and poly(vinyl alcohol)-based hydrogels for wound dressings and soft tissue implants and in hydroxyapatite-based coatings for hard tissue implants, and it emphasizes fundamental concepts of biomaterials structure–property relationships, processing methods, and biological responses. The pharmacokinetics of drug release is of great importance in medical treatments; therefore, special attention is devoted to the modeling of the drug release process. Fractional-order models are found to be more adequate for compartmental analysis in many cases especially when, in a process under consideration, memory effects are pronounced. Applications of fractional calculus used for medical and health science are included. Mathematical results provide a solid basis for an accurate explanation of real-life problems.

State-of-the-art novel biomaterials design, synthesis, and testing and application of fractional calculus in the drug release process are written by experts at the forefront of interdisciplinary areas. Thus, the book is intended for research professionals and students in various research areas, including materials science and engineering, chemical engineering, polymer engineering, ceramic engineering, biomedical engineering, health care, medicine, pharmacy, and mathematics. It is recommended as an academic or a training text for various courses in biomaterials, tissue engineering, medical devices, implants, pharmacokinetics, fractional calculus, diffusion transport, etc.

This book aims to help readers both in academia and in industry to better understand advanced biomaterials for medical treatments and relevant related technologies. A discussion of the utility of different biomaterial types for creating the optimal fabrication is provided. Finally, current trends influencing the future of advanced biomaterial sectors for human and veterinary medical devices in pharmaceutical industry are highlighted.

The authors wish to thank the collaborators who contributed to the experimental results presented in this book. Their names are provided in publications listed in the references.

November 2023
Belgrade, Novi Sad, Serbia

Vesna Mišković-Stanković
Teodor Atanackovic

1 Introduction

Biomaterials are interesting in tissue engineering and wound dressing because of their advantages, including controlled chemical composition, thickness and morphology, "green"- producing technology without using harmful chemical agents, controlled release of a long-lasting antibacterial agent, and local *in situ* use of an antibacterial agent instead of systemic antibiotic treatment to avoid bacterial resistance. Numerous problems associated with infections could occur in the postoperative recovery period of patients after surgery, injuries, or various diseases when systemic antibiotics administration could lead to bacterial resistance due to long-term use of antibiotics. Topical application of antibacterial agents is usually more convenient because it allows faster delivery of the drug to the site of infection, with the use of lower doses to achieve the same or stronger effect. Therefore, this book presents environmentally friendly production processes and a characterization of two groups of advanced biomaterial: polymer hydrogels, based on alginate and poly(vinyl alcohol) with silver nanoparticles and gentamicin (Chapter 2), for wound dressing and soft tissue implants, and bioceramic composite coatings on titanium, based on hydroxyapatite with silver nanoparticles and gentamicin (Chapter 3), for hard tissue implants.

Chronic wound healing and care is a major area of medical and biomaterials science research, as frequent and persistent infections (often caused by multidrug-resistant microbial strains) and ever-rising numbers of antibiotic-resistant bacterial strains have become a serious concern in recent years. Traditional, mostly cotton-based dressing materials (gauzes, bandages, etc.) have many shortcomings, including susceptibility to bacterial infection, poor moisture regulation, dryness, and the tendency to stick to the wound tissue, causing a need for frequent replacement. Current practice and expert consensus recommend the use of silver-loaded wound dressings in acute, surgical, traumatic, and chronic wounds for both prophylaxis and treatment of localized, spreading, and systemic infections (the latter, of course, in combination with antibiotic therapy). However, the existing commercial silver-based dressings have their own shortcomings – they are quite expensive and this could render them inaccessible for sensitive groups of patients, such as low-income individuals, minorities, or elderly citizens. Moreover, these wound dressing materials are often classified as "medical aid" or "medical device," and, therefore, they are required to pass more lenient safety controls in comparison to drugs. This could cause concerns regarding their safety, and, indeed, some research studies showed a worryingly high *in vitro* cytotoxicity effect of some commercial silver-loaded dressings. Furthermore, the existing commercial wound dressings rely on loading excessive amounts of silver in order to achieve sustained wound protection for several days. A variety of silver-containing and antibiotic-containing products have been developed and utilized especially for treatments of infections in burns, open wounds,

DOI: 10.1201/9781032668895-1

and chronic ulcers. The synthesis of silver nanoparticles (AgNPs) became popular for applications in biomedicine since nanocrystalline silver has proved to be the most efficient antimicrobial agent with a wide inhibiting spectrum toward different types of microorganisms. However, one of the key problems for application of AgNPs is a strong tendency of these particles to agglomerate due to a high specific surface area and surface energy. To overcome this problem, polymers are used not only as capping agents to prevent AgNPs agglomeration, but also as their carriers, in the hydrogel form. The hydrogel form is applicable as wound dressing or soft tissue implant. AgNPs embedded in hydrogel matrices are attractive for biomedical applications due to the possibility of their controlled release, resulting in antimicrobial activity. These gels are hydrophilic, biocompatible, biodegradable, easily processed into different shapes, and approved for medical use. Thus, a combination of AgNPs with biocompatible hydrogels, like alginate, poly(vinyl alcohol) (PVA), poly(vinyl pyrolidone) (PVP), and chitosan (CHI, CS), provides the potential for design of improved medical treatments and devices (antimicrobial wound dressings, soft tissue implants). Beside the physico-chemical, two electrochemical methods for material fabrication were used: (1) electrochemical synthesis of AgNPs in the polymer solution under galvanostatic conditions and (2) electrochemical reduction of Ag^+ ions into AgNPs inside the polymer hydrogel, with a variation of applied voltage and implementation time. The electrochemical procedures exhibit advantages over chemical methods for the synthesis of small metal particles: the high purity of the metal, particularly important for biomedical applications, and the possibility of a precise particle size control, which can be achieved by adjusting deposition current density, voltage, and potential. Based on a cytotoxicity test, antibacterial test, and *in vivo* test, the results demonstrated that novel electrochemically produced polymer hydrogels with silver nanoparticles, as well as gentamicin-loaded polymer hydrogels produced by freezing-thawing method (Chapter 2), for wound dressing and soft tissue implants are excellent candidates for future biomedical applications.

Synthetic hydroxyapatite (HAP), as the most promising ceramic material used for biomedical applications such as hard tissues implant, has excellent bioactivity and biocompatibility and has a chemical composition similar to that of the bone. The development of synthetic materials with close resemblance to the biological and mechanical properties of natural bone tissue is required to overcome the load-bearing problem. Titanium has found wide application as a basic metal material for manufacturing bioceramic coatings such as hydroxyapatite due to its attributes of strength, stiffness, toughness, impact resistance, and corrosion resistance. However, HAP is very brittle, and, for this reason, much attention has been focused on the development of composite HAP coatings. Natural biodegradable polymer lignin (Lig), chitosan (CHI, CS), and synthetic poly(vinyl alcohol) (PVA) is considered as an alternative for the development of advanced biocomposite coating. On the other hand, the general idea of using graphene (Gr) as nanofiller is to minimize the brittleness of HAP and gain improved mechanical properties of biocomposite coating. However, in recent years problems regarding bacterial infection of bone implants have resulted in body rejection. To stop bacterial infection it is crucial to inhibit bacterial adhesion since biofilm can be very resistant to systematic administration of antibiotics. Hence, the possibility of preventing the implant infections using the antimicrobial properties of silver nanoparticles or antibiotic *in situ* has generated great interest in the development of silver-loaded and antibiotic-loaded composite hydroxyapatite coatings. As a producing method of HAP biocomposite coatings with lignin, PVA, CHI, and graphene doped with silver and antibiotic gentamicin (Chapter 3) on titanium substrate, the electrophoretic deposition (EPD) method was used due to its numerous advantages. EPD allows the formation of thin films of controlled thickness and morphology by changing the deposition parameters (voltage, time), with no additional reduction agents, and representing "green" technology of hard tissue implants production. Based on a cytotoxicity test, antibacterial test, and *in vitro* bioactivity test, the results demonstrated that novel electrophoretically produced coatings for hard tissue implants are an excellent candidate for biomedical applications.

The pharmacokinetics of drug release is of great importance in medical treatments; therefore, special attention is devoted to modeling the drug release process (Chapter 4). In pharmacokinetics, a popular choice is that of compartmental models, due to their simplicity and ease of understanding in relation to the mass balance equations and to assumptions for uniform distribution, homogeneous transient times, and immediate response to drug bolus administration. Numerous works have identified, and decades of research have tailored, their applicability for optimal drug delivery–assist devices in several domains of medical applications, e.g., diabetes, cancer, anesthesia, immune deficiency, leukemia, hormonal treatment, implants, and wound dressing. Selecting appropriate models is a crucial step in capturing complex biological and physiological phenomena. Any choice of a model structure implies a simplified view of the interaction among the various elements that may characterize a dynamical system. In many cases, fractional-order models are found to be more adequate for compartmental analysis, especially when, in a process under consideration, memory effects are pronounced.

The latest developments and trends in the application of fractional calculus (FC) were found in biomedicine and biology. Diffusion of substances in the human body, e.g., drug diffusion, is also a phenomenon well known to be captured with such mathematical models. Drug release that influences biocompatibility and antibacterial activity, and compartmental models are often used in pharmacokinetics to describe the response to drug bolus administration in different medical treatments (Chapter 4). In addition, for the first time, applications of general fractional derivatives to models of drug release in poly(vinyl alcohol)-based hydrogels for wound dressings and soft tissue implants and hydroxyapatite-based coatings aimed for hard tissue implants are explored. The results obtained by the use of models presented in this book are compared with other diffusion models used for drug release in surrounding tissue.

2 Hydrogels Aimed for Wound Dressings and Soft Tissue Implants

Recent developments in biomaterials science have seen increasing interest in research for novel solutions for new generation wound dressing materials. In-hospital wound infections and overwhelming emergence of antibiotic-resistant bacterial strains are an ever-looming threat in medicine and patient care. Infected wounds can be very difficult to treat and are a major cause of patient mortality. Traditional wound dressings, e.g., gauzes, bandages, etc., are ill equipped for this purpose, especially for more severe wounds due to many shortcomings such as low absorption ability, the need for frequent replacing, high adhesiveness, and sticking to the wound tissue, which could cause damage to the newly formed epidermis. Commonly used dressings and bandages are able to provide only a physical protection of the wound during the healing process and, as such, they have many drawbacks (Stashak, Farstvedt, and Othic 2004). For one, although sterile initially, they are very prone to bacterial infection and therefore carry with their usage inherent risks for patients, especially during chronic wound treatment. Further, the usual dressings are mostly cotton-based materials that tend to dry out quickly and provide poor moisture regulation, which is crucial for wound healing. This also carries another shortcoming, which is sticking to the wound tissue and damage upon replacement. The proneness to bacterial infection, on the other hand, dictates the need to frequently change these dressings, which could enhance the risk of wound tissue damage and thus could impede the normal healing process. On a related note, the susceptibility to bacterial adhesion mandates the local/topical application of drugs, usually antibiotics, to prevent infection. The widespread use of antibiotics has led to resistance developing in many bacterial strains, which has become a very common and a very serious problem (Blair et al. 2015).

Wound healing is a complex process occurring over several phases, including hemostasis, inflammation, epithelial cells migration, and proliferation, followed by remodeling of epithelial tissue and wound healing. Hemostasis and inflammation phases are the first line of defense when the organism is battling bacterial infection; they occur almost simultaneously, usually lasting anywhere from 24 hours to three days. During this initial period, it is critically important to prevent bacterial migration and adhesion to the wound, so it is desirable for a wound dressing to contain an active antibacterial component that should impede biofilm formation in the first 24 to 48 hours. An ideal wound dressing should provide protection and support to the wound during the entire remodeling and healing process, and, in this regard, it needs

DOI: 10.1201/9781032668895-2

to fulfill many strict prerequisites, such as biocompatibility and non-toxicity, oxygen and water vapor permeability, ability to maintain local moisture to prevent drying of the wound, ability to absorb wound exudates, and low adhesiveness to alleviate the danger of wound trauma during dressing replacement (Naseri-Nosar and Ziora 2018; Caló and Khutoryanskiy 2015). As mentioned, together with being a physical barrier for bacterial colonization, wound dressings often need to contain an antibacterial agent for active infection protection, which would be released gradually to maintain wound sterility (Simões et al. 2018). Hydrogels, highly porous cross-linked polymer matrices containing up to 90 % liquid phase, are potentially excellent wound dressing materials as they could be tailored to successfully meet all the aforementioned requirements. High water content in the hydrogel enables effective moisture regulation; the swelling ability of polymer hydrogels is advantageous for exudate absorption and removal of necrotic tissue from the wound surface, whereas the porosity of the matrix assures good O_2 and CO_2 permeability. Additionally, the structure of the hydrogel matrix resembles the extracellular matrix (ECM) structure, facilitating cell migration and proliferation and accelerating tissue remodeling and wound healing (Koehler, Brandl, and Goepferich 2018).

In an effort to alleviate the inherent risks connected with traditional wound dressings, gauzes, and bandages, novel materials, predominantly biopolymer-based hydrogels and films, have been the focus of many researchers around the world during the last several decades (Caló and Khutoryanskiy 2015). The most "popular" wound dressing polymers are natural-origin ones, such as alginate (Sun and Tan 2013; Diniz et al. 2020), cellulose (Hebeish et al. 2013), chitin, and chitosan (Jayakumar et al. 2011), but also synthetic biopolymers, including poly(vinyl alcohol) (Bhowmick and Koul 2016; Hong 2007) and poly(vinyl pyrrolidone) (Jovanović et al. 2011; Torres-Giner, Pérez-Masiá, and Lagaron 2016). A frequent focus of wound dressing materials studies is also on blends, copolymers, and grafts of the aforementioned polymers (T. T. T. Nguyen, Tae, and Park 2011; Bal et al. 2015) as well as their chemically modified derivatives (Zhou et al. 2017; D. Zhang et al. 2015).

These new materials need to possess a number of properties that correspond to the requirements of wound care. Some of these properties are (Koehler, Brandl, and Goepferich 2018; Boateng et al. 2008; Broussard and Powers 2013; Biancheraet al. 2020): biocompatibility and non-toxicity toward healthy tissue, good wound exudate absorption ability, good gas permeability (O_2, CO_2, water vapor), the ability to maintain moist wound environment and to prevent the drying of the wound, sterility and barrier properties against microorganisms, the ability to maintain optimal wound temperature, low adhesiveness to the wound tissue, etc. Next generation biomaterials, especially biopolymer-based hydrogels, have for quite some time been at the forefront of wound dressing research (Caló and Khutoryanskiy 2015; Koehler, Brandl, and Goepferich 2018; Boateng et al. 2008; Biancheraet al. 2020; Powers, Morton, and Phillips 2013; Naseri-Nosar and Ziora 2018; Nešović and Mišković-Stanković 2020). This is hardly surprising because of their exceptional tailorability and the ability to address some or all of the issues listed above (Caló and Khutoryanskiy 2015; Koehler, Brandl, and Goepferich 2018). A wide array of polymers have been used for active wound dressing applications, both synthetic and natural origin. The polymers derived from natural resources include various polysaccharides, such as cellulose (Gupta et al. 2020; Koivuniemi et al. 2020), starch (Xiao Yang et al. 2019), dextran (Gharibi et al. 2019; Innocenti Malini et al. 2019), chitosan (Matica et al. 2019; Kenawy et al. 2019; Rubina et al. 2019), alginates (Jasmina Stojkovska et al. 2018; Ying et al. 2019), and hyaluronic acid (Ying et al. 2019; S. Zhang et al. 2020; Lin et al. 2019), but also some protein-based biopolymers, including keratin (W. Li et al. 2019) and collagen (Rubina et al. 2019; Ying et al. 2019; Lin et al. 2019), gelatin (Chuysinuan et al. 2019; Du et al. 2020), silk fibroin and sericin (Gholipourmalekabadi et al. 2020). On the other hand, bioactive or bioinert synthetic polymers used in wound dressing research encompass some hydrophobic materials, such as polycaprolactone (Salehi-Abari, Koupaei, and Hassanzadeh-Tabrizi 2020), polypropylene (Fages et al. 2011), and poly(lactic acid) (Pankongadisak et al. 2019; Ghaffari-Bohlouli et al. 2020; Maleki, Mathur, and Klein 2020), and different hydrophilic synthetic polymers, e.g., poly(vinyl alcohol) (M.-S. Kim et al. 2020; Alipour et al. 2019; Augustine et al. 2018), poly(methacrylic acid) (Bajpai, Chand, and Mahendra 2013) and poly(ethylene glycol) (Salehi-Abari, Koupaei, and Hassanzadeh-Tabrizi 2020; Zhu et al. 2018). Both natural origin and synthetic polymers are also rarely used "stand-alone" to produce wound dressing materials, as blending, grafting, and copolymerization open a much wider spectrum of structures and properties and provide the pathway to controlled production of tailor-made materials. This is why the wound dressings are usually made from blends or copolymers of the above-mentioned polymers. The choice of antibacterial agent, however, also to some degree dictates the choice of polymer components, and especially in the case of silver nanoparticles it is important to carefully choose the polymers that will exert excellent stabilization effect, while at the same time providing sustained, and preferably controllable, release of AgNPs into the wound area to achieve maximum protection against bacterial and other infections.

PVA is one of the most frequently used and the oldest synthetic polymer that has been employed as wound dressings. However, PVA hydrogel has inadequate elasticity, stiff membrane, a relatively poor barrier property to bacterial penetration, sometimes poor mechanical stability, and incomplete hydrophilic characteristics, which restrict its use alone as the wound dressing polymeric membranes. Among the various hydrogels described in the literature, hydrogels prepared using PVA blended with some natural polysaccharides and some other synthetic ones, including chitosan, graphene, and Ag nanoparticles (AgNPs), are attractive and the most widespread route of membranes synthesis because of the abundance of such polymers, easily for chemical derivatization or modification, and usually good biocompatible. However, these nanomaterials may potentially be risky for human health. Therefore, it is necessary to thoroughly examine their biocompatibility under *in vivo* conditions.

The simple structure and unique properties of PVA polymers, such as adhesion, strength, film formation, hydrophilicity but very low swelling capacity (due to their sensitivity to hydrogen bonding and over-crystallization), biocompatibility, safety and non-cancerous properties, make them desirable for specific biomedical applications. To date, many uses of PVA hydrogels have been proposed in biomedicine, including as soft materials for building contact lenses, artificial cornea, artificial cartilage and meniscus, tendon and bone regenerations, hydrogel coating humeral head surface in shoulder joint prosthesis, and for decreasing formation of adhesions in peritonitis, a carrier for the medicaments, including prolonged release of antibiotics in veterinary medicine, cell growth substrate for prostate brachytherapy preparations (P. Li et al. 2015), cardiovascular grafts (Alexandre et al. 2017), and others. It is necessary to look with great optimism at the results of the first clinical study with long-term follow-up (5 to 8 years) of the commercial PVA (Cortiva, RTI Surgical Inc., FL, USA) implant success in focal cartilage defects. These results showed that synthetic PVA hydrogel implants guarantee functional recovery of a knee joint in mid-life patients with focal lesions of the cartilage (Sciarretta 2013). The first preliminary results of a clinical study on repairing the human joint surface metacarpal bone by implantation of PVA in patients with osteoarthritis were published (Taleb, Berner, and Mantovani Ruggiero 2014). Also, excellent clinical results five years after PVA hydrogel hemiarthroplasty of the first metatarso-phalangeal joint in advanced hallux rigidus were obtained (Daniels et al. 2017).

However, physical properties of PVA hydrogels are generally reversible and that disrupts their stability. The viscosity, the degree of crystallization, and pH sensitivity of PVA cryogels changes over time, which leads to decrease of mechanical properties. Also, in comparison with other hydrogels, PVA hydrogels weakly adsorb the proteins, resulting in low cell adhesion, which, in the opinion of some authors, makes them less effective in the treatment of cartilage defect by the matrix-associated autologous chondrocyte transplantation (Baker et al. 2012). Therefore, many PVA copolymers have been synthesized. Chitosan (CHI, CS) is especially interesting as the only natural polycationic polysaccharide and a biopolymer with intrinsic antibacterial properties that make it an excellent choice for wound dressing applications. A polysaccharide of natural origin, it is usually obtained by partial or complete deacetylation of chitin (Croisier and Jérôme 2013). It has gained considerable attention in biomaterials research, including wound dressings and drug delivery (Hamedi et al. 2018; Sur et al. 2019; Matshetshe et al. 2018), due to its remarkable properties, such asits intrinsic antibacterial activity, biocompatibility, and biodegradability (Croisier and Jérôme 2013). As a result of partial chitin deacetylation, CHI contains many amino ($-NH_2$) groups on its chain, which are subject to protonation in acidic media, gaining positive charge and becoming $-NH_3^+$ (Croisier and Jérôme 2013). Thus, CHI is soluble in acidic, but not in alkaline, media, and its pH-dependent solubility has been used to tailor the properties of biomaterials. Another consequence of pH-dependent solubility is the fact that CHI is the only natural polycation, which enables formation of polyelectrolyte complexes with other polymers, such as alginate. Some studies have argued that precisely the presence of $-NH_3^+$ on chitosan chain is the reason for its antibacterial properties, as they allow interactions with negatively charged bacterial cytoplasmic membranes, disrupting their functions and interfering with respiratory and other processes, which leads to cell death (Croisier and Jérôme 2013; Kong et al. 2010; Paul, Sharma, and Tirunal 2004; H. Liu et al. 2004; Zheng and Zhu 2003; Fei Liu et al. 2001; Chung et al. 2004). Chitosan has also been shown to possess the ability to promote wound healing (Paul, Sharma, and Tirunal 2004; Ueno, Mori, and Fujinaga 2001). Due to the presence of polar $-OH$ and $-NH_2$ groups, chitosan has been identified as an efficient stabilizing agent for metallic nanoparticles, and many research works were dedicated to obtaining chitosan-based biomaterials containing AgNPs (T. T. T. Nguyen, Tae, and Park 2011; Agnihotri, Mukherji, and Mukherji 2012; Tran et al. 2010; Abdelgawad, Hudson, and Rojas 2014). In addition, CHI is also a mild reducing agent, thus enabling green synthesis of AgNPs without other chemical reducents (Kozicki et al. 2016). However, one drawback of pure chitosan hydrogels is the fact that they have poor mechanical properties, especially those prepared by physical cross- linking methods (Croisier and Jérôme 2013). For this reason, chitosan is rarely used in pure form; rather, it is utilized to form blends with other polymers, such as alginate or PVA (Venkatesan et al. 2017; Mozalewska et al. 2017). PVA/CHI blends are especially interesting as the presence of PVA facilitates physical hydrogel formation through freezing-thawing and provides structural integrity to the matrix, whereas chitosan improves antibacterial properties and enables better immobilization of AgNPs inside the hydrogel (Nešović et al. 2018). However, chitosan has been successfully utilized in combination with other polymer materials to prepare wound dressings with improved properties. The production of the hydrogel can be achieved via different methods, and chitosan is most frequently applied as a blend or a copolymer with different polymeric materials, such as gelatin (Tyliszczak et al. 2017; N. T.-P. Nguyen et al. 2019; Rehman et al. 2019), dextran (Shi et al. 2019), alginate (Khampieng et al. 2018; Gómez Chabala, Cuartas, and López 2017), hyaluronic acid (B. Lu et al. 2017), polyacrylamide (Ferfera-Harrar, Berdous, and Benhalima 2018), or PVA (Nešović, Janković, Radetić et al. 2019; Gholamali, Asnaashariisfahani, and Alipour 2019; Hiep et al. 2016); however, some studies report free-standing AgNP-containing pure chitosan hydrogels (Xie et al. 2018; Pérez-Díaz et al. 2016; Mekkawy et al. 2017; C.-H. Yang et al. 2016).

The formation of the hydrogel can be achieved by physical or chemical cross-linking, depending on the properties of the chosen polymer(s), and the desired properties of the obtained hydrogel, such as degree of cross-linking, swelling ability, mechanical properties, etc. The chemical cross-linking involves gelation using chemical agents, and the obtained product is irreversible, meaning that it is insoluble and cannot be returned to sol state without breaking of chemical bonds. Chemical cross- linking is relatively easy and quick and allows facile control of the obtained hydrogel characteristics (Maitra and Shukla 2014). However, a major problem with this method in the field of biomedical materials science is the threat of toxicity when using chemical cross linkers, which are usually some organic solvents. For example, a very well-known cross-linking agent for chitosan is glutaraldehyde, along with other aldehyde-based cross linkers, which are toxic and must be carefully washed out or extracted from the obtained hydrogel (Hoffmann et al. 2009). A viable alternative are physical cross-linking methods, which have also been shown to be very effective and efficient for obtaining hydrogel biomaterials (Maitra and Shukla 2014). The main advantages of physical methods are non-toxicity of the obtained product as well as reversibility of the hydrogels, which could be easily returned back to sol state under the right conditions, facilitating the biodegradability of the material (Maitra and Shukla 2014). For example, PVP is usually cross-linked by radiation (Mozalewska et al. 2017), yielding highly structurally and mechanically stable hydrogels with excellent properties (Duygu Sütekin and Güven 2019). The cross-linking is achieved by exposing the liquid polymer solution or dispersion to gamma radiation, which causes braking of chemical bonds within the polymer and the formation of free radicals, and their reactions with polymer chains create new intermolecular chemical bonds (Jovanović et al. 2011). Varying the irradiation dose and other parameters enables very accurate control of cross-linking degree, as well as hydrogel properties (Duygu Sütekin and Güven 2019).

The simplest physical cross-linking method to obtain hydrogels of certain polymers (such as PVA), is freezing and thawing in several cycles (Fukumori and Nakaoki 2014; Hassan and Peppas 2000). During freezing and thawing, the cross links between polymer chains are formed through hydrogen bonding, orientation into microcrystalline regions, and by semi-permanent entanglements (Peppas and Stauffer 1991). Thus, a physically cross-linked hydrogel matrix is formed, which can be easily returned to the sol state – e.g., PVA hydrogels can be dissolved in plain distilled water by heating to 80 °C–90 °C (Nešović et al. 2018). However, not all polymers can form hydrogels by this method. It has been shown that pure PVP (Obradovic et al. 2012) hydrogels cannot be obtained by freezing and thawing, but PVP and CHI hydrogel blends with PVA can (Nešović et al. 2018; Obradovic et al. 2012; Figueroa-Pizano et al. 2018).

Apart from hydrogels, the polymer-based wound dressings can be prepared in the form of thin films, which involves preparation of colloid solutions or dispersions, addition of antibacterial component, and finally casting and drying the solution to obtain free-standing films. This method was used to prepare PVA films (Surudžić, Janković, Bibić et al. 2016; Surudžić, Janković, Mitrić et al. 2016), chitosan films (Wei et al. 2009), and alginate films (Lawrie et al. 2007). Hydrogels and films are two of the most frequent choices of wound dressing form because of their facile preparation, easy incorporation of antibacterial agent, long-term immobilization inside the polymer matrix, and sustained and controlled release to the wound site.

2.1 HYDROGELS WITH SILVER NANOPARTICLES AIMED FOR WOUND DRESSINGS AND SOFT TISSUE IMPLANTS

The introduction of AgNPs into polymer/copolymer hydrogels increases their antimicrobial activity, while the incorporation of graphene increases their mechanical properties. However, these materials do not have biodegradability, so their use is recommended for surface wound treatment or as soft tissue implants. It was found that out of all metals with antimicrobial properties, silver had the most effective antibacterial action and lower toxicity to animal cells. AgNPs antimicrobial properties are associated with (1) ability to strongly react with a thiol group of compounds found in respiratory enzymes of bacterial cells; (2) non-coupling of oxidative phosphorylation in the bacterial cell; (3) induction of bacterial death by release of free oxygen radicals; (4) interference with the respiratory chain at the cytochrome C level, and components of the electron transport system; (5) interaction with sulfurone groups in bacterial membranes, thereby damaging the bacterial wrap; (6) interaction with phosphorous groups in DNA, thereby causing damage to the chromosomal material of the cells. As a result, AgNPs are effective antiseptic agents for controlling broad-spectrum microbial and antibiotic-resistant bacteria, and therefore their use significantly reduces the ability of bacterial resistance to antibiotics. However, the potential toxic effects of AgNPs on the circulatory, respiratory, central nervous system, and liver and skin should not be forgotten. There is an increased trend for reduced usage of antibiotics in both humans and animals, as well as antibiotics in animal production. Numerous studies on the properties and possibilities of the application of the hybrid PVA/AgNPs material (Moretto et al. 2004; Pencheva, Bryaskova, and Kantardjiev 2012) proved its advantages for a topical therapeutic use in the experimental creamy formula with silver, suitable for recovery of the microbial homeostasis in animals.

Along with improved physical properties of the dressing, the aim is to incorporate an antibacterial agent in order to achieve active protection from bacterial infection. In this sense, recent research has seen a significant shift away from antibiotics and toward other active components that will provide similar or better antibacterial activity without the risk of bacterial resistance. Among the most common alternative antibacterial agents are metal and especially silver nanoparticles (AgNPs) due to their wide spectrum activity and low susceptibility to bacterial resistance (Rai, Yadav, and Gade 2009). The mechanism of AgNPs antibacterial action have been widely explored but not yet conclusively determined, as they include cytoplasmic membrane damage, disruption of DNA replication through binding to sulfur- and phosphorus-containing groups, inhibition of respiratory processes, as well as reactive oxygen species (ROS) generation, causing membrane and protein damage (Rai, Yadav, and Gade 2009; Durán et al. 2016; Feng et al. 2000). Due to their very potent and diverse antibacterial activity, AgNPs have become a popular choice of antibacterial component in polymer-based wound dressings (Konop et al. 2016). There are various possibilities for AgNPs synthesis and immobilization, along with tuning their sizes and size distributions, shapes, and morphologies. Silver nanoparticle-incorporated hydrogels could be obtained by *in situ* AgNPs synthesis or by synthesizing AgNPs first and then incorporating them in the polymer matrix. The synthesis itself is most commonly achieved *via* reduction from an ionic Ag^+ precursor, usually silver nitrate solution. Most frequently applied methods in the literature are chemical reduction (with a strong reducing agent such as $NaBH_4$) (Dai et al. 2016), or γ -irradiation technique, which enables reduction of silver ions to Ag^0 with free radicals (Jovanović et al. 2011; Jovanović, Radosavljević et al. 2012; Jovanović et al. 2013; Spasojević et al. 2017). Both of these methods have their advantages, but both also have their drawbacks. The chemical reduction method is attractive because it is relatively easy to perform, enables high yield of the synthesis, and facilitates the control of AgNPs size and homogeneous distribution (L. Lu et al. 2006). On the other hand, the use of potentially toxic chemical agents could compromise biocompatibility of the material and special care must be taken to wash out and extract leftover chemicals (Caló and Khutoryanskiy 2015; Montoro, Medeiros, and Alves 2014). Gamma irradiation is a greener method that helps avoid potential chemical toxicity, allowing simultaneous cross-linking and sterilization of hydrogel (Caló and Khutoryanskiy 2015). Recently, interest has grown in electrochemical routes for AgNPs synthesis, as this method provides both green reduction without the use of chemicals (apart from ionic precursor) as well as use of inexpensive equipment that is accessible and easy to handle. AgNPs could be electrochemically synthesized galvanostatically or at constant voltage, *in* or *ex situ*, in colloid solutions of polymers (Jovanović, Stojkovska et al. 2012; Obradović et al. 2015; Jasmina Stojkovska et al. 2014; Surudžić, Janković, Bibić et al. 2016; Jasmina Stojkovska et al. 2012; Obradovic and Miskovic-Stankovic 2013) or directly inside the hydrogel (Mohamed M Abudabbus et al. 2018; M M Abudabbus et al. 2016; Nešović, Abudabbus et al. 2017; Nešović, Kojić et al. 2017; Nešović et al. 2018; Nešović, Janković, Perić-Grujić et al. 2019; Nešović, Janković, Radetić et al. 2019; Nešović et al. 2020).

There are different AgNPs syntheses routes, with the most common methods including chemical synthesis using either trisodium citrate (Xie et al. 2018; Pereira et al. 2020; Choudhury et al. 2019), ascorbic acid (Mohanty and Swain 2019; Escobar-Hernández and Escobar-Remolina 2019), or sodium tetrahydroborate (Tyliszczak et al. 2017; Gholamali, Asnaashariisfahani, and Alipour 2020; Chitra et al. 2018) as a reducing agent, but also biosynthesis using natural extracts such as hyacinth plant leaves (Oluwafemi et al. 2019), *Combretum erythrophyllum* (Jemilugba et al. 2019), *Crinum latifolium* (Vo et al. 2019), *Curcuma longa* (Ferfera-Harrar, Berdous, and Benhalima 2018), *F. verticillioides* (Mekkawy et al. 2017), or *Sanghuangporus sanghuang* (Ran et al. 2019). On the other hand, a frequently applied route to obtain silver nanoparticles is simply mixing a precursor (such as silver nitrate) into the polymer solution where simultaneous reduction of Ag^+, formation of AgNPs and their stabilization takes place (Gómez Chabala, Cuartas, and López 2017; B. Lu et al. 2017; Masood et al. 2019; Verma et al. 2017; Ryan et al. 2017) due to the well-known ability of chitosan to reduce silver and to form a hydrogel with AgNPs at the same time (Kozicki et al. 2016; Wahid et al. 2017). Aside from the obvious advantages of this method being simplicity and the avoidance of any reducing agents, one disadvantage could be the long reaction times (24 hours and more) needed to complete the synthesis. Electrochemical synthesis provides an *in situ* and completely green method to reduce Ag^+, while also allowing for additional reduction with chitosan to improve the yield of AgNPs in a much shorter timeframe (Nešović et al. 2018; Nešović, Janković, Perić-Grujić et al. 2019; Nešović, Janković, Radetić et al. 2019). All of the hydrogel formulations have exhibited very potent antibacterial activity range against a variety of bacteria, such as *Staphylococcus aureus* (both methicillin-resistant and methicillin-susceptible), *Escherichia coli*, *Pseudomonas aeruginosa*, which was confirmed by various tests such as agar diffusion, LIVE/DEAD staining, minimum inhibitory and bactericidal concentration (MIC/MBC) as well as quantitative tests by counting colony forming units after exposure to tested samples. Several studies have even confirmed the applicability of chitosan-based hydrogels as wound dressings through *in vivo* tests that confirmed accelerated healing of the wounds treated with these materials (B. Lu et al. 2017; Hiep et al. 2016; Xie et al. 2018; Ran et al. 2019; Masood et al. 2019; Verma et al. 2017). Cytotoxicity, as an important factor for the potential clinical use of an antibacterial material, has also been tested against various cell lines (mostly fibroblasts or cancer-derived cells), and the results showed generally good biocompatibility of chitosan-based wound dressings. An interesting study (Khampieng et al. 2018) also compared the antibacterial activity and cytotoxicity effects of chitosan-PVP-AgNPs hydrogels to some commercial silver-based wound dressing materials such as ACTICOAT™, Algivon®, and Suprasorb® A+Ag. This research indicated that, although the commercial coatings achieved the same or similar antibacterial activity against methicillin-resistant *S. aureus* (MRSA) and *E. coli* to the prepared hydrogel samples, their biocompatibility was much worse, and the viability of L929, HaCaT, and HDFa cells even dropped below 20 to 30 %. Thus, it can be observed that there is a vast potential to improve current proprietary and commercially available wound dressing materials with significantly better ones. These are very good results as they indicate that the potential toxicity of AgNPs as a potent antibacterial agent can be circumvented by using a lower Ag concentration and leaning on its synergistic effect together with chitosan (Nešović, Janković, Radetić et al. 2019; Shi et al. 2019). Further, the controllability of the release behavior of AgNPs from chitosan-based hydrogels could also be an important factor, as seen in a recent paper where even the hydrogels with higher AgNPs concentration exhibited no cytotoxicity (Nešović, Janković, Radetić et al. 2019), unlike previously tested PVA-based hydrogels without chitosan, which showed serious dose-dependent cytotoxicity with increased AgNPs content (M M Abudabbus et al. 2016). This could be explained by better stabilization of AgNPs by chitosan and their controlled release over longer time periods, which not only enables prolonged antibacterial effect, but also helps curb the cytotoxicity issues (Nešović et al. 2018; Nešović, Janković, Perić-Grujić et al. 2019; Nešović, Janković, Radetić et al. 2019).

2.1.1 Electrochemical Synthesis of Silver Nanoparticles as a Green Reducing Method

Electrochemical synthesis of silver nanoparticles offers several advantages over other reduction methods, including simple setup, facile control of reaction conditions, as well as non-toxicity of the used chemicals. Different methods for electrochemical synthesis of AgNPs have been reported in the literature. The first method involves the AgNPs synthesis in the colloid solution of polymers, with subsequent preparation of the desired forms (films, hydrogels, microbeads, microfibers), whereas in the second method hydrogels are prepared first, then swollen in the solution of Ag^+ precursor, and subsequently subjected to electrical current to synthesize the AgNPs inside the hydrogel.

2.1.1.1 Galvanostatic Method

The first method (Figure 2.1a) performed in colloid polymer solutions, with added $AgNO_3$ as an ionic precursor, involves synthesis in galvanostatic regime, i.e., applying constant current density to the working electrode over a short period of time. The electrochemical cell is filled with the colloid solution mixed with $AgNO_3$ at desired concentration, along with KNO_3, which serves as a base electrolyte to improve conductivity. The cell contains working and auxiliary electrodes and a reference electrode (e.g. a saturated calomel electrode, SCE) connected to a potentiostat used to supply constant current density. The reaction is carried out under N_2 flow to remove

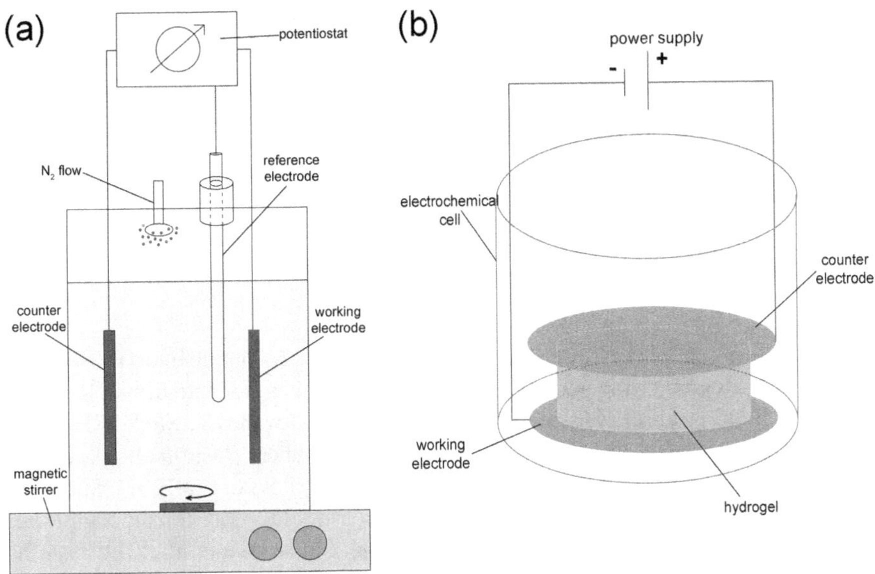

FIGURE 2.1 Schematic representation of the electrochemical synthesis of silver nanoparticles in polymer-based colloid solutions, hydrogels, and films: (a) galvanostatic method, (b) constant-voltage method (reprinted from Nešović and Mišković-Stanković 2020 with permission from John Wiley & Sons)

the oxygen from the cell, while being constantly stirred on a magnetic stirrer in order to ensure uniformity of the concentrations in the colloid bulk. As the electrolyte is an aqueous solution, electrochemical reactions always include water electrolysis, i.e., hydrogen evolution at the cathode (Eq. 2.1) and oxygen evolution at the anode (Eq. 2.2). The working electrode is a cathode; therefore, the synthesis of AgNPs is achieved *via* cathodic reduction of silver ions (Eq. 2.3). When the galvanostatic electrochemical synthesis is performed in aqueous solution around neutral pH and in the absence of stabilizing agents, the thermodynamically favored process is the electrochemical deposition of a macroscopic Ag layer on the cathode surface. This process is, of course, undesirable as it prevents formation and dispersion of AgNPs and diminishes their yield in the solution. Therefore, to prevent this bulk cathodic deposition and to achieve a stable AgNP dispersion, stabilization agents are added – the electrolyte is therefore an aqueous colloid solution of a polymer such as PVA or alginate. It has also been shown that other anodic side-reactions could occur due to the presence of polymers in the electrolyte, e.g., to include oxidation of polymer components and their slight deposition on the anode surface, besides the oxygen evolution reaction (Jovanović, Stojkovska et al. 2012; Jasmina Stojkovska et al. 2012). On the cathode, however, the reactions are the same, i.e., hydrogen evolution (Eq. 2.1) and silver reduction (Eq. 2.3). But now, due to the presence of stabilizing agents, the Ag atom clusters that form at the cathode can interact with polymer chains and move into the solution, which is why the synthesis is usually performed in an electrochemical cell with continuous stirring – to achieve uniform mass transfer and homogeneous distribution of the synthesized AgNPs across the electrolyte volume.

$$2H_3O^+ + 2e^- \rightarrow H_2 + 2H_2O \quad (2.1)$$

$$2H_2O \rightarrow O_2 + 4H^+ + 4e^- \quad (2.2)$$

$$nAg^+ + ne^- \rightarrow \left(Ag\right)_n \quad (2.3)$$

Thus obtained colloid contains AgNPs that are shielded by polymers in the solution and are stable for long time periods. The colloid can then be cast into films (Surudžić, Janković, Bibić et al. 2016), extruded to microbeads (Jovanović, Stojkovska et al. 2012; Jasmina, Stojkovska et al. 2012, 2014) and microfibers (Jasmina Stojkovska et al. 2018), or cross-linked to form hydrogels (Jasmina Stojkovska et al. 2014; Surudžić, Janković, Bibić et al. 2016). This method has been used to obtain nanocomposites of different polymers, such as alginate (Jovanović, Stojkovska et al. 2012; Jasmina Stojkovska et al. 2012, 2014), PVP (Obradovic et al. 2012), PVA (Surudžić, Janković, Bibić et al. 2016), and their blends (Obradovic et al. 2012).

2.1.1.2 Constant-Voltage Method

The second electrochemical route of AgNPs synthesis involves first preparing the hydrogel by some of the above-mentioned cross-linking methods, followed by swelling of the obtained hydrogel in the $AgNO_3$ solution (with KNO_3 added to improve the electrical conductivity). Equilibrium-swollen hydrogel is then placed between two platinum plates (working and counter electrodes) in a glass electrochemical cell, depicted in Figure 2.1b. The electrodes are connected to a DC power source, which supplies a constant voltage needed for the electrochemical synthesis of AgNPs. Thus, the swollen hydrogel serves as an electrolyte, and as the $AgNO_3$ swelling medium is an aqueous solution, the main reaction is again water electrolysis, described by Eqs. 2.1 and 2.2. The synthesis of AgNPs takes place by the reduction of Ag^+ ions; however, the process itself is likely slightly different from the first method. As the hydrogel can be viewed mostly as a solid electrolyte, the reduction of silver ions by electrical current is most likely to result in a deposition of a bulk Ag layer on the cathode surface (Eq. 2.4). This is an undesirable reaction, as the deposition of silver on platinum surface inevitably depletes the hydrogel of silver ions and lowers the yield of the synthesis. This is why the polarity of the electrodes during the synthesis is often reversed, as upon the polarity reversal the cathode becomes an anode, the bulk Ag layer on its surface is dissolved and the Ag^+ ions are replenished inside the hydrogel. Further, due to intensive hydrogen evolution on the cathode (Eq. 2.1), the most likely formation of AgNP nucleation sites is achieved *via* reduction with H_2 molecules inside the hydrogel (Eq. 2.5) (Merga et al. 2007).

$$Ag^+ + e^- \rightarrow \left(Ag\right)_{bulk} \quad (2.4)$$

$$2Ag^{+} + H_2 \rightarrow 2(Ag)_{np} + 2H^{+} \qquad (2.5)$$

The AgNPs obtained by this method are stabilized inside the hydrogel matrix by interactions with polymer chains and incorporation in the matrix pores, which enables their long-term stabilization. The constant-voltage *in situ* electrochemical method was used to obtain AgNP-hydrogel nanocomposites with PVP (Jovanović et al. 2014), PVA (Mohamed M Abudabbus et al. 2018; M M Abudabbus et al. 2016; Nešović, Abudabbus et al. 2017), and PVA/CHI (Nešović, Kojić et al. 2017; Nešović et al. 2018; Nešović, Janković, Perić-Grujić et al. 2019; Nešović, Janković, Radetić et al. 2019).

2.1.2 Alginate-Based Hydrogels with Silver Nanoparticles

Alginate is especially attractive biomaterial since it is a naturally derived linear copolymer that easily forms biocompatible hydrogels, which are already in medical use. It is composed of 1,4-linked β-d-mannuronic acid (M-block) and α-l-guluronic acid (G-block) units. Aqueous solutions of alginates are known to form hydrogels in the presence of divalent cations such as Ca^{2+}, via ionic interactions between acid groups on G blocks and the gelating ions. As a result, calcium-alginate gels are physically cross-linked polymers with mechanical and structural properties that depend on alginate composition. These gels are hydrophilic, biocompatible, biodegradable, and easily processed into different shapes, which make them attractive for a variety of applications in biotechnology and biomedicine, such as gelling agents in food products, substrates for immobilization of cells and bioactive molecules, tissue engineering scaffolds, and carriers for drug delivery as well as for wound dressings.

Wound dressings based on alginate, mostly as Ca-alginate hydrogel, are in commercial use, providing biocompatibility and high sorption capacity and, thus, regulation of moisture levels that leads to rapid granulation and reepithelization of the damaged tissue. Supplementation of silver to alginate dressings offers the advantage of an additional feature of antimicrobial activity, so that a number of products based on alginate fibers with incorporated silver ions were produced (Qin 2005). These dressings are easily removed and replaced without causing much trauma due to the highly hydrophilic alginate gel nature. In addition, alginate hydrogels are widely investigated for regeneration and engineering of a number of tissues and organs, including skeletal muscle, blood vessels, nerve, pancreas, liver, and cartilage. High water content in these gels supports efficient transport of nutrients and gases and provides an aqueous environment comparable to that in soft tissues. Also, alginate gels can be introduced into the body to fill irregularly shaped defects by a minimally invasive procedure. All of these properties make alginate hydrogels attractive and potentially applicable as soft tissue implants.

However, incorporation of AgNPs within alginate solutions and/or hydrogels provides possibilities for controlled and prolonged release of Ag nanoparticles and/or ions and production of a variety of formulations with different compositions and forms. Alginate as an anionic polymer with high charge density can stabilize nanoparticles by a negative charge, resulting in stability against agglomeration. There are several approaches investigated for synthesis of AgNPs in combination with alginate, which will be overviewed in this chapter with the special attention to electrochemical synthesis of AgNPs. Chemical reduction is one of the most used methods for production of AgNPs as colloidal dispersions in water or organic solvents. This method was also applied in alginate solutions supplemented with silver salts (e.g., nitrate, sulfate) using sodium borohydride as the reductant (Dubas and Pimpan 2008; Marie Arockianathan et al. 2012). Alginate was shown to be a good capping agent of AgNPs, which were in the size range 3–20 nm as determined in different studies, while the obtained colloid solutions were investigated for several potential applications. It was shown to be possible to form nanocomposite thin films by using a layer-by-layer dipping technique alternating between anionic colloid alginate solution and cationic poly(diallyldimethylammonium chloride) (PDADMAC) solution (Dubas and Pimpan 2008). The obtained nanocomposite films displayed fast color change upon exposure to water or to a less polar solvent such as ethanol, making them attractive for potential sensing applications or optical switches. Another advantage of using alginate solutions is that they can be easily mixed with solutions of other polymers in order to obtained final products with improved properties as compared to using either polymer alone. Alginate colloid solution with chemically synthesized AgNPs was successfully mixed with sago starch and ethylene glycol and the obtained mixture was casted and dried so to produce nanocomposite films attractive for potential use as wound dressings (Marie Arockianathan et al. 2012). The obtained films exhibited enhanced wound healing patterns as compared to untreated controls in *in vivo* studies in rats. In another study, dialyzed alginate colloid solution with chemically synthesized AgNPs was freeze-dried for three days and cross-linked by dipping in 0.2 M $CaCl_2$ solution, resulting in formation of a nanocomposite Ca-alginate sponge (Seo et al. 2012). Obtained sponge exhibited antimicrobial activity against *E. coli* and *K. pneumonia*, but also cytotoxicity toward human fibroblasts. On the other hand, the amounts of proinflammatory cytokines released from macrophages treated with the nanocomposite Ca-alginate sponge were lower as compared to the control, indicating potential anti-inflammatory activity of this product if medically used (Seo et al. 2012). To avoid the addition of chemical reductants and the need for purification of the obtained colloid solution, radiation techniques can be used. Gamma irradiation of the alginate solution supplemented with silver nitrate and isopropanol resulted in formation of a colloid solution containing AgNPs in the size range 5–30 nm and stable for six months (Yusheng Liu et al. 2009).[6] Finally, a simpler, method for production of AgNPs using alginate both as a reducing agent and as a stabilizer was developed based on just heating the solution of silver nitrate and alginate at 90° C for 1 hour (S. Sharma et al. 2012). The obtained colloid solution contained AgNPs in the size range 5–21 nm and was further mixed with chitosan solution. The mixture was then cast and dried, resulting in the formation of nanocomposite films that exhibited antibacterial activity against both Gram-negative and Gram-positive bacteria, having stronger effects on the latter group (S. Sharma et al. 2012).

2.1.2.1 Electrochemical Synthesis and Characterization of Silver/Alginate Solutions

Electrochemical synthesis of metal nanoparticles, as compared to conventional chemical methods, offers advantages especially attractive for biomedical applications, such as high purity of the particles and the possibility for a precise particle size control achieved by adjusting current density or applied potential.

Ag/alginate colloid solutions were obtained from 2 % w/v Na-alginate, 0.1 M KNO_3 and $AgNO_3$ in the concentration range between 0.5 and 3.9 mM by electrochemical synthesis performed galvanostatically. Current density was varied between 5 and 50 mA cm^{-2}, while the time varied between 0.5 and 10 minutes (Jovanović, Stojkovska et al. 2012). Ag/alginate colloid solutions obtained under various experimental conditions were analyzed using transmission electron microscopy. The nanoparticles obtained were all spherical in shape, approximately 10–30 nm in diameter, independently of applied current density. The nanoparticles synthesized at current density of 5 mA cm^{-2} seemed to be slightly smaller, but formed larger aggregates, so it can be considered that applied current density does not affect the size of Ag nanoparticles. It is known from the literature (Jovanović, Stojkovska et al. 2012; Murali Mohan et al. 2007; Sambhy et al. 2006) that nanoparticles of the dimensions obtained exhibit antimicrobial characteristics.

Regardless of the parameters of synthesis, UV-Vis analysis has shown that Ag/alginate colloid solutions exhibited surface plasmon absorption band peaking in the wavelength range of 405–440 nm, corresponding to particles whose radii are smaller than ~30 nm. (Jovanović, Stojkovska et al. 2012; Slistan-Grijalva et al. 2005b, 2005a). In addition, absorption spectra of Ag/alginate colloid solution corresponded to Lorentzian fit, implying monodispersity of the nanoparticles (Angelescu et al. 2010), which is consistent with TEM measurements. On the contrary, UV-Vis spectra of pure alginate solution and dissolved control alginate microbeads did not exhibit the absorbance peak in the examined range of wavelengths, as shown in Figure 2.2. These results correspond to a plasmon resonance effect originating from the quantum size of AgNPs (Mulvaney 1996) and thus confirmed the presence of Ag nanoparticles in Ag/alginate colloid solutions, as well as in Ag/alginate microbeads.

UV-Vis spectra were used also to determine the effects of $AgNO_3$ concentration in the alginate solution, applied current density and time on the amount and relative size of silver nanoparticles formed, i.e., on the absorbance maximum, A_{max}, and the wavelength of the absorbance maximum, λ_{max}, in different Ag/alginate colloid solutions (Jovanović, Stojkovska et al. 2012). It was observed that the increase in $AgNO_3$ concentration in the alginate solution, applied current density, and time decreases the λ_{max} arriving at the value of 405 nm in the solution synthesized at $c = 3.9$ mM, $j = 50$ mA cm^{-2}, $t = 10$ min. Lower λ_{max} values were reported to correspond to smaller nanoparticles (Šileikaitė et al. 2006; X. Li et al. 2010). Linear increase in A_{max} with the increase of $AgNO_3$ concentration in the initial alginate solution is expected, since the absorbance is proportional to the concentration of silver nanoparticles formed. The higher concentrations of Ag^+ ions in the alginate solution resulted in higher concentrations of nanoparticles. Similarly, it could be expected that higher values

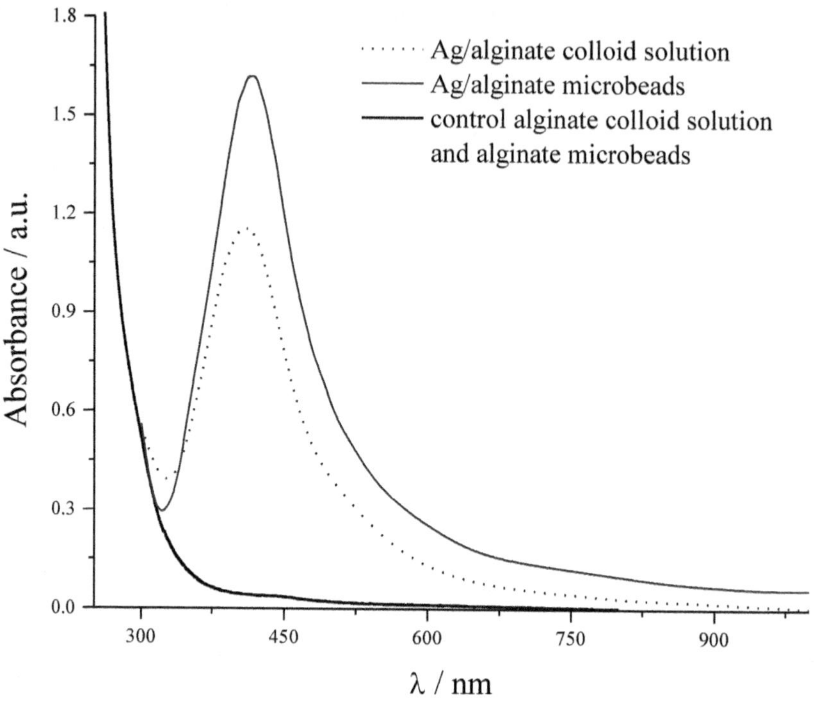

FIGURE 2.2 Absorption spectra of control alginate solution and alginate microbeads, Ag/alginate colloid solution (c = 3.9 mM, j = 50 mA cm^{-2}, t = 10 min), and Ag/alginate microbeads (reprinted from Jovanović, Stojkovska et al. 2012 with permission from Elsevier)

of current density and longer times will result in more intensive nanoparticle formation as observed up to the current density of 25 mA cm^{-2} and time of 6 minutes. However, further increases in these parameters had a slight effect on AgNP concentration although they induced shift of the absorbance maxima toward 405 nm. As a consequence, the Ag/alginate colloid solution, synthesized at 50 mA cm^{-2}, for 10 minutes, with $AgNO_3$ concentration in the initial alginate solution of 3.9 mM, was chosen for further investigations as well as for the production of Ag/alginate hydrogel microbeads, due to the higher concentration and smaller dimensions of Ag nanoparticles obtained.

Cyclic voltammetry was used in order to obtain a better insight into the silver reduction process (Jovanović, Stojkovska et al. 2012). Figure 2.3a shows stationary cyclic voltammograms for Pt electrode in 1.9 w/v % alginate solution containing 0.1 M KNO_3 + 3.9 mM $AgNO_3$ and in Ag/alginate solution, which exhibited anodic peaks, appearing at around 450 and 465 mV, respectively. As the corresponding counterpart, one cathodic peak appeared at about 165 mV (in 1.9 w/v % alginate solution containing 0.1 M KNO_3 + 3.9 mM $AgNO_3$), and around 25 mV (in Ag/alginate colloid solution), which corresponded to the reduction of silver. The shift of this cathodic peak in Ag/alginate colloid solution toward more negative potential

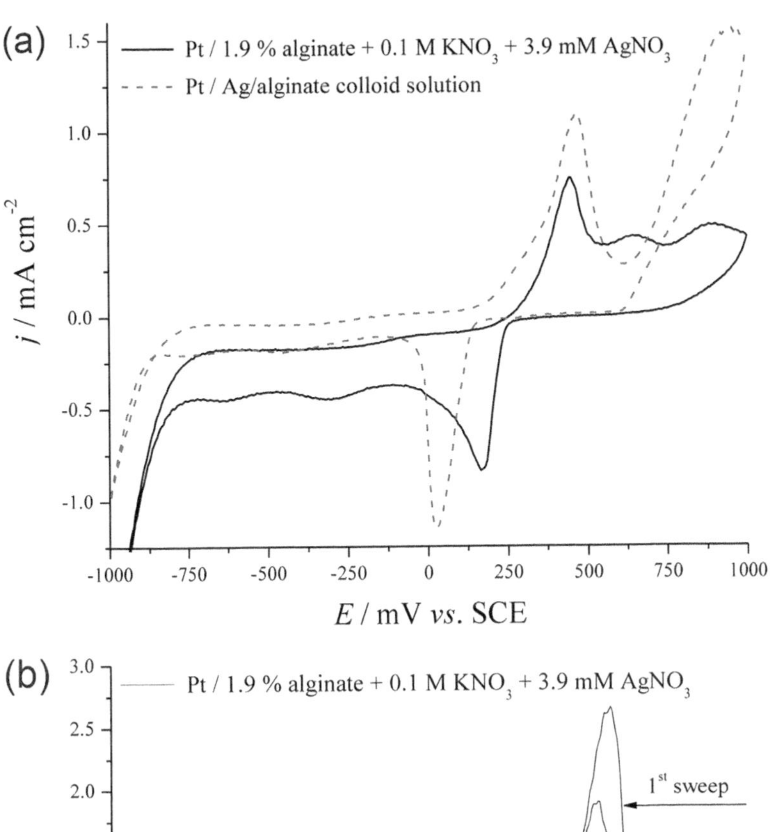

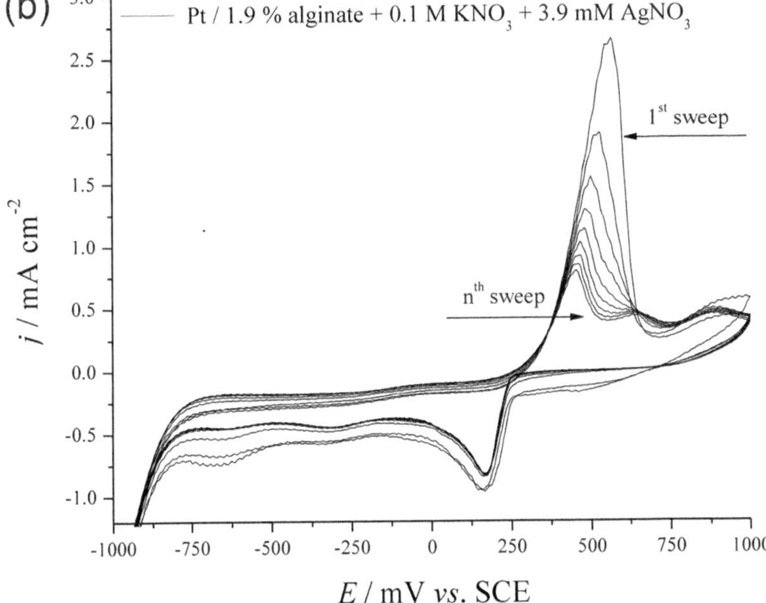

FIGURE 2.3 (a) Stationary cyclic voltammograms for Pt electrode in 1.9 w/v % alginate solution containing 0.1 M KNO_3 + 3.9 mM $AgNO_3$ and in Ag/alginate colloid solution and (b) cyclic voltammograms for Pt electrode in 1.9 w/v % alginate solution containing 0.1 M KNO_3 + 3.9 mM $AgNO_3$ (reprinted from Jovanović, Stojkovska et al. 2012 with permission from Elsevier)

indicates differences in the reduction process. In 1.9 w/v % alginate solution containing 0.1 M KNO_3 + 3.9 mM $AgNO_3$, Ag^+ reduction appears as formation of silver nanoparticles. On the other hand, in Ag/alginate colloid solutions, the appearance of the cathodic peak can probably be explained due to the further growth of already formed silver nanoparticles (somewhat restricted by the presence of alginate molecules) and the re-synthesis of silver nanoparticles from eventually present residual silver ions.

In the stationary cyclic voltammogram for Pt electrode in 1.9 w/v % alginate solution containing 0.1 M KNO_3 + 3.9 mM $AgNO_3$, the second anodic peak is observed at around 645 mV (Figure 2.3a). Since this peak does not have a related counterpart, all sweeps of cyclic voltammetry analysis obtained for Pt electrode in this solution (Figure 2.3b) should be concerned. At Figure 2.3b, the anodic peak is observed at around 565 mV, which decreased with every following sweep, and also changed the peaking position toward more negative potentials, arriving at the value of 450 mV in the nth sweep, as it can be seen in Figure 2.3a. At some point between the 6th and 7th sweep, a new anodic peak appeared at around 645 mV as a result of the separation/disjunction of the corresponding peak (at 565 mV). The absence of the cathodic counterpart for this anodic peak appearing at 645 mV indicates that the reduction process is not affected by further influence of the applied current, and it continues due to the synthesis of silver nanoparticles from Ag^+ ions. On the other hand, the decrease in the current peak intensity at 565 mV indicates lowering of the content of silver available for oxidation, due to the synthesis of silver nanoparticles. The appearance of the second anodic peak at a more positive potential value suggests that a certain amount of silver becomes even less susceptible for oxidation (X. Li et al. 2010), probably as a consequence of the entrapment of silver nanoparticles by alginate molecules during this process, suggesting that synthesized silver nanoparticles are very stable. This result points to the validity of alginate as a choice for the electrochemical synthesis of silver nanoparticles in the solution, considering that more stable nanoparticles are formed in solutions of capping agents that exhibit a certain level of bonding with silver ions and silver nanoparticles formed.

Interactions of alginate molecules with Ag nanoparticles were investigated using FT-IR spectroscopy, performed on alginate and Ag/alginate thin films. The films were obtained by solvent evaporation from alginate solution and Ag/alginate colloid solution. Pure alginate spectrum showed the following absorption bands: broad absorption band peaking in the region of 3250 – 3400 cm^{-1} (at 3257 cm^{-1}) indicating the weak H–bonding of hydroxyl groups, followed by a peak at 2927 cm^{-1}, which can be assigned to vibration of the CH group. The alginate spectrum also displayed absorption peaks at 1712, 1593, and 1406 cm^{-1} corresponding to the H–O–C=O stretching vibrations, asymmetric and symmetric stretching of carboxylate vibrations, respectively, followed by characteristic absorption bands of polysaccharide structure appearing at 1367 and 1296 cm^{-1} (C–C–H and O–C–H bending), 1124 cm^{-1} (C–O stretching), 1082 cm^{-1} (both C–O and C–C stretching of pyranose rings,) and at 1024 cm^{-1} (C–O stretching). Also, the characteristic bands of uronic acid residues peak at 9 cm^{-1} (C–O stretching vibration), 887 cm^{-1} (C1–H deformation vibration of the β -mannuronic acid residues), and 814 cm^{-1} (C1–H deformation vibration of the α -guluronic acid residues) (Jovanović, Stojkovska et al. 2012). These results are in accordance with the results found in the literature for pure alginate (Šileikaitė et al. 2006). On the other hand, Ag/alginate spectrum exhibited several differences in peak positions compared to the pure alginate spectrum, suggesting possible bonding between alginate molecules and Ag nanoparticles. The most important differences observed are in two spectral ranges, i.e., between 1370 – 1205 cm^{-1} and between 1160 – 1015 cm^{-1}. Absorption bands of the pure alginate appearing in the first specified range at 1367 cm^{-1} and 1296 cm^{-1} shift toward 1358 cm^{-1} and 1298 cm^{-1}, respectively, in the Ag/alginate spectrum. This possibly indicates interactions of Ag nanoparticles with OH groups in uronic acid residues, observed as a shift of the C–OH bending vibration. In the second spectral range, the vibration frequency shifted from 1082 cm^{-1}, recorded for pure alginate, to 1078 cm^{-1}, recorded in Ag/alginate spectrum as a result of the coordination of both OH and ether groups to Ag nanoparticles, which weakened the strength of C–O bond in these two functional groups. Moreover, the C–O frequency slightly shifted from 1024 cm^{-1} recorded for pure alginate to 1026 cm^{-1} recorded for Ag/alginate spectrum, pointing out to interactions of the ring C(5) oxygen atoms of both, guluronic and mannuronic acid residues with Ag nanoparticles. Overall, the comparison of peak positions in pure alginate and Ag/alginate thin film spectra indicates the bonding of hydroxyl and ether groups as well as ring oxygen atoms in uronic acid residues of alginate molecules by coordination with Ag nanoparticles.

The findings obtained by FT-IR spectroscopy are in accordance with cyclic voltammetry results and indicate the bonding of alginate molecules with Ag nanoparticles, which prove alginate to be a good choice for the electrochemical synthesis of silver nanoparticles. Namely, the synthesis process of metal nanoparticles is shown to be a competition between two different cathode surface processes, i.e., the particle formation, by reduction and stabilization of metal ions by the capping agent, and the metallic film deposition at the cathode surface (Rodríguez-Sánchez, Blanco, and López-Quintela 2000). The metal deposition on the cathode limits the yield of the particle synthesis, because when the electrode surface is totally covered by the metallic deposit, the only process that occurs is further deposition of metal coating. Therefore, deposition process must be minimized. So, the role of the capping agent is to accelerate metal nanoparticle formation, and lower the metal deposition on the cathode (Yin et al. 2003). Furthermore, efficiency of the capping agent is in tight connection with its potential to bond to the metal nanoparticle surfaces.

2.1.2.2 Synthesis and Characterization of Silver/Alginate Hydrogels

Alginate hydrogel with incorporated AgNPs in the form of microbeads were obtained by electrostatic extrusion of Ag/alginate solutions (Jovanović, Stojkovska et al. 2012; Obradovic et al. 2012) at a constant flow rate of 25.2 ml h^{-1} through a blunt edge, stainless steel needle using a 5 ml syringe and a syringe pump as described previously (Nedović et al. 2001). The needle was connected to a positive electrode of a high voltage d.c. generator at applied electrostatic potential of 6 kV and positioned 2.5 cm above the gelling bath containing 1.5 % w/v $Ca(NO_3)_2 \times 2H_2O$, which was grounded. At the tip of the needle, a stream of droplets was formed and collected in the bath, which provided exchange of Na^+ and Ca^{2+} ions and alginate gelling. The obtained microbeads were left in the bath for additional 30 minutes in order to complete gelling. Electrostatic extrusion of Ag/alginate solution resulted in the formation of uniform hydrogel microbeads incorporated with AgNPs, which colored the beads in yellow. At the optimal experimental conditions for Ag/alginate solution synthesis ($c = 3.9$ mM, $j = 50$ mA cm^{-2}, $t = 10$ min), the microbead size was found to be 487.75 ± 16.5 μm. The presence of AgNPs was confirmed by UV-Vis spectroscopy of dissolved microbeads (Figure 2.2). It can be observed that the absorption maximum wavelength remained at 405 nm verifying that nanoparticle aggregation did not occur during the production process. In addition, a somewhat higher absorption maximum was observed for microbeads as compared to Ag/alginate solution due to further Ag^+ ions reduction during the electrostatic extrusion. Thus, it can be concluded that all AgNPs in alginate solution were preserved and incorporated in the microbeads.

Furthermore, nanocomposite hydrogels in the form of microbeads (<1 mm in diameter) are suitable for controlled release of AgNPs and/or ions due to the large specific surface area and short internal diffusion distances. Alginate microbeads were shown to be suitable for immobilization of variety of cell types such as insect and mammalian cells (Goosen et al. 1997) as well as brewing yeast cells (Nedovic et al. 2001). It was previously shown that alginate microbeads could be also used for cartilage tissue engineering as supports for chondrogenic cells (e.g., bone marrow stromal cells (Osmokrović et al. 2006) and bovine calf chondrocytes (Jasmina Stojkovska, Bugarski, and Obradovic 2010) coupled with biomimetic bioreactors that imitate physiological conditions in articular cartilage. Supplementation of AgNPs within alginate microbeads could potentially provide an additional feature of prolonged sterility of the engineered implant.

As confirmed, one of the techniques for controlled production of uniform hydrogel microbeads is electrostatic droplet generation based on extrusion of alginate solution under the action of electrostatic forces that disrupt the liquid filament at the capillary/needle tip to form a charged stream of small droplets collected in a gelling bath (Bugarski et al. 1994). As Na^+ ions are exchanged with Ca^{2+} ions from the gelling solution, droplets solidify, forming microbeads down to 50 μm in diameter (Bugarski et al. 1994; Manojlovic et al. 2006). The process of electrostatic droplet formation is a complex function of a number of parameters (Poncelet et al. 1999; Jasmina Stojkovska et al. 2012), while for a chosen electrode setup and the polymer, the applied electrostatic potential was shown to be the key determinant of the droplet and, consequently, also the microbead size (Poncelet et al. 1999). For potential biomedical utilization of nanocomposite hydrogels, it is required that the production procedure be simple, precisely regulated, and scalable while the final products are pure, sterile, and with controlled properties. Specifically, the possibilities for sterilization and manipulation of Ag/alginate colloid solutions with retention of AgNPs have been investigated (Jasmina Stojkovska et al. 2012) as well as the production of nanocomposite microbeads regarding the effects of electrostatic extrusion parameters on the microbead size and AgNP concentration.

2.1.2.3 Biomechanical Properties

Biomechanical properties of packed beds of alginate microbeads with different concentrations of incorporated AgNPs (1, 1.5 and 3.9 mM concentrations in the source solutions) were examined in a biomimetic bioreactor while packed bed of 1.9 % w/v Ca-alginate microbeads served as a control (Jasmina Stojkovska et al. 2012). The experiments were performed under dynamic compression at 10 % strain in two regimes: at a loading rate of 337.5 μm/s and at sequential increments of 50 μm displacement every 30 min. All microbeads exhibited similar linear responses to the dynamic loading, although the values determined for the control alginate microbeads were slightly lower than those of Ag/alginate microbeads. Values of compression moduli determined from the slopes of the best stress-strain linear fits were 141 ± 2 kPa and 154 ± 4 kPa, for packed beds of the alginate and Ag/alginate microbeads, respectively. On the other hand, equilibrium stresses determined at sequential strains after 30 minutes pauses were significantly different for the alginate and Ag/alginate microbeads, yielding equilibrium unconfined compression moduli of 47 ± 0.5 and 34 ± 2 kPa, respectively.

Slight effects of AgNP on mechanical properties of alginate microbeads are consistent with weak interactions of the nanoparticles with polymer chains, so that phase transition, thermosensitivity, and viscoelasticity of the polymer gel were reported to remain unchanged (Schexnailder and Schmidt 2009). The presence of AgNPs in alginate microbeads apparently induced a slight increase in dynamic compression modulus while the decrease in the equilibrium unconfined compression modulus. These results imply that under dynamic conditions AgNPs induced higher retention of water within the hydrogel matrix while when the hydrogels were provided with time to relax, negative effects of AgNPs on the hydrogel strength were revealed. In addition, although the influence of the nanoparticle presence could be distinguished with respect to the control alginate hydrogel, the effects of AgNP concentration in the investigated range (1.5 – 3.9 mM) could not be perceived. These results are in agreement with reported effects of AgNPs at low concentrations (< 1 wt. %) incorporated within poly(vinyl alcohol) (PVA) hydrogels (Mbhele et al. 2003). Specifically, addition of AgNPs was shown to induce an abrupt increase in the hydrogel elastic modulus, which then remained constant as the AgNP concentration was increased up to 0.8 wt. %. On the contrary, during the stress relaxation, Ag/PVA nanocomposites exhibited reduced stability as compared to pure PVA hydrogels. These results were explained by interactions of nanoparticles with polymer chains inducing immobilization of interfacial regions and enhanced stiffness during loading. However, loading also induced debonding of nanoparticles, which allowed easier structural rearrangements of polymer chains during the stress relaxation (Mbhele et al. 2003) consistent with the lower equilibrium unconfined compression modulus determined for Ag/alginate microbeads as compared to that of the pure alginate microbeads.

2.1.2.4 Cytotoxicity

In order to evaluate *in vitro* cytotoxicity of Ag/alginate microbeads, two types of experimental studies were carried out: monolayer cultures of bovine calf chondrocytes and 3D cultures of the same cell type immobilized in alginate microbeads in perfusion bioreactors (Jasmina Stojkovska et al. 2014). Full thickness articular cartilage was harvested aseptically from the femoropatellar grooves of either 6- or 12-month-old bovine calves within 8 hours of slaughter. Primary chondrocytes obtained from the cartilage of 6-month-old calves were used for cytotoxicity studies in monolayer cultures. Primary chondrocytes isolated from the cartilage of 12-month-old calves were directly immobilized in alginate microbeads and used for 3D cell cultures in perfusion bioreactors.

Cytotoxicity of Ag/alginate microbeads with different concentrations of AgNPs was determined first in monolayer chondrocyte cultures using the standard MTT test (Mosmann 1983). Cultures with pure Ca-alginate microbeads without AgNPs were also established in order to verify alginate biocompatibility, while monolayer cultures alone served as a control. Cell survival is defined as the ratio of the number of cells grown in the presence of the investigated agent and the number of cells in the control. Since the number of live cells is directly proportional to the absorbance, the cell survival, S, can be calculated as:

$$S = A_u / A_c \cdot 100 \quad (2.6)$$

where A_u is the absorbance of cells grown in the presence of alginate or Ag/alginate microbeads and A_c is the absorbance of control cells. Cytotoxicity was rated as following: non-cytotoxic (> 90 % cell survival), slightly cytotoxic (60 %–90 % cell survival), moderately cytotoxic (30 %–59 % cell survival), and severely cytotoxic (≤ 30 % cell survival) (Meriç, Dahl, and Ruyter 2008).

The cell viability was determined after 48 hours and the effects of AgNP concentrations on the cell survival, S, in the presence of alginate and Ag/alginate microbeads is presented in Figure 2.4. It could be seen that the presence of alginate and Ag/alginate microbeads with released silver concentrations of up to 5 μg ml^{-1} induced negligible effects on bovine calf chondrocyte survival (S > 90 %). However, when released silver concentration was increased to about 7 μg ml^{-1}, it induced severe cytotoxicity (S = 13.9 ± 0.8 %). The obtained results are in agreement with other studies of the effects of different systems containing AgNPs on various mammalian cell types, where cytotoxic concentrations of AgNPs were reported to range from 1.6 to 50 μg/ml (Hussain et al. 2005; Park, Yi et al. 2010). Overall, results of Ag/alginate microbead cytotoxicity studies in monolayer cell cultures have shown that Ag/alginate microbeads released approximately 40 %–50 % of the initial AgNP amount and that the released silver concentrations in the culture medium up to 5 μg ml^{-1} were not cytotoxic for chondrocytes (Jasmina Stojkovska et al. 2014).

To examine cytotoxicity of Ag/alginate microbeads under conditions that imitate the physiological environment upon potential implantation *in vivo*, the 3D cultures of bovine calf chondrocytes immobilized in alginate microbeads were established in perfusion bioreactors (Jasmina Stojkovska et al. 2014). Cell loaded microbeads were mixed with Ag/alginate microbeads in the approximate ratio 3:1 and cultivated in perfusion bioreactors under continuous medium flow of 0.38 ml/min. The applied

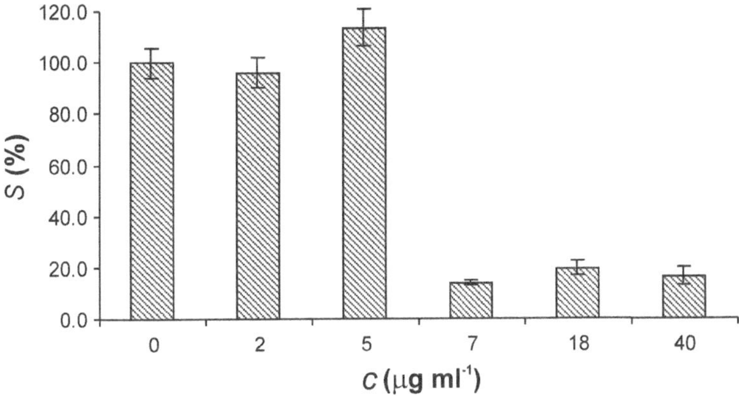

FIGURE 2.4 Survival, *S*, of bovine calf chondrocytes cultured in the presence of alginate or Ag/alginate microbeads with different AgNP concentrations normalized to the control sample as a function of total released silver concentrations in the medium, *c* (reprinted from Jasmina Stojkovska et al. 2014 with permission from Elsevier)

flow rate corresponded to the superficial medium velocity of ~100 μm/s, which is in the range of blood velocities in capillaries. After two weeks of bioreactor cultivation, microbeads slightly deformed, while the concentration of immobilized cells slightly but not significantly decreased with the viability preserved at 78 %, implying slight cytotoxic effects. To determine the maximal concentration of the released AgNPs and/or ions in the medium to which the cells were exposed, corresponding to the first medium exchange (i.e., 72 hours), a parallel experiment was performed using Ag/alginate microbeads (5.5 ± 0.4 mM AgNPs concentration), pure alginate microbeads instead of cell loaded microbeads, and saline solution instead of the cultivation medium. The concentration of free Ag^+ ions in the saline solution was 0.9 ± 0.3 μg ml^{-1}, not significantly different from measured Ag^+ concentrations in the monolayer studies. Thus, the total amount of released AgNPs and/or ions from Ag/alginate microbeads was determined based on measured silver concentrations in initial microbeads and after the experiment (5.5 ± 0.4 mM and 102 ± 16 μM, respectively). Based on the mass of Ag/alginate microbeads and measured saline solution volumes, the total silver concentration in the saline solution can be calculated as 9.3 ± 0.9 μg ml^{-1}. This concentration corresponds to strong cytotoxicity as determined in monolayer cultures (Figure 2.4). However, under *in vivo*–like settings in perfusion bioreactors and 3D environment, this concentration had only a negligible effect on cell viability. Consequently, cells in monolayers could be regarded as more sensitive to AgNPs and Ag^+ than cells surrounded by the alginate matrix in a 3D environment. Thus, these results stress the importance of the comprehensive biomaterial assessment, including different aspects and settings, and demonstrate the utility of biomimetic bioreactors for functional biomaterial evaluation under *in vivo*–like conditions.

TABLE 2.1
Colonies Count of *Staphylococcus aureus* TL and *Escherichia coli* ATCC 25922 in the Control Suspension and Suspensions with Wet and Dried Ag/Alginate Microbeads at the Concentration of 0.4 g/ml Based on the Microbead Wet Weight (Adapted from Jasmina Stojkovska et al. 2014 with Permission from Elsevier)

	Initial	1h
Staphylococcus aureus TL		
Control (CFU/ml)	3.8×10^5	6.6×10^5
Wet Microbeads (CFU/ml)	3.8×10^5	$(9.5 \pm 2.1) \times 10^4$
Dried Microbeads (CFU/ml)	$(3.7 \pm 0.3) \times 10^5$	$(9.5 \pm 4.9) \times 10^4$
Escherichia coli ATCC 25922		
Control (CFU/ml)	2.8×10^6	7.6×10^6
Wet Microbeads (CFU/ml)	$(1.7 \pm 0.2) \times 10^6$	$(8.3 \pm 0.3) \times 10^4$
Dried Microbeads (CFU/ml)	$(2.2 \pm 0.4) \times 10^6$	$(5.0 \pm 3.7) \times 10^5$

2.1.2.5 Antibacterial Activity

Antibacterial activity of wet and dried Ag/alginate microbeads was estimated against *S. aureus* TL and *E. coli* ATCC 25922 (Jasmina Stojkovska et al. 2014). Both microbead types demonstrated the release of AgNPs and/or ions inducing growth delay of both *S. aureus* and *E. coli* (Table 2.1). After 1 hour of incubation bacterial concentrations in both microbeads, groups were lower than the initial concentrations. It is interesting to note that wet and dried microbeads exhibited similar antibacterial activity against both investigated bacterial strains.

The obtained results are in agreement with other studies of different systems containing AgNPs against *S. aureus* and *E. coli*, where the minimum inhibitory concentrations of AgNPs were reported to range from 0.34 to 120 μg ml^{-1} for *S. aureus* and 0.26 to 180 μg ml^{-1} for *E.* coli (Panáček et al. 2006; Morones et al. 2005; Petráš and Magin 2011), considering that antibacterial activity could be attributed mainly to the release of AgNPs and/or ions. If the results of antibacterial activity of Ag/alginate microbeads are compared to the results of cytotoxicity studies, it can be assumed that the release of silver nanoparticles and/or ions can be tuned so to induce antibacterial activity without causing cytotoxic effects. Overall, it could be assumed that wet Ag/alginate microbeads could be attractive for tissue engineering applications in combinations with cell scaffolds, constructs, or soft tissue implants providing a sterile environment, either *in vitro* or *in vivo*. On the other hand, dried Ag/alginate microbeads could be applied as antibacterial powders in wound treatments, providing moisture capture by rapid alginate matrix reswelling and antibacterial effects due to the release of AgNPs and/or ions.

2.1.2.6 *In Vivo* Studies

Deep, necrotic, infected, and heavily exuding wounds (e.g., burns, ulcers) present a serious clinical problem since conventional wound treatment methods do not promote healing. Dressings based on alginate effectively regulate moisture levels in wounds, leading to rapid granulation and reepithelization of the damaged tissue (Paul, Sharma, and Tirunal 2004; Queen et al. 2004). These dressings are also easily removed and replaced without causing much trauma due to the hydrophilic nature of the hydrogel. Various medical products containing silver were developed, such as antimicrobial wound dressings, ointments, and coatings. Furthermore, silver nanoparticles were reported to be even more potent than silver ions due to attachment and interactions with the bacterial cell membrane, release of silver ions, and, possibly, penetration into the cell interior (V. K. Sharma, Yngard, and Lin 2009).

Ag/alginate colloid solutions containing 1 mM AgNPs, 1.73 % w/v alginate and 0.1 g dm^{-3} ascorbic acid were used in wound treatment studies on rats, as well as Ag/alginate microfibers produced by extrusion of the colloid solution containing 1.4 mM AgNPs and 1.73 % w/v alginate. The resulting microfibers had a mean diameter of 250 ± 40 μm and exhibited the UV-Vis absorption maximum at ~410 nm. Male Wistar rats were used for studies of effectiveness of nanocomposite Ag/alginate solutions and microfibers for wound treatments in a rat burn model (J Stojkovska et al. 2013). Thermal burn injuries were standardized as reported in the literature (dos Santos Tavares Pereira et al. 2012) in order to obtain deep second-degree burns of the same size. The animals were divided randomly into three groups: control group (G1, n = 9), group treated with 1 mM Ag/alginate colloid solution (G2, n = 9), and group treated with Ag/alginate microfibers (G3, n = 9). Wound contraction is a parameter used for assessment of wound healing. After one day of thermal injuries, wound areas in all three groups were not significantly different and were ~ 2-fold higher as compared to the initial burns. Then the wounds started to continuously contract in all groups until complete restoration (Figure 2.5). The wound contraction was consistently faster in treated groups, whereas significant differences as compared to the control were observed 11 days after the thermal injury induction and this trend was maintained until the end of experiment. The scabs fell off between 10 and 12 days after the injury induction in treated groups (G2 and G3) and between 15 and 16 days in the control. It is interesting to note that wound contraction appeared slightly slower in the group treated with microfibers (G3) as compared to the group treated with Ag/alginate solutions (G2) until the scabs fell off. However, thereafter wounds in the group G3 rapidly contracted and completely healed at day 19 as compared to day 21 in the group G2. In the same time, wounds in the control group G1, on day 21 were still visible. Clinical evaluations have proved the complete wound healing in treated groups (G2 and G3) on days 21 and 19, respectively, while in the control group even after 21 days the wounds did not completely heal. The obtained results indicated that both Ag/alginate solutions and microfibers significantly enhanced healing of second-degree burns in rats. These macroscopic findings were also supported by the results of histological analyses, which have shown enhanced granulation and reepithelization, reduced inflammation, and improved organization of the extracellular matrix in both treated groups. It should be pointed out that silver concentrations were 0.011 % w/w for the Ag/alginate colloid solution and 0.016 % w/w for Ag/alginate microfibers, which is more than two orders of magnitude lower than those in commercial silver-containing alginate dressings (Qin 2005).

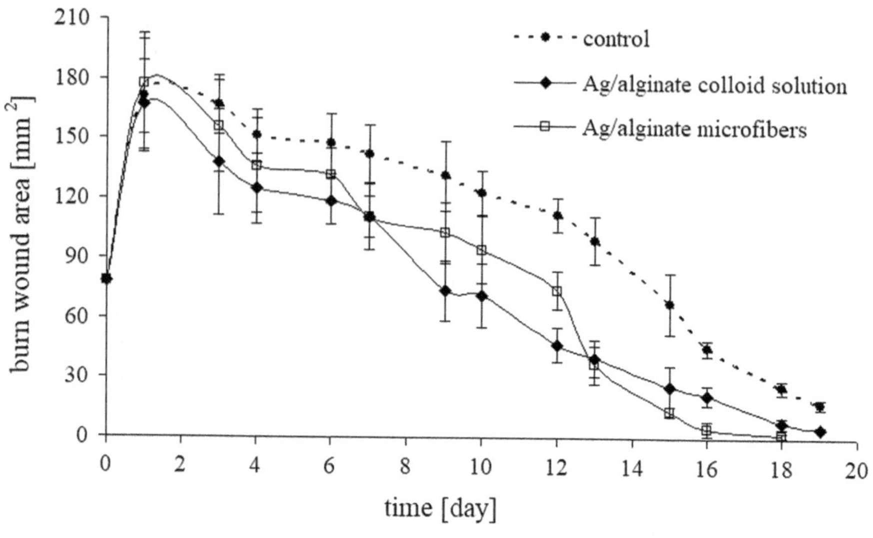

FIGURE 2.5 Burn wound area as a function of time for the control group, group treated with Ag/alginate colloid solution and the group treated with Ag/alginate microfibers (adapted from Jasmina Stojkovska et al. 2018 with permission from SAGE Publications)

2.1.3 Poly(vinyl Pyroliddone)-Based Hydrogels with Silver Nanoparticles

2.1.3.1 Electrochemical Synthesis and Characterization of Silver/Poly(Vinyl Pyrrolidone) Hydrogels

Ag/PVP hydrogels were successfully obtained by electrochemical synthesis of silver nanoparticles inside a PVP hydrogel. First, the PVP hydrogels have been obtained by gamma irradiation, followed by swelling in 3.9×10^{-3} M $AgNO_3$ solution. The electrochemical synthesis of Ag nanoparticles was performed by imposing a constant voltage, in the range of 15 – 300 V during different times (Jovanović et al. 2014). The absorption spectra of the Ag/PVP nanocomposites exhibited a surface plasmon band with absorbance maxima at ≈416 nm, confirming the formation of AgNPs (Figure 2.6). The absorbance intensity, which is related to the concentration of AgNPs, increased with increasing applied voltage and time, up to the values of 200 V and 4 minutes, respectively (Figures 2.6a and 2.6b), while further increases in both applied voltage and time did not follow this trend.

To evaluate the optimum conditions for the synthesis of the silver nanoparticles inside the PVP hydrogel network, the values of absorbance maximum wavelength, λ_{max}, and the full width at half-maximum absorbance, β, for the absorption spectra of Ag/PVP hydrogel obtained under different experimental conditions have been measured. Bearing in mind that lower values of the wavelength of the absorbance maximum and of the full width at half-maximum (fwhm) absorbance correspond to smaller silver nanoparticles (Hövel et al. 1993), at applied voltage of 200 V and time of 4 minutes were chosen as the optimal conditions for the synthesis of the AgNPs,

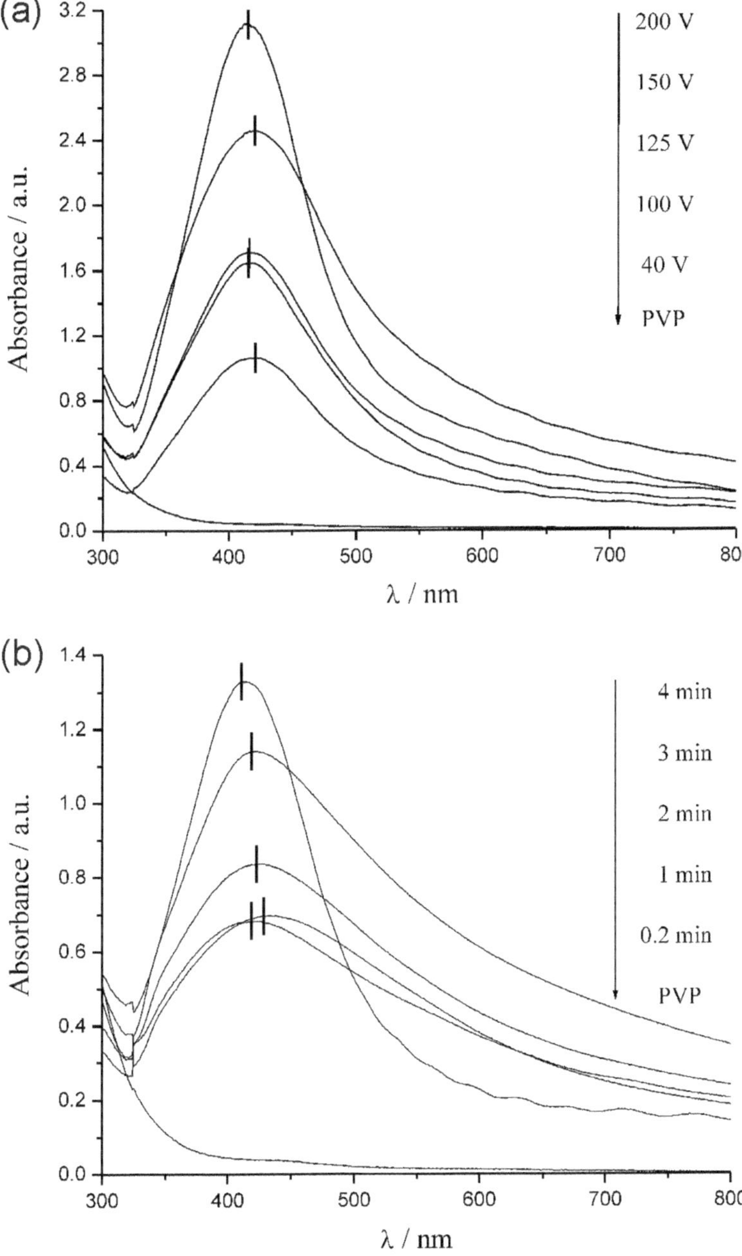

FIGURE 2.6 Absorption spectra of PVP and Ag/PVP hydrogels obtained at (a) different values of the applied voltage during four minutes, and (b) different times at 30 V, 72 hours after the synthesis (reprinted from Jovanović et al. 2014 with permission from John Wiley & Sons)

and the further investigations were performed on Ag/PVP hydrogel obtained under these conditions.

Theoretical predictions of the UV-Vis spectra for monodisperse nanoparticles should follow a Lorentzian plasmon resonance band, while a Gaussian distribution should indicate polydispersity (He et al. 2002). Here, the absorption spectrum of the Ag/PVP hydrogel nanocomposite was more in agreement with a Lorentzian than with a Gaussian fit, which suggests monodispersity of the silver nanoparticles in the Ag/PVP hydrogel. The same result was obtained for Ag/alginate colloid solution. However, the existence of silver nanoparticles inside the PVP hydrogel was not evident during and immediately after synthesis; the complete yellow coloration of the Ag/PVP hydrogel occurred 24 hours after the synthesis. This suggested the synthesis of silver nanoparticles was a gradual process. Namely, the first step of AgNPs synthesis would be the reduction of Ag^+ ions into Ag atoms inside the PVP network, which occurred as a cathodic reaction. The as-formed Ag atoms became seeds or nuclei for the further growth and the formation of AgNPs, which gave a yellow color to Ag/PVP hydrogel nanocomposites. It is reported in the literature that AgNPs formation, presuming nucleation and growth, is the result of classical nucleation and growth, aggregative nucleation and growth, and Ostwald ripening processes, which can occur either in consecutive or in parallel regimes (Richards, Rath, and Buhro 2010). It is generally considered that the nanoparticles obtained from molecular (atom) precursors grow by classical nucleation and growth, while nanoparticles originated from smaller nanocrystals grow by Ostwald ripening. There are also reports that aggregative growth contributes in both growing processes. A previous study, concerning the synthesis of silver nanoparticles in alginate solutions, confirmed the growth of AgNPs for three days after the synthesis by aggregative mechanism and Ostwald ripening. After that period, Ag/alginate colloid solution remained stable for an additional 30 – 40 days (Jovanović, Stojkovska et al. 2012). Using FE-SEM microphotographs of Ag/PVP hydrogel and a histogram presenting particle size distribution of AgNPs, the size of AgNPs was measured to be 75 ± 19 nm, and the average cluster size was 209 ± 33 nm. Comparing the UV-Vis spectroscopy results with FE-SEM imaging, it is observed that the spectroscopy "sees" small particles rather than clusters, suggesting that the absorption peak position of 416 nm corresponds to the 75 nm AgNPs. This is in agreement with the literature data, where the absorption peak positions of 416 nm and 418 nm correspond to AgNPs of 55 nm and 60 nm in size, respectively (Kora, Sashidhar, and Arunachalam 2010, 2012).

To obtain more information about the reduction of silver ions into AgNPs inside PVP hydrogel network, and to evaluate eventual side effects of the synthesis, Ag/PVP hydrogel was investigated by cyclic voltammetry (Jovanović et al. 2014). The monitoring was performed immediately after synthesis and after drying and reswelling in 0.1 M KNO_3 because of the visual observation that the freshly prepared Ag/PVP hydrogel was not colored, while the re-swollen one was dark yellow. Actually, the freshly obtained, colorless Ag/PVP hydrogel becomes dark yellow only 24 hours after the synthesis. Higher current intensity, corresponding to the greater mobility of the system components, indicates that the majority of the silver present in newly synthesized Ag/PVP hydrogel was still in the form of Ag atoms, and that the growth processes had not yet started. On the other hand, cyclic voltammograms of the re-swollen Ag/PVP hydrogels exhibited peaks with significantly lower current intensity, confirming the entrapment of AgNPs inside the PVP network. Ag/PVP hydrogel immediately after the synthesis caused an anodic peak at around 490 mV and one (broad and unusually shaped) at 900 mV; both could originate from the oxidation of Ag particles and those trapped in PVP hydrogel. Theirs counterparts, two cathodic peaks at ≈115 and ≈265 mV, correspondingly suggest the reduction of silver ions, and those inside the PVP network. In the case of the re-swollen Ag/PVP hydrogel, all currents are considerably smaller, suggesting the entrapment of AgNPs inside the PVP network. There are now three anodic peaks at around 390 mV, 545 mV, and 800 mV that can be related to the different oxidation processes of silver nanoparticles in the Ag/PVP hydrogel. The corresponding cathodic peaks were observed at ≈70, ≈185, and ≈370 mV. Since there is an appearance of the third pair of peaks, it was checked if there was an influence of the side effect of the synthesis, meaning the Ag layer deposited at the surface of the hydrogel. The cyclic voltammetry of Ag/PVP hydrogel, from which the outer layer is removed by cutting, was also monitored. This cyclic voltammogram exhibited neither the anodic peak at 545 mV nor its counterpart at 185 mV. This suggests that those peaks could be attributed to the oxidation/reduction processes of the Ag surface layer deposited during the synthesis. Similarly, to the peaks observed for the Ag/PVP hydrogel immediately after the synthesis, the pair of peaks 390 mV/70 mV can be attributed to the oxidation/reduction of AgNPs inside the hydrogel, and the pair of peaks 800 mV/370 mV can also suggest the oxidation/reduction of AgNPs inside the hydrogel, but of those firmly entrapped inside, and coordinately bonded to PVP molecules. The results suggest that there are two types of AgNPs inside the hydrogel, those that are relatively free and susceptible to the oxidation, as well as those that are already bonded to PVP molecules and, hence, less reactive. Since FE-SEM imaging shown the formation of clusters of small nanoparticles, the "free" nanoparticles could be those attached between themselves, only, and the less reactive ones those nanoparticles at the interface with the PVP hydrogel.

2.1.3.2 Biomechanical Properties

Evaluation of the potential biomedical use for Ag/PVP hydrogels was performed in a bioreactor with mechanical stimulation and interstitial medium flow under physiological regimes simulating *in vivo* conditions in articular cartilage (dynamic compression at 10 % strain, 0.42 Hz, 1 h on / 1 h off, medium flow rate 5×10^{-3} cm^3 s^{-1} corresponding to superficial medium velocity of 25 μm s^{-1} – these conditions were set to mimic walking, and blood velocities found in capillaries (superficial medium velocity ranges from 10 – 100 μm s^{-1}) (Jovanović et al. 2014). The PVP and Ag/PVP hydrogels were tested at the 10 % strain in two regimes: (a) at a loading rate of 337.5 μm s^{-1} and (b) at sequential increments of 100 μm displacement at the same loading rate with pauses of 30 minutes. In all experiments, the stress was shown to be an almost linear function of the applied strain for both hydrogel types. Values of the compression module for PVP and Ag/PVP hydrogels were calculated from the slopes of the best linear fits of the experimental stress-strain curves.

The value of compression module obtained at the loading rate of 337.5 μm s^{-1} for PVP was 37.6 kPa, and for Ag/PVP was about 22.3 % higher (48.4 kPa), indicating that the presence of AgNPs led to a slight decrease in hydrogel elasticity. One of the factors contributing to different biomechanical behavior of the Ag/PVP hydrogel compared to the PVP hydrogel could be the possibility of fluid retention. A slower SBF release from Ag/PVP hydrogel could be explained by the entrapment of ions originating from SBF in the hydrogel voids that are already occupied with AgNPs, making the transit of these ions through the Ag/PVP hydrogel more difficult. In addition, the charging of the AgNPs over time, as a result of the interactions with the polyelectrolyte SBF solution, may change the swelling affinity of the hydrogels and, consequently, the mechanical properties by retaining a certain amount of liquid for a longer time than pure PVP, probably by solvation of the charged AgNPs.

The second experiment in the bioreactor, performed at sequential increments of 100 μm displacements with pauses of 30 minutes, enabled the evaluation of the equilibrium unconfined compression (Young's) modules for the PVP and Ag/PVP hydrogels. The period of 30 minutes was provided for stress relaxation, i.e., to relax the PVP polymer network. The equilibrium stress-strain relationships, as well as those obtained at a loading rate of 337.5 μm s^{-1}, followed linear trends and the equilibrium unconfined compression modules were also calculated from the slopes of the best linear fits of the experimental stress-strain curves. The values of equilibrium unconfined compression modules were found to be quite similar, 31.1 kPa for the PVP disk and 32.0 kPa for the Ag/PVP disk. The difference between these values for the pure PVP and the Ag/PVP hydrogels (2.8 %) was significantly lower than that obtained at a loading rate of 337.5 μm s^{-1} (22.3 %). This may suggest that the presence of AgNPs has no influence on the biomechanical properties of the PVP hydrogels since the equilibrium unconfined compression module values are obtained after the period of polymer relaxation. The possibility of measuring the mechanical properties of hydrogels using this bioreactor system was proven by the obtained values of the equilibrium unconfined compression modules. For both PVP and Ag/PVP hydrogels, these values were in agreement with the values of the Young's module reported for chemically cross-linked PVP hydrogels (Davis, Huglin, and Yip 1988), ranging from 19 kPa to 504 kPa. In addition, the application of PVP and Ag/PVP hydrogels in medicine is rather promising, since the minimal values of the Young's modulus found in the literature required for the application of hydrogels as wound dressings were in the range of 1.5 kPa – 150 kPa (Nickerson et al. 2006; Rattanaruengsrikul, Pimpha, and Supaphol 2009). This suggests that, regarding the mechanical properties, both types of investigated hydrogels could potentially be applicable in medicine.

2.1.3.3 Cytotoxicity

Survivals of target peripheral blood mononuclear cells (PBMC) and human cervix carcinoma cells (HeLa) cells grown in the presence of PVP and Ag/PVP hydrogel swollen in 3.9 mmol dm^{-3} $AgNO_3$ solution were determined by MTT test (Jovanović et al. 2013). The presence of PVP hydrogel caused only a slight decrease in the target cell survival, i.e., 84 ± 9 % for PBMC and 73 ± 9 % for HeLa cells as compared to controls. On the other hand, in the presence of Ag/PVP hydrogel there was a

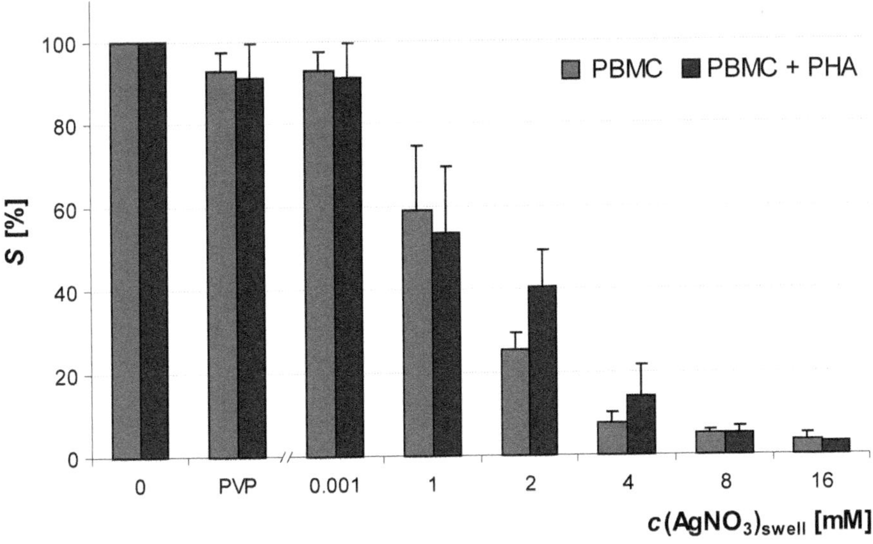

FIGURE 2.7 Survival, *S*, of non-stimulated and PHA-stimulated PBMC cultured for 72 hours in the presence of pure PVP and Ag/PVP hydrogels with different $AgNO_3$ concentrations, $c(AgNO_3)_{swell}$, compared to the control (data represent the average of three measurements; error bars represent standard deviations) (reprinted from Jovanović et al. 2013 with permission from Elsevier)

notable decrease in cell survival, i.e., 60 ± 7 % for PBMC, and 56 ± 8 % for HeLa cells as compared to controls. These results indicated that the sensitivity of normal PBMC and malignant HeLa cells to the presence of PVP and Ag/PVP hydrogels was not significantly different and the subsequent experiments were performed using PBMC only. After the preliminary experiments, cytotoxicity of both hydrogels in PBMC cultures was further studied as a function of AgNP concentration in hydrogel and compared to cytotoxicity of Ag^+ ions originating from addition of $AgNO_3$ solutions. Figure 2.7 presents survival, *S*, of non-stimulated and PHA-stimulated PBMC exposed to PVP and Ag/PVP hydrogels swollen in solutions of different $AgNO_3$ concentrations (1- 16 mmol dm^{-3}) compared to the control.

It should be noted that the presence of PVP hydrogel leads only to a slight decrease in the survival of non-stimulated and PHA-stimulated PBMC, i.e., 92.6 ± 4.7 % and 91.0 ± 8.5 %, respectively, referring to the control sample. On the other hand, survival of PBMC remarkably decreased in the presence of Ag/PVP hydrogel. It can be deduced that the release of silver from Ag/PVP hydrogel swollen in 1 mmol dm^{-3} $AgNO_3$ exerted slight cytotoxicity in non-stimulated PBMC culture, while Ag/PVP hydrogel swollen in more concentrated $AgNO_3$ solutions exerted pronounced cytotoxicity. In addition, cytotoxic effects were not significantly different in non-stimulated and PBMC cultures stimulated for proliferation. It can be seen that the presence of Ag^+ ions in the concentrations up to 1 μmol dm^{-3} induced only a low decrease in PBMC survival, corresponding to slight cytotoxicity. However, Ag^+ concentration of

10 μmol dm^{-3} produced significant decrease in PBMC survival, down to less than 20 %. Again, the presence of PHA had negligible effects on cell survival in all cultures.

IC_{50} values, defined as the concentration of an agent inhibiting cell survival by 50 % as compared to the control, for Ag^+ ions were 4.8 μmol dm^{-3} and 5.6 μmol dm^{-3}, for non-stimulated and PHA-stimulated PBMC, respectively. These results are comparable with the previous report of Hidalgo and Domínguez (Hidalgo and Domínguez 1998), where human dermal fibroblasts were exposed to $AgNO_3$ at concentrations of 4.12 – 82.4 μmol dm^{-3} for 8 and 24 hours. After 24 hours, Ag^+ ions at the concentration of 16.5 μmol dm^{-3} caused 50 % decrease in protein content, in the presence of 10 % of fetal calf serum (FCS). Slightly higher IC_{50} values obtained in this study after 72 hours exposure of PBMC to Ag^+ ions, confirm that silver cytotoxicity to human cells is dependent not only on the ion concentration and exposure period but also on the cell type.

From the *in vitro* experiments here presented, it was observed that AgNPs and Ag^+ ions exhibited dose-dependent cytotoxicity in PBMC cultures. In addition, there were no remarkable differences in cytotoxicity of the investigated agents in non-stimulated and PHA-stimulated PBMC cultures. The results suggest that the same slight cytotoxic effects are induced in 1 μmol dm^{-3} $AgNO_3$ solution as in the presence of Ag/PVP hydrogel swollen in the $AgNO_3$ solution of three orders of magnitude higher concentration (1 mmol dm^{-3}). Furthermore, the antibacterial activity of Ag/PVP hydrogels against *S. aureus* was performed by the agar diffusion test (Jovanović et al. 2014). After 24 hours of incubation, an obvious clear zone of $\approx$1 mm appeared around the disk specimens, indicating the absence of bacterial growth. This suggests the reaching of the minimum inhibitory concentrations of released silver around the Ag/PVP hydrogel. After removal of Ag/PVP hydrogel from the Petri dishes, the zone of the bacterial growth inhibition was also observed on the agar surface at the locations of previous specimen positions, suggesting acceleration of the top-down diffusion of silver. These results demonstrated that the Ag/PVP hydrogel efficiently released AgNPs and/or Ag^+ ions and induced bactericidal effects against *S. aureus*.

2.1.3.4 Silver Release

The decrease in silver concentrations within Ag/PVP hydrogel under static conditions, in perfusion bioreactors and in the bioreactor with dynamic compression coupled with SBF perfusion, up to 42 days, is presented in Figure 2.8. The initial concentration of AgNPs in Ag/PVP hydrogel swollen in 3.9 mmol dm^{-3} $AgNO_3$ solution was determined to be 206.2 ± 62.2 mg dm^{-3}. This value yields approximately 50 % of the value that would be expected if the reduction of all Ag^+ ions present in the swollen hydrogel were complete. The experimentally determined value was used in further calculations in the diffusion model that is later discussed. Differences in the silver release profiles obtained in the three investigated systems were statistically insignificant (under 3 %), which implies that under all investigated conditions the governing mass transport phenomenon was internal diffusion. This finding suggests that the flow of SBF both in perfusion bioreactors as well as in the bioreactor with dynamic compression coupled with SBF perfusion is carried out mostly around and not through the samples, leaving diffusion as the sole silver release mechanism.

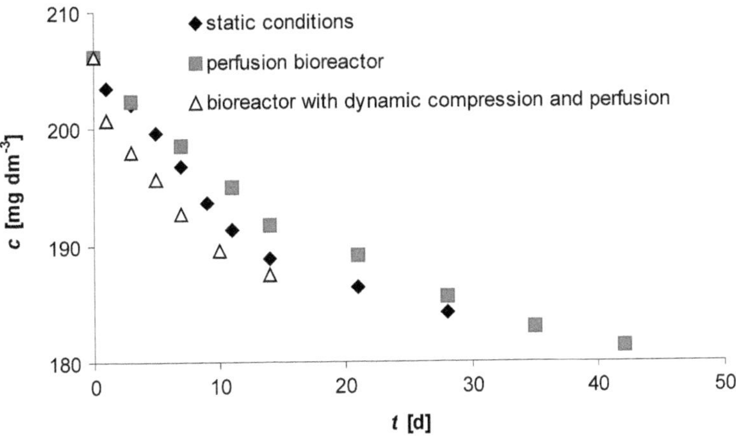

FIGURE 2.8 Silver concentrations in Ag/PVP hydrogels during release studies under static conditions, in perfusion bioreactors and in the bioreactor with dynamic compression coupled with SBF perfusion (data represent the average of three measurements; standard deviations are within 10% but error bars are omitted for the figure clarity) (reprinted from Jovanović et al. 2013 with permission from Elsevier)

Also, surface washout of silver in the bioreactors as compared to static conditions did not contribute to the amounts of silver released, suggesting that the Ag/PVP hydrogel surfaces were not significant sources of silver, which was indeed the aim of the nanocomposite synthesizing procedure. It should be noted that a slightly lower release rate observed in perfusion bioreactors as compared to static conditions was probably due to the more frequent medium exchange and, thus, the slightly increased diffusion driving force in the latter system. On the other hand, silver concentrations in Ag/PVP hydrogel in the bioreactor with dynamic compression coupled with SBF perfusion were consistently lower than those in the other two systems, indicating a slightly higher silver release rate in the former system (Figure 2.8), probably as a result of dynamic compression. Namely, dynamic compression was performed at the 10 % strain and a loading rate of 337.5 $\mu m\ s^{-1}$ (yielding the frequency of 0.37 Hz) in a 1 hour on / 1 hour off regime, which enabled slight intensification of the silver release. The amount of released silver over the 14 day bioreactor study yielded ~ 9 % of the total initial content. It is also important to note that the effects of dynamic compression on the silver release rate are not highly pronounced as may be expected, due to the reverse medium flow inside the hydrogel during the decompression phase. Thus, the overall effect is insignificantly different as compared to pure diffusion observed under static conditions.

Regardless of the experimental conditions, silver concentration decrease in Ag/PVP hydrogel is rather low, up to 12 % that was determined after 42 days under static conditions. Minor influences of hydrodynamic bioreactor conditions on the silver release rate is most likely the consequence of the stability of silver nanoparticles inside the highly cross-linked PVP hydrogel network, since they coordinate with amide-carbonyl groups of PVP molecules (Jovanović et al. 2011). As a result, these Ag/PVP hydrogels could be used for a prolonged period of time, preserving the sterility of a soft tissue implant for example.

The influence of different experimental conditions (static, SBF perfusion, dynamic compression coupled with SBF perfusion) on the silver release from Ag/PVP hydrogels was quantified by application of the diffusion model. To distinguish the slight influence of dynamic compression, results obtained under these conditions were modeled separately from the results obtained in the other two systems. Initial linear dependences between the ratio m_t/m_∞ vs. $t^{1/2}$ confirmed the diffusion mechanism that obeys the second Fick's law of diffusion (Crank 1970).

$$\frac{m_t}{m_\infty} = \frac{4}{\delta} \frac{D^{1/2}}{\pi^{1/2}} t^{1/2} \quad (2.7)$$

where m_t is the amount of silver released at time t, m_∞ is the amount of silver released at equilibrium, D is the diffusion coefficient of AgNPs through pure the hydrogel, and δ is the thickness of the hydrogel sample. Diffusion coefficient of AgNPs through Ag/PVP hydrogel network of 1.64 x 10^{-10} cm^2 s^{-1} was calculated from the initial liner slope of the m_t/m_∞ vs time for static and SBF perfusion bioreactor conditions, while the apparent diffusion coefficient of 2.79 x 10^{-10} cm^2 s^{-1} was calculated for silver release in the bioreactor with dynamic compression coupled with SBF perfusion. As it can be observed, dynamic compression induced for ~ 40 % higher silver release rate compared to static conditions and SBF perfusion as determined by the value of the apparent diffusion coefficient.

The diffusion model can be used in conjunction with results of cytotoxicity studies to predict performance and the possible lifetime of Ag/PVP hydrogels applied in different environments. Namely, it was shown (Jovanović et al. 2013) that the final concentration of released silver in medium after 72 hours is calculated to be 0.4 μmol dm^{-3}. Considering that the slight cytotoxicity of Ag/PVP hydrogel is achieved after 72 hours, this should be the time after which the wound dressing is to be removed/changed. On the other hand, the system that simulates physiological conditions in articular cartilage (bioreactor with dynamic compression coupled with SBF perfusion) would correspond to a soft tissue implant in a synovial joint, e.g., knee. The volume of synovial fluid (SF) in normal human joints is approximately 0.5 – 2.0 cm^3 (Moskowitz et al. 2001; Levick et al. 1999). However, since SF undergoes continuous turnover by trans-synovial flow into synovial lymph vessels, water and proteins in the SF are replaced within a period of 2 hours or less (Levick et al. 1999). Now, the diffusion model can be used to calculate the amount of silver released from the same Ag/PVP hydrogel swollen in 1 mmol dm^{-3} $AgNO_3$ solution if potentially implanted in the knee for 2 hours needed for the complete replacement of SBF. The diffusion coefficient of 2.79 x 10^{-10} cm^2 s^{-1} was determined for the bioreactor with dynamic compression coupled with SBF perfusion, the total amount of silver in Ag/PVP hydrogel and the amount of the released silver after 2 h was calculated to be 0.1 μmol dm^{-3} and 0.03 μmol dm^{-3}, for the volume of SF in normal human joints of 0.5

cm^3 and 2 cm^3, respectively. These results mean that during the time needed for the complete replacement of SBF in the knee joint of 2 hours, silver concentrations will be below the value that was determined in this study to induce only slight cytotoxicity (0.4 μmol dm^{-3}). The other benefit is that the implanted Ag/PVP hydrogel would preserve its sterility for a prolonged time. Model predictions thus imply that Ag/PVP hydrogels could be used both as wound dressings and as cartilage implants without harming effects to the surrounding tissue.

2.1.4 Poly(Vinyl Alcohol)-Based Hydrogels with Silver Nanoparticles

2.1.4.1 Electrochemical Synthesis and Characterization of Silver/Poly(Vinyl Alcohol) and Silver/Poly(Vinyl Alcohol)/Graphene Solutions and Films

Poly(vinyl alcohol) (PVA) is a widely used synthetic polymer. The benefits of its use lie in its properties: non-toxicity, water solubility, biocompatibility and biodegradability. Also, its low price and wide availability makes PVA a polymer of choice in a large number of applications. Hydrogels made of PVA have become attractive as matrices for repairing and regenerating several types of tissues and organs in the fields of tissue engineering and regenerative medicine (Georgieva, Bryaskova, and Tzoneva 2012; Gonzalez et al. 2012; Maiolo et al. 2012; Jiang, Liu, and Feng 2011; Nacer Khodja et al. 2013; M.-H. Huang and Yang 2008). The significant swelling capacity of PVA hydrogels, which enables the absorption of exudates generated during the process of wound healing, makes them adequate biomaterials for wound dressings (Jiang, Liu, and Feng 2011; Singh and Pal 2012; Păduraru et al. 2012; Salarizadeh et al. 2013; Ahmad, Yusuf, and Ooi 2012). As a result of its extraordinary structure, graphene (Gr), a single-layered hexagonal honeycomb lattice consisting solely of sp^2-bonded carbon atoms, has very unique properties, such as high mechanical strength, electrical conductivity, and a large specific surface area, and it possesses enhanced transport characteristics. Graphene can significantly improve poor mechanical properties or even facilitate drug delivery and targeting of cells. The general aim of using graphene nanosheets as nanofillers is to significantly improve mechanical properties while retaining the original biocompatibility (Surudžić, Janković, Mitrić et al. 2016).

Silver nanoparticles were electrochemically synthesized by reduction of silver ions, using PVA as a capping agent (Surudžić et al. 2013; Surudžić, Janković, Bibić et al. 2016; M. M. Abudabbus et al. 2016; Mohamed M. Abudabbus et al. 2018). In general, formation of metal nanoparticles by electrolysis starts with the reduction of their ions at the cathode. Stabilization agents are being introduced to speed up the formation of AgNPs, reduce the metal layer deposition on the cathode surface, and limit the agglomeration of nanoparticles in the solution. The reduction of water and Ag^+ ions occurs at the cathode (Eqs. 2.1 and 2.3), respectively, while water oxidation occurs at the anode (Eq. 2.2). Since Pt electrode was used as the anode, another possible anodic reaction is the oxidation of Pt:

$$Pt + O_2 \rightarrow PtO_2 + 4e^- \quad (2.8)$$

Silver layer electrodeposition at the cathode surface occurs simultaneously, decreasing the effective surface for silver nanoparticle production. Based on previously reported mechanisms found in the literature for AgNPs production in a polymer matrix (Rudko et al. 2015), the following mechanism can be proposed. The possible anchoring sites for Ag-PVA complexation are the C=O groups in the acetate residuals and exposed -OH groups in PVA. Lone pairs on the oxygen atoms can occupy two sp orbitals of Ag^+ to form a metal complex. The first step is the formation Ag_m^{m+}-PVA complex, where m is the number of Ag^+ bounded with PVA molecule. The second step is the electrochemical reduction of Ag_m^{m+}-PVA complex at the cathode surface, followed by formation of Ag_m^0-PVA adatoms stabilized with PVA chains. The presence of PVA ensures that the Ag_m^{m+}-PVA complex is being reduced rather than individual Ag^+ ions. Consequently, the deposition of a metallic silver layer at the cathode surface is lowered. In the succeeding step, PVA promotes silver nucleation. The final stage involves AgNPs growth with particle aggregation being restricted by the presence of PVA.

Ag/PVA colloid dispersions were obtained by electrochemical reduction of silver ions in PVA solutions containing 5 or 10 wt. % PVA, 0.1 M KNO_3, and 3.9 mM $AgNO_3$. Applied current density was 25 mA cm^{-2} and synthesis time was 10 minutes (Surudžić et al. 2013). UV-Vis spectroscopy was employed to monitor the silver nanoparticles formation. The first absorption peak at ~400 nm confirms the formation of silver nanoparticles. The second absorption band peaking at nearly 650 nm can be explained by aggregation or agglomeration of silver nanoparticles present in the colloid dispersion. The difference between the spectra of Ag/PVA colloid dispersions containing 5 and 10 wt. % PVA was in the absorbance intensity, where higher absorbance exhibited the solution with higher PVA concentration. This suggests that a higher concentration of silver nanoparticles was obtained with a higher concentration of PVA in the initial solution, since the silver nanoparticles concentration is proportional to the absorbance intensity.

UV-Vis analysis was also used to determine the effect of PVA concentration on the amount and relative size of silver nanoparticles. An increase in PVA concentration increases the absorbance maximum, indicating the greater amount of silver nanoparticles in Ag/PVA colloid dispersion. For both Ag/PVA colloid solutions A_{max} increases up to 20th day and remains almost constant up to day 30, while further increase in A_{max} is a consequence of gelation. It can be said that the absorbance maximum is reached 20 days after the synthesis when the silver nanoparticles growth is terminated. It was noticed for both Ag/PVA dispersions that the λ_{max} increases up to day 20, and then remains almost constant, as well as the concentration of PVA solution does not affect the size of synthesized silver nanoparticles. This is in accordance with the previous assumption that the growth of silver nanoparticles terminated around 20 days after the synthesis. Since it was proved that the higher concentration of silver nanoparticles in Ag/PVP solution were synthesized from 10 wt.% PVA solution (UV-Vis measurements) as well as more stable silver nanoparticles were formed (CV measurements), all further characterizations were performed on Ag/PVA solution synthesized from 10 wt. % PVA.

To study the effect of graphene, Ag/PVA and Ag/PVA/Gr (0.01 wt.% Gr) colloid dispersions were obtained by electrochemical reduction of silver ions in PVA and PVA/Gr solutions, respectively, containing 10 wt. % PVA, 0.1 M KNO_3, 3.9 mM $AgNO_3$ and in the case of Ag/PVA/Gr 0.01 wt.% Gr additionally. The applied current density was 40 mA cm^{-2} and the reaction time was 30 minutes. (Surudžić, Janković, Bibić et al. 2016). The absorption spectra of pure PVA solution and Ag/PVA and Ag/PVA/Gr colloid dispersions are shown in Figure 2.9. The PVA spectrum did not exhibit an absorbance peak in the examined range of wavelengths. Both Ag/PVA and Ag/PVA/Gr colloid dispersions exhibited absorption spectra with two bands peaking at around 400 and around 650 nm. The first absorption peak at ≈400 nm confirmed the formation of AgNPs, while the second absorption band peaking at nearly 650 nm indicated aggregation or agglomeration of the AgNPs. Because the concentration of AgNPs is proportional to the absorbance intensity, it was concluded that that presence of graphene slightly decreased the amount of AgNPs in the Ag/PVA/Gr colloid dispersion.

UV-Vis analysis was also used to determine the effect of aging time on the amount and relative size of AgNPs in the colloid dispersions. The presence of graphene decreased the absorbance maximum, A_{max}, indicating a smaller amount of AgNPs in the Ag/PVA/Gr colloid dispersion. For both Ag/PVA and Ag/PVA/Gr colloid dispersions, A_{max}, increased up to day 15 and then increased slowly up to day 20, while a

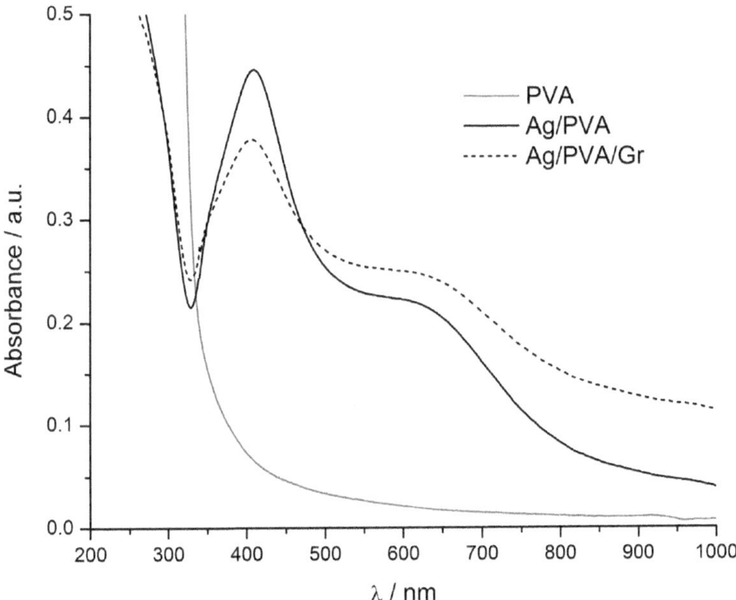

FIGURE 2.9 UV-Vis spectra of 10 wt.% PVA solution and Ag/PVA and Ag/PVA/Gr colloid dispersions at day 14 after synthesis (reprinted from Surudžić, Janković, Bibić et al. 2016 with permission from Elsevier)

further increase in A_{max} with time was the consequence of gelation. The absorbance maximum was attained 15 days after the synthesis, when the growth of the silver nanoparticles terminated. For both Ag/PVA and Ag/PVA/Gr colloid dispersions, the wavelength of the absorbance maximum, λ_{max}, increased with time, reaching a value of 407 nm for Ag/PVA/Gr, and 410 nm for Ag/PVA on day 15 (Surudžić, Janković, Bibić et al. 2016). A lower λ_{max} values has been reported to correspond to smaller nanoparticles; the results therefore suggested that AgNPs in the Ag/PVA/Gr colloid dispersions had smaller dimensions than those in the Ag/PVA colloid dispersions, indicating that graphene sheets situated between the polymer chains prevented the further growth and aggregation or agglomeration of AgNPs.

TEM micrographs proved the sphere-like morphologies of AgNPs at the nanoscale level (Surudžić, Janković, Bibić et al. 2016). Diameter of AgNPs was approximately 10–40 nm for both Ag/PVA and Ag/PVA/Gr colloidal dispersions. It was assumed that the following three-step mechanism of particle assembly occurred: (1) silver ions interacted with the hydroxyl groups of PVA, (2) nearby silver atoms that had been reduced electrochemically aggregated at close range (primary nanoparticles), and (3) nearby primary nanoparticles coalesced with other primary nanoparticles or interacted with PVA molecules to form larger aggregates (secondary nanoparticles). As a consequence, entrapment of silver nanoparticles by PVA molecules occurred; this implied that the AgNPs had enhanced stability. The small dimensions and low aggregation of AgNPs in the Ag/PVA/Gr dispersion due to the presence of transparent graphene sheets situated between the PVA polymer chains prevented further growth and aggregation or agglomeration of AgNPs. This is in agreement with the results obtained from UV-Vis.

Cyclic voltammogram of the Pt electrode in 10 wt. % PVA solution exhibited a broad cathodic peak at about –100 mV, originating from reduction of the Pt oxide formed during the anodic sweep. The anodic counterpart of this peak at about 850 mV, corresponding to Pt oxide formation, was slightly visible due to an overlap with the oxidation current at potentials more positive than 400 mV (Surudžić, Janković, Bibić et al. 2016). The shift of the cathodic peak from -250 mV to -100 mV, as well as the slightly visible anodic peak at about 850 mV with respect to the reference solution containing 3.9 mM $AgNO_3$ and 0.1 M KNO_3 (Jovanović et al. 2014), was attributed to the presence of PVA polymer chains that impeded oxidation/reduction processes on the Pt electrode. Cyclic voltammogram of the Pt electrode in the Ag/PVA colloid dispersion exhibited two anodic peaks: a main peak at around 680 mV, which originated from the oxidation of AgNPs, and a small, slightly visible anodic peak at around 870 mV due to oxidation of free Pt surfaces and Pt oxide formation. Two cathodic counterparts were observed: a peak at around 180 mV corresponding to the reduction of AgNPs, and a peak at around – 300 mV originating from reduction of Pt oxide. Shifts of the anodic peak due to AgNP oxidation and the cathodic peak due to AgNP reduction toward more positive potentials (680 and 180 mV, respectively) in comparison with reference solution containing 3.9 mM $AgNO_3$ and 0.1 M KNO_3 (600 and 160 mV, respectively) was a consequence of PVA polymer chains that impeded oxidation/reduction processes on the Pt electrodes. In the cyclic voltammogram of the Pt electrode in Ag/PVA/Gr colloid dispersion, two anodic peaks were obvious – one at around 650 mV due to AgNP oxidation and the second at around 950 mV due to oxidation of free Pt surfaces and Pt oxide formation. Two cathodic counterparts were observed: a peak at around 130 mV corresponding to AgNPs reduction and a peak at around – 370 mV due to reduction of the Pt oxide. The shift of the anodic peak of AgNP oxidation and the cathodic peak of AgNPs reduction toward more negative potentials (650 and 130 mV, respectively) in comparison with Ag/PVA colloid dispersion (680 and 180 mV, respectively) indicated that the AgNPs in the Ag/PVA/Gr dispersion had smaller dimensions and/or lower aggregation due to graphene sheets situated between the polymer chains that prevented the further growth and aggregation or agglomeration of AgNPs. This is in agreement with the results obtained from UV-Vis and TEM.

Ag/PVA and Ag/PVA/Gr nanocomposite films were obtained from colloid dispersions by solvent evaporation at 60 °C, and these films were characterized by FE-SEM, Raman spectroscopy, FT-IR, XRD, XPS, TGA, and tensile tests (Surudžić, Janković, Bibić et al. 2016). FE-SEM microphotographs showed that AgNPs in the Ag/PVA/Gr film had smaller dimensions and/or lower aggregation than AgNPs in the Ag/PVA film due to graphene sheets between the polymer chains that prevented the further growth and aggregation or agglomeration of AgNPs in the Ag/PVA/Gr film. Raman analysis was performed to verify the incorporation of graphene in Ag/PVA/Gr film (Surudžić, Janković, Bibić et al. 2016). Raman spectroscopy of graphene is generally characterized by two main features: the G-peak, which arises from first order scattering of the E_{2g} phonon from sp^2 carbon atoms (in the range of 1500–1600 cm^{-1}), and the D-peak (in the range of 1200–1500 cm^{-1}), which arises from the breathing mode of k-point photons with A1g symmetry. D-peak at 1379 cm^{-1} represents edges, other defects, disordered sp^3-bonded carbon atoms, and impurities, while the G-band at 1618 cm^{-1} corresponds to ordered sp^2-bonded carbon atoms. The low intensity of both D and G peaks was attributed to the low concentration of graphene in the Ag/PVA/Gr composite film.

FT-IR measurements of Ag/PVA and Ag/PVA/Gr films were performed to characterize the interactions among PVA molecules, AgNPs, and graphene, exhibiting a few differences compared to that of pure PVA. Important changes were observed for bands peaking at 1418 cm^{-1} and 1323 cm^{-1} in the PVA spectrum corresponding to coupling of the –OH in-plane vibration with C–H wagging vibrations. The shift of the band peaking at 1418 cm^{-1} in PVA to 1371 cm^{-1} in Ag/PVA and 1353 cm^{-1} in Ag/PVA/Gr spectra, and the disappearance of the band peaking at 1323 cm^{-1} in Ag/PVA and Ag/PVA/Gr spectra, suggested in both cases an interaction between the AgNPs and the hydroxyl groups of the PVA molecules through decoupling between the corresponding vibrations. The greater shift of the band at 1418 cm^{-1} (for PVA) to 1353 cm^{-1} (for Ag/PVA/Gr) than for Ag/PVA (1371 cm^{-1}) indicated the occurrence of additional hydrogen bonding interactions between the OH^- groups present in PVA and oxygen containing groups in graphene sheets situated between the polymer chains in the Ag/PVA/Gr film that prevented further growth and aggregation or agglomeration of AgNPs, as proven by the FE-SEM microphotographs.

XRD patterns of Ag/PVA and Ag/PVA/Gr films have shown the broad peaks at 2θ =19.65° and 19.45°, respectively, corresponding to the (002) lattice plane, are related to the characteristic peak of PVA at 2θ =19.3° due to the semi-crystalline structure of PVA (Bryaskova et al. 2010). It was clear that the five diffraction peaks for Ag/PVA and Ag/PVA/Gr films at 2θ of 38.2°, 44.4°, 64.6°, 77.4°, and 81.5° corresponded to Bragg's reflections from the (111), (200), (220), (311), and (222) crystal planes of Ag. A weak broad peak near 25° indicated that graphene was present in the Ag/PVA/Gr films. Average crystallite domain size, D_p, was calculated from the half height width ($\beta_{1/2}$) of the XRD reflection of the (002) plane, using the Scherer equation:

$$D_p = \frac{K\lambda}{\beta_{1/2} \cos\theta} \tag{2.9}$$

where λ is the wavelength of the X-ray radiation of 1.5418 Å, K is the shape coefficient equal to 0.9 and θ is the diffraction angle. The average crystallite domain size, D_p, of 0.2782 nm for PVA has been changed upon incorporation of AgNPs and graphene sheets to 0.2880 nm and 0.2602 nm, for Ag/PVA and Ag/PVA/Gr film, respectively, indicating in both cases interactions between the AgNPs and the hydroxyl groups of PVA molecules, as well as additional interactions between PVA molecules and graphene sheets situated between the polymer chains in the Ag/PVA/Gr film. Single layer graphene comprises carbon atoms arranged periodically in a hexagonal manner, and the nearest distance between two carbon atoms is 0.142 nm. Multilayer graphene sheets contain several graphene monolayers with an interwall distance of 0.340 nm (Yi Liu, Huang, and Li 2013). However, the average crystallite domain size of the (002) lattice plane in Ag/PVA/Gr was calculated to be 0.2602 nm, indicating the occurrence of hydrogen bonding interactions between the OH^- groups present in PVA and oxygen containing groups in graphene. This confirmed the hypothesis (Surudžić, Janković, Bibić et al. 2016) that graphene sheets situated between the polymer chains prevented the further growth and aggregation or agglomeration of AgNPs as observed by FT-IR and FE-SEM.

Elemental compositions of Ag/PVA and Ag/PVA/Gr films were investigated via surface analysis by XPS, respectively (Surudžić, Janković, Bibić et al. 2016). XPS survey spectra of both films revealed the presence of carbon (C1s), oxygen (O1s), and silver (Ag3d). The C1s peak may have originated from the PVA itself (binding energy (BE) of 285.02 eV) or from added graphene with a BE of 284.95 eV because the C1s peak corresponding to the BE of 285.0 eV could be attributed to aromatic hydrocarbons, actually C=C (sp^2 bond) in the graphitic network. The BE of the Ag3d peak (≈ 368 eV) agreed with that reported in the literature, indicating formation of a nanocomposite with silver (Joshi, Markad, and Haram 2015). The O1s peak may have originated from PVA itself with a BE of 533.0 eV or from added graphene with a binding energy of 532.9 eV due to C-O bonds, which are characteristics of C-O stretches of graphene sheets (Bon et al. 2009). Survey spectra of the Ag/PVA/Gr film revealed indisputable evidence of graphene incorporation, namely, an increased C1s content (77.38 at% in respect to 56.54 at% in Ag/PVA) and decreased O1s content (22.30 at% in respect to 41.36 at% in Ag/PVA). The smaller atomic percentage of silver in Ag/PVA/Gr film (0.32 at%) than Ag/PVA film (2.10 at%) indicated smaller AgNPs, as was observed by FE-SEM.

Thermogravimetric analysis (TGA) and corresponding differential thermogravimetric analysis (DTG) were performed to investigate the effect of incorporation of graphene sheets on the thermal stability of the polymer matrix (Surudžić, Janković, Bibić et al. 2016). Both Ag/PVA and Ag/PVA/Gr films showed a three-step weight loss process. The small weight loss in the first step at about 70 °C – 120 °C was attributed to the loss of absorbed water. The weight loss at about 230 °C –320 °C during the second step suggested the degradation of PVA (in Ag/PVA film) or PVA and graphene (in Ag/PVA/Gr film). The third weight loss step at about 350 °C – 600 °C was attributed to further decomposition of the remaining composites. The peak temperature of the DTG curve represents the temperature at which the maximum weight loss rate was reached. The peak temperature of the Ag/PVA/Gr film was about 282 °C, 8 °C higher than that of the Ag/PVA film; this confirmed bonding between PVA molecules and graphene sheets (Yuan 2011; Gong et al. 2015). Similarly, the smaller weight loss at 450 °C for Ag/PVA/Gr (77.26 wt. %) than for Ag/PVA (80.21 wt. %) demonstrated that the Ag/PVA/Gr film was more stable than the Ag/PVA film due to stronger interactions between molecules in the former.

To evaluate the mechanical properties of Ag/PVA and Ag/PVA/Gr films, tensile tests were performed (Surudžić, Janković, Bibić et al. 2016). Tensile strength of the Ag/PVA/Gr film relative to that of Ag/PVA film increased by 16.4% from 121.2 to 141.1 MPa, and the Young's modulus increased by 126.9 % from 0.309 to 0.701 GPa. The elongation at break of the Ag/PVA film was the same as that of the Ag/PVA/Gr film. The enhanced mechanical properties, i.e., greater values of tensile strength and Young's modulus of the Ag/PVA/Gr film are the consequences of incorporation of Gr into the PVA matrix and bonding between PVA molecules and graphene sheets.

2.1.4.2 Cytotoxicity

Ag/PVA and Ag/PVA/Gr hydrogels were obtained from colloid dispersions by the freeze-thaw method in five cycles of successive freezing and thawing (one cycle involved freezing for 16 hours at -18 °C and thawing for 8 hours at 4 °C) (Surudžić, Janković, Bibić et al. 2016). Determining dose-dependent cytotoxicity of AgNPs and Ag^+ ions incorporated into hydrogels was the primary concern in the quest for the best-suited composite (M M Abudabbus et al. 2016). The cell survival, *S*, of non-stimulated and PHA-stimulated PBMCs exposed to pure PVA hydrogel and Ag/PVA hydrogels swollen in solutions of different $AgNO_3$ concentrations (0.25, 0.5,1, and 3.9 mM) was determined. It could be observed that the increase in silver concentration in $AgNO_3$ solutions induced decrease in target cell survival. It should be noted that the presence of pure PVA hydrogel leads only to a slight decrease in the survival of non-stimulated and PHA-stimulated PBMC, i.e., 90.77 ± 0.88 % and 84.01 ± 7.86 %, respectively. On the other hand, survival of PBMC remarkably decreased in the presence of high dosage of AgNPs in Ag/PVA hydrogels. It can be deduced that the release of silver from Ag/PVA hydrogels swollen in 0.25 mM $AgNO_3$ solutions demonstrated the lowest cytotoxicity in non-stimulated PBMC culture, while Ag/PVA hydrogels swollen in more concentrated $AgNO_3$ solutions exerted pronounced cytotoxicity. It should be also noted that when stimulated to proliferation (induced PHA into the culture medium) cells retained high survival rate as cytotoxic effects of hydrogels were not significantly different in non-stimulated and stimulated for proliferation PBMC cells.

In the case of Ag/PVA/Gr hydrogel, dose-dependent cytotoxicity of AgNPs and Ag^+ ions after the preliminary experiments and cytotoxicity of PVA/Gr and Ag/PVA/Gr hydrogels seeded by PBMC cultures was further studied as a function of AgNPs concentration in composites. Survival of PBMC remarkably decreased in the presence of Ag/PVA/Gr when the loading of Ag increased. The release of silver from Ag/PVA/Gr hydrogel swollen in 0.25 mM $AgNO_3$ solution exerted the lowest cytotoxicity toward non-stimulated PBMC culture, while Ag/PVA/Gr hydrogels swollen in more concentrated $AgNO_3$ solutions exerted pronounced cytotoxicity. The presence of PHA had negligible effects on the overall cell survival since cytotoxic effects were not significantly different in non-stimulated and proliferated PBMC cells. The results suggest that slight cytotoxic effect was observed for both Ag/PVA and Ag/PVA/Gr hydrogels swollen in 0.25 mM $AgNO_3$ solution.

2.1.4.3 Antibacterial Activity

Antibacterial activities of the Ag/PVA and Ag/PVA/Gr hydrogels against *S. aureus* TL and *E. coli* in PB, were evaluated quantitatively by monitoring the changes in the number of viable bacterial cells in suspension (Figure 2.10).

Both Ag/PVA and Ag/PVA/Gr hydrogels significantly reduced bacterial cell viability after just 1 hour of incubation when compared to the initial number of cells in suspension. Ag/PVA resulted in a 3 logarithmic unit reduction of *S. aureus* colonies and a 2 logarithmic unit reduction of *E. coli* colonies, while Ag/PVA/Gr resulted in complete reduction of *S. aureus* and a 5 logarithmic unit reduction of *E. coli* colonies Ag/PVA killed all *S. aureus* colonies after 24 hours and all *E. coli* colonies after 3 hours. In contrast, Ag/PVA/Gr completely destroyed all *S. aureus* TL and *E. coli* colonies after 3 hours and 24 hours, respectively. Greater antibacterial activity of Ag/PVA/Gr than Ag/PVA could be a consequence of the smaller dimensions of the AgNPs embedded in the hydrogel network, as discussed earlier. Additionally, the antibacterial activity of Ag/PVA/Gr hydrogel can be explained by the presence of graphene affecting bacterial cell membrane and/or by oxidative stress it causes, i.e., by synergistic action of both silver and graphene. Physical damage on bacterial membranes occurs upon direct contact by graphene-based materials e.g., low thickness graphene sharp edges cut through membranes resulting in release of intracellular contents (Santos et al. 2012; S. Liu et al. 2011). Graphene may also chemically increase cellular oxidative stress through formation of reactive oxygen species (ROS). However, graphene-based materials may disrupt a specific microbial process or a vital cellular structure or component by disturbing or oxidizing them, but without producing ROS. These effects are more pronounced in the case of pure graphene due to a stronger interaction between sharp sheet edges and the bacteria's cell membrane and/or better charge transfer between the bacteria and the graphene-based material itself (S. Liu et al. 2011).

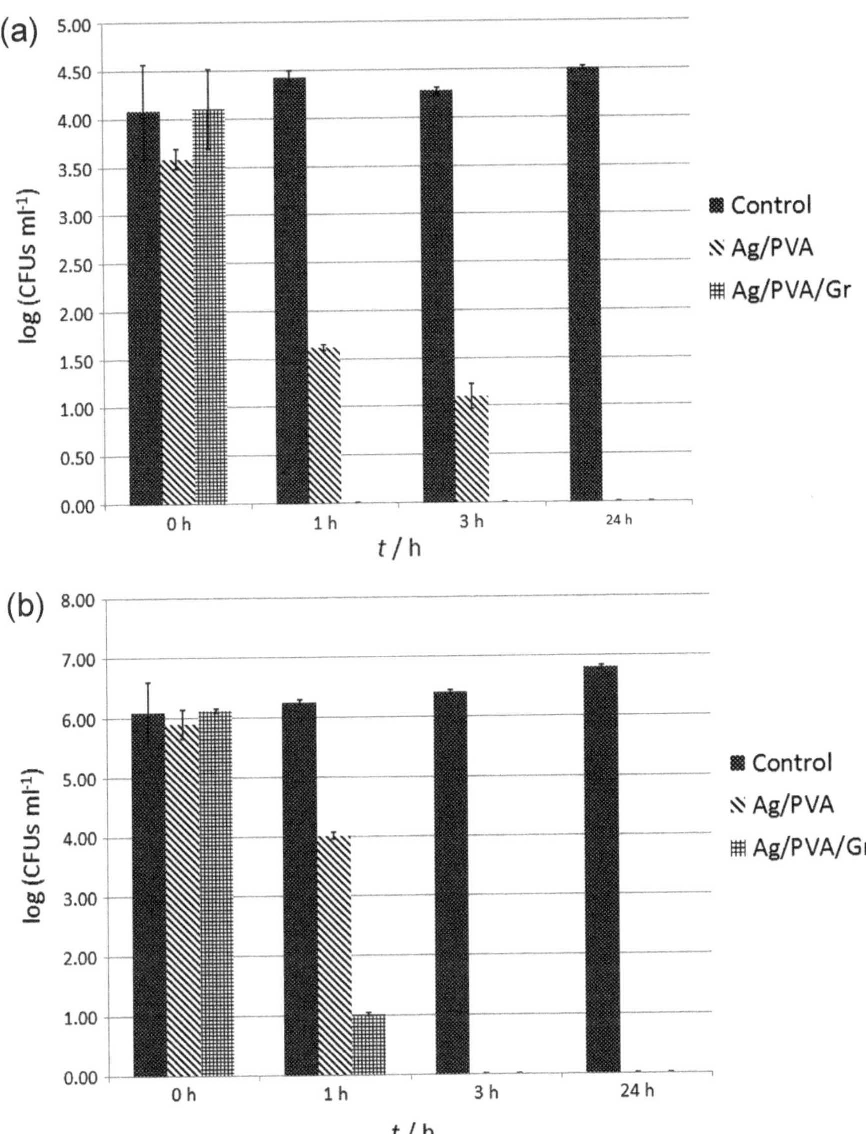

FIGURE 2.10 Reduction of viable cell number of (a) *S. aureus* and (b) *E. coli* after contact with Ag/PVA and Ag/PVA/Gr hydrogels for 0, 1, 3, and 24 hours in PB as compared to the control w/o samples (reprinted from Surudžić, Janković, Bibić et al. 2016 with permission from Elsevier)

2.1.4.4 Silver Release

The kinetics of antibacterial agent release is very important for the applications of antibacterial medical devices, as it influences their antibacterial efficiency and life cycle. The release of silver nanoparticles was monitored over the time period of 28 days in modified phosphate buffered solution (PB, pH 7.4) at 37 °C, for Ag/PVA and Ag/PVA/Gr hydrogels with different concentrations of silver (0.25 mM, 0.5 mM, 1.0 mM, and 3.9 mM). Based on the obtained experimental data it was found that, during the initial period hydrogels exhibited "burst release," marked by a sharp decrease in Ag content, but the release profiles reached a plateau after around two to five days, and further release was significantly slower (Nešović and Mišković-Stanković 2022). Table 2.2 represents the obtained data for the initial concentration of silver in the hydrogel, $c_{Ag,0}$, and the concentration of silver remained in the hydrogel, $c_{Ag,gel}$, after 28 days release, measured by atomic absorption spectroscopy (AAS) for different hydrogels, as well as the percentages of the released silver during a 28-day period. This release behavior is especially important for wound dressings, as the high initial release of antibacterial agent to the wound and surrounding tissue ensures prevention of adhesion of bacteria and biofilm formation. Subsequent slow and steady release can preserve the sterility of the wound and prevent infection over a prolonged application period. It is obvious that all hydrogels retained a certain amount of silver in

TABLE 2.2
Initial Concentration of Silver in the Hydrogel, $c_{Ag,0}$, and the Concentration of Silver Remained in the Hydrogel, $c_{Ag,gel}$, After 28 Days Release in the PB Medium at 37 °C, the Percentages of Released Silver and Silver Diffusion Coefficients, D_{Ag}, Calculated from the Standard and Modified ETA Models (Adapted from Nešović and Mišković-Stanković 2022 with Permission from John Wiley & Sons)

Hydrogel	$c_{Ag,0}$/ mg dm^{-3}	$c_{Ag,gel}$/ mg dm^{-3}	silver released/%	D_{Ag}/10^{-8}cm^2 s^{-1} (Standard ETA)	D_{Ag}/10^{-8} cm^2 s^{-1} (Modified ETA)
0.25Ag/PVA	41.3±8.0	13.3±3.8	68	1.60	0.53
0.5Ag/PVA	50.8±7.2	26.6±2.7	48	1.40	0.38
1.0Ag/PVA	81.4±15.8	27.9±4.3	66	6.79	2.75
3.9Ag/PVA	247.5±27.9	65.4±3.4	74	12.7	5.92
0.25Ag/PVA/Gr	28.2±1.7	9.7±3.6	66	1.71	0.49
0.5Ag/PVA/Gr	64.8±5.6	28.3±7.8	56	1.40	0.53
1.0Ag/PVA/Gr	70.6±14.7	15.2±6.1	78	10.9	4.38
3.9Ag/PVA/Gr	273.1±19.5	59.4±12.2	78	15.6	7.07

their matrices after prolonged release, attesting to their longevity as potential wound dressings. However, a high percentage (60 %–80 %) of the total initial amount of AgNPs was released during the monitored period, confirming that these materials could provide sustained infection protection to the wound. The results of silver release indicated that Ag/PVA and Ag/PVA/Gr hydrogels can be applied for prolonged periods, providing a sufficient amount of antibacterial agent to preserve the sterility of the wound dressing or soft tissue implant.

The generated release profiles were fitted with several theoretical models in order to investigate the kinetics of the silver release. The models were chosen among those most frequently found in literature to describe the diffusion mechanisms behind the drug release processes. One of these models deals with the so-called burst release effect that is often observed during release of drugs and other active substances from polymer carriers, and, as such, it is used to describe the diffusion in the early phase of release; thus, it is called the early time approximation (ETA). For ETA, two equations were used to compare the appropriateness of the model for experimental data. Specifically, a widely used standard ETA (Eq. (2.10)), and a modified ETA (Eq. (2.11)) proposed by Ritger and Peppas (Ritger and Peppas 1987) were applied. In these equations, $c_{Ag,t}/c_{Ag,0}$ denotes the fraction of released silver at the time t, D_{Ag} is the diffusion coefficient of silver, t is the time of release, δ is the hydrogel thickness, and r is the radius of the hydrogel disc.

$$\frac{c_{Ag,t}}{c_{Ag,0}} = 4 \cdot \left(\frac{D_{Ag} \cdot t}{\pi \cdot \delta^2} \right)^{1/2} \tag{2.10}$$

$$\begin{aligned} \frac{c_{Ag,t}}{c_{Ag,0}} = {} & 4 \cdot \left(\frac{D_{Ag} \cdot t}{\pi \cdot r^2} \right)^{1/2} - \pi \cdot \left(\frac{D_{Ag} \cdot t}{\pi \cdot r^2} \right) - \frac{\pi}{3} \cdot \left(\frac{D_{Ag} \cdot t}{\pi \cdot r^2} \right)^{3/2} + 4 \cdot \left(\frac{D_{Ag} \cdot t}{\pi \cdot \delta^2} \right)^{1/2} \\ & - \frac{2r}{\delta} \cdot \left[8 \cdot \left(\frac{D_{Ag} \cdot t}{\pi \cdot r^2} \right) - 2\pi \cdot \left(\frac{D_{Ag} \cdot t}{\pi \cdot r^2} \right)^{3/2} - \frac{2\pi}{3} \cdot \left(\frac{D_{Ag} \cdot t}{\pi \cdot r^2} \right)^2 \right] \end{aligned} \tag{2.11}$$

The ETA models represent the dependence of the fraction of released silver on the square root of the release time, according to both the Eqs. 2.10 and 2.11; however, the Eq. 2.10 implies that this dependence should be linear, whereas the Eq. 2.11 suggests non-linear relationship for the release from thick hydrogel disks and slabs. Figures. 2.11 and 2.12 represent the ETA models for silver release from Ag/PVA and Ag/PVA/Gr hydrogels, respectively. From the obtained results, it can be observed that the modified ETA model provided better correlation with the experimental data. It is also obvious that the best correlation, spanning almost the entire release periods, were achieved for hydrogels with lower AgNPs concentrations, i.e., 0.25Ag/PVA, 0.5Ag/PVA, 0.25Ag/PVA/Gr and 0.5Ag/PVA/Gr. On the other hand, hydrogels with higher amounts of silver (1.0Ag/PVA, 3.9Ag/PVA, 1.0Ag/PVA/Gr and 3.9Ag/PVA/Gr) exhibited a narrower timespan over which the ETA model could be applied, which could be due to the fact that the burst release effect was much more

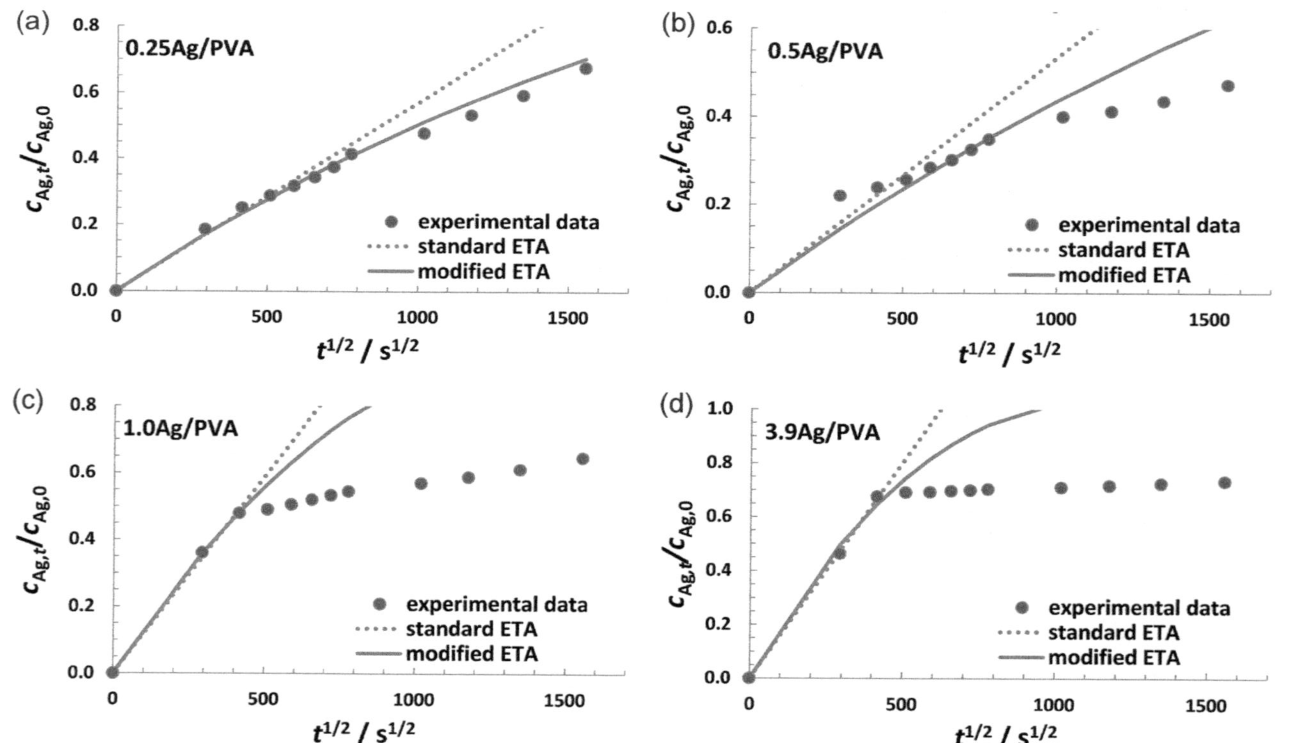

FIGURE 2.11 Early time approximations (ETA) for silver release from (a) 0.25Ag/PVA, (b) 0.5Ag/PVA, (c) 1.0Ag/PVA, and (d) 3.9Ag/PVA hydrogels (reprinted from Nešović and Mišković-Stanković 2022 with permission from John Wiley & Sons)

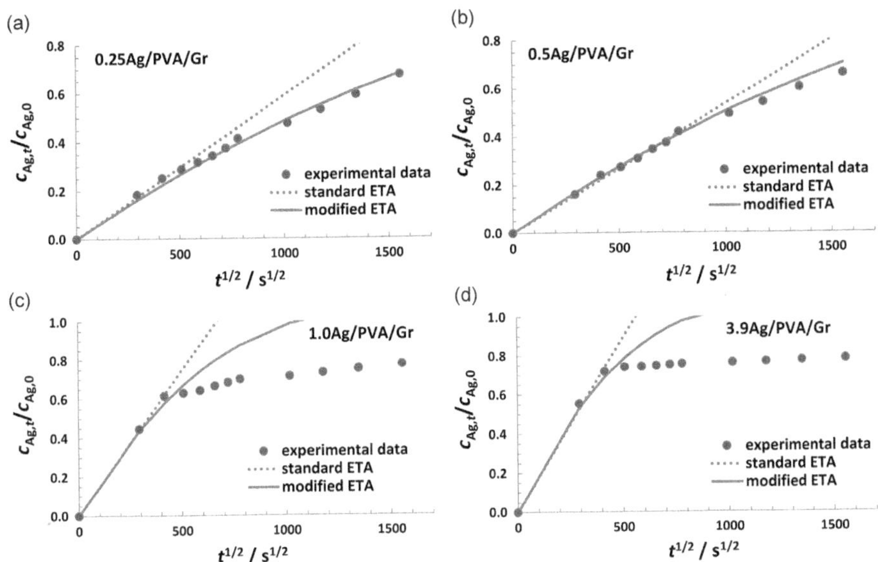

FIGURE 2.12 Early time approximations (ETA) for silver release from (a) 0.25Ag/PVA/Gr, (b) 0.5Ag/PVA/Gr, (c) 1.0Ag/PVA/Gr, and (d) 3.9Ag/PVA/Gr hydrogels (reprinted from Mišković-Stanković 2022 with permission from John Wiley & Sons)

pronounced for these hydrogels – more than 60 % of silver was released within the first 48 hours. The quantitative results for the silver diffusion coefficients, D_{Ag}, calculated from both the standard and the modified ETA models, are listed in Table 2.2. The obtained D_{Ag} data provide another interesting observation, that the values calculated by the standard ETA models are always significantly higher than the corresponding D_{Ag} values from the modified ETA fit. This implies that the standard ETA model usually overestimates the rate of drug release from cylindrical samples, and thus it should be used with caution, and replaced with the modified model whenever possible.

Further, another three models were applied to the release data, in order to elucidate the diffusion parameters over the entire release period, and to quantitatively compare silver release behavior of different hydrogels. The models applied were Makoid-Banakar (Makoid, Dufour, and Banakar 1993), Korsmeyer-Peppas (Korsmeyer et al. 1983), and Kopcha (Kopcha, Lordi, and Tojo 1991), which are described by Eqs. 2.12, 2.13, and 2.14, respectively.

$$\frac{c_{\mathrm{Ag,t}}}{c_{\mathrm{Ag,0}}} = \mathrm{k_{MB}} \cdot t^{n} \cdot \exp\left(-\mathrm{c} \cdot t\right) \tag{2.12}$$

$$\frac{c_{\mathrm{Ag,t}}}{c_{\mathrm{Ag,0}}} = k_{\mathrm{KP}} \cdot t^{n} \tag{2.13}$$

$$\frac{c_{Ag,t}}{c_{Ag,0}} = A \cdot t^{1/2} + B \cdot t \tag{2.14}$$

where $c_{Ag,t}$ is the concentration of silver released at time t, $c_{Ag,0}$ is the initial concentration of silver in the hydrogel, k_{MB} is the Makoid-Banakar constant, c is the Makoid-Banakar parameter (related to dissolution limitations as the function approaches maximum value), k_{KP} is the Korsmeyer-Peppas constant, and n is the coefficient that describes release transport mechanism ($n < 0.5$ – Fickian diffusion, $n > 0.5$ – non-Fickian/anomalous diffusion, $n = 1$ – Case II transport (Korsmeyer et al. 1983)). A and B are the Kopcha's constants that depend on the dominant transport phenomenon during release.

The release profiles representing the dependence of the fraction of released silver, $c_{Ag,t}/c_{Ag,0}$, on the time of release, t, for Ag/PVA and Ag/PVA/Gr hydrogels are presented in Figures 2.13 and 2.14, respectively. Additionally, the values for different fit parameters and constants for all three models are listed in Table 2.3. Analyzing the experimental release profiles, the first observation is that the hydrogels with higher AgNPs contents (1.0Ag/PVA, 3.9Ag/PVA, 1.0Ag/PVA/Gr, and 3.9Ag/PVA/Gr) exhibited very quick initial release within the first 48 hours or so, corresponding with the so-called burst effect that was also noticed during fitting with early time approximations. From Figures 2.13b, d, f and 2.14b, d, f, it could be concluded that the burst effect resulted in the release of ≈50 % of the initial silver concentration, for the hydrogels with 1.0 mM $AgNO_3$, i.e., nearly 70 % in the case of hydrogels with 3.9 mM $AgNO_3$. The hydrogels with lower AgNPs concentrations also exhibited the burst effect, but, in those cases, it was noted as the release of ≈20 % of silver within the initial 24 hours, which was followed by more gradual release, and the release rate consistently slowed down toward the end of the monitored 28-day period. Comparing the values of the coefficient R^2 (Table 2.3) as a measure of how well the models correspond to the experimental data, and which was always higher for hydrogels with 0.25 mM and 0.5 mM $AgNO_3$, often even >0.99, it can be concluded the release profile for hydrogels with lower AgNP contents resulted in better overall correlation of all models with the experimental data, compared to the hydrogels with 1.0 mM and 3.9 mM $AgNO_3$. Comparing different models among themselves, the Korsmeyer-Peppas and the Makoid-Banakar models provided notably better correlation with the experimental data, compared to the Kopcha model, which was especially pronounced in the case of hydrogels with higher silver contents. On the other hand, the Korsmeyer-Peppas and the Makoid-Banakar models did not differ significantly, which was not surprising, as the Korsmeyer-Peppas model (Eq. 2.13) can be seen as an approximation of the Makoid-Banakar equation (Eq. 2.12), in the edge case when $c \to 0$. From Table 2.3, it is obvious that the c parameter from the Makoid-Banakar model was indeed very small, indicating that the Makoid-Banakar and Korsmeyer-Peppas models were very similar for AgNP-loaded hydrogels, which was further confirmed by the fact that parameters n, as well as k_{KP} and k_{MB} constants, had very similar values. As already mentioned, the time exponent n is an indication of the dominant diffusion mechanism, and, as its values were always <0.5, it can be concluded that the release of silver from all of the hydrogels conformed to the

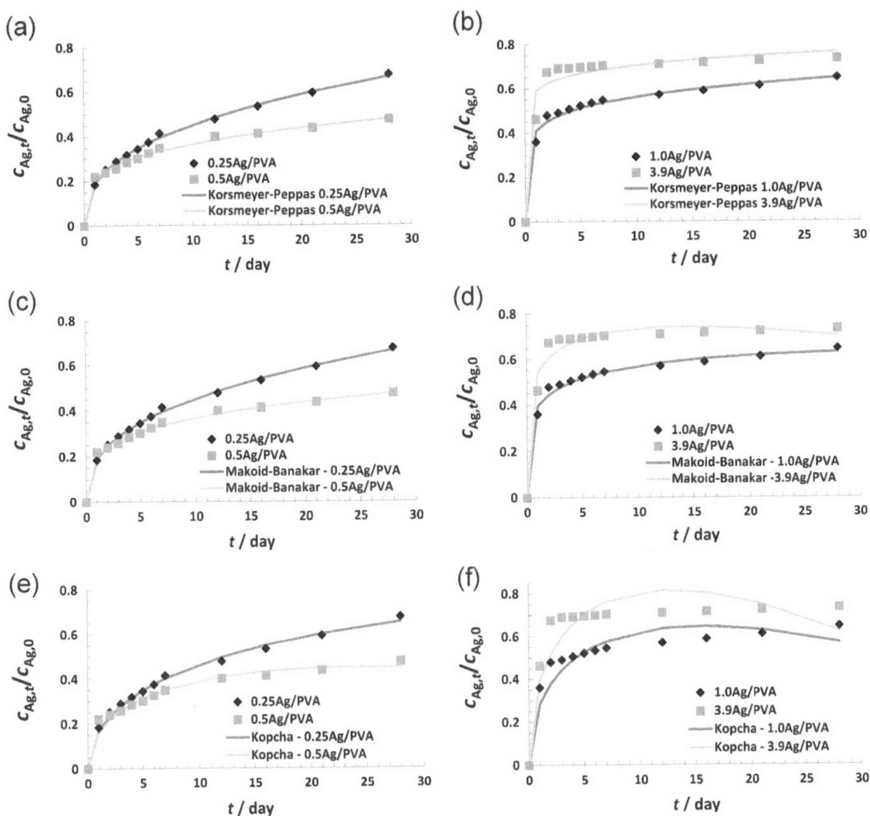

FIGURE 2.13 Models of silver release from 0.25Ag/PVA, 0.5Ag/PVA, 1.0Ag/PVA, and 3.9Ag/PVA hydrogels: (a) and (b) Korsmeyer-Peppas, (c) and (d) Makoid-Banakar, (e) and (f) Kopcha (reprinted from Nešović and Mišković-Stanković 2022 with permission from John Wiley & Sons)

Fickian diffusion behavior (Korsmeyer et al. 1983) and was governed mainly by the concentration gradient of released silver. This was also confirmed by the Kopcha model, as the absolute values of the parameter A were higher compared to |B|, indicating that the predominant driving force for the release is the diffusion, and not the polymer matrix relaxation.

The Higuchi model (Higuchi 1961, 1963) was also applied in order to compare it with other models and to gain insight into the governing phenomena during release. The Higuchi model is based on several assumptions for the derivation of the mathematical model, including time- and concentration-independent diffusion coefficients, perfect sink conditions, steady-state release, insolubility of the carrier matrix, and one-dimensional geometry as well as the condition that the initial concentration of the drug is significantly greater than its solubility in the release medium (Higuchi 1961, 1963; J Siepmann and Peppas 2001). The mathematical expression for the Higuchi model (Eq. 2.15) is quite simple and equivalent to the aforementioned

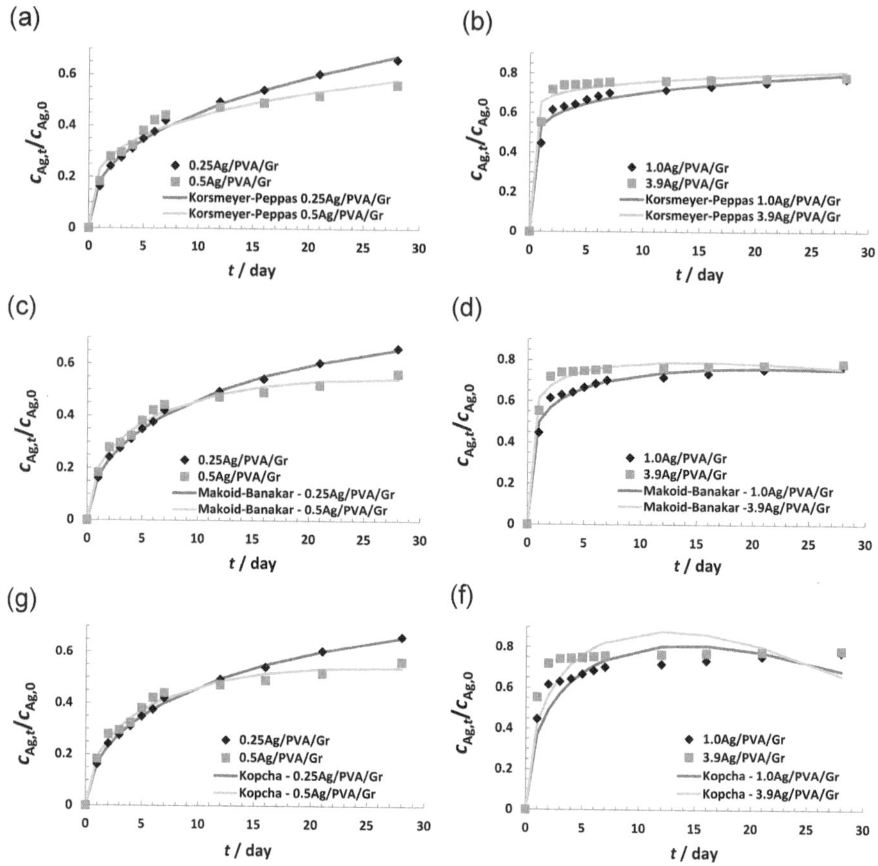

FIGURE 2.14 Models of silver release from 0.25Ag/PVA/Gr, 0.5Ag/PVA/Gr, 1.0Ag/PVA/Gr, and 3.9Ag/PVA/Gr hydrogels: (a) and (b) Korsmeyer-Peppas, (c) and (d) Makoid-Banakar, (e) and (f) Kopcha (reprinted from Nešović and Mišković-Stanković 2022 with permission from John Wiley & Sons)

standard ETA model (Eq. 2.10), as they both imply the linear dependence of the fraction of released drug and square root of time, although the proportionality constant, the so-called Higuchi constant, k_H, has a slightly different meaning than in the ETA model (Juergen Siepmann and Peppas 2011). Based on these considerations, it could be anticipated that the Higuchi model would not provide an appropriate description of silver release from the investigated Ag/PVA and Ag/PVA/Gr hydrogels, as some of the basic assumptions are too simplified for the given system, most important of which is neglecting the radial diffusion of silver along the hydrogel edges. Thus, as expected, Figure 2.15 reveals that the Higuchi equation is appropriate only in the initial period of release, whereas this model significantly overestimates the amount of released silver during prolonged exposure to PB, much like the standard ETA model

TABLE 2.3
Fitting Parameters Obtained from Korsmeyer-Peppas, Makoid-Banakar, and Kopcha Models of Silver Release from the Hydrogel Matrices (Reprinted from Nešović and Mišković-Stanković 2022 with Permission from John Wiley & Sons)

	Korsmeyer-Peppas			Makoid-Banakar				Kopcha		
Hydrogel	k_{KP} / s^{-n}	n	R^2	k_{MB} / s^{-n}	n	c / 10^{-7} s^{-1}	R^2	A / 10^{-3} $s^{-1/2}$	B / 10^{-7} s^{-1}	R^2
0.25Ag/PVA	0.003	0.376	0.998	0.003	0.376	0.000034	0.998	0.61	-1.24	0.995
0.5Ag/PVA	0.012	0.251	0.994	0.011	0.261	0.12	0.994	0.61	-2.06	0.970
1.0Ag/PVA	0.087	0.136	0.987	0.055	0.174	0.51	0.989	1.12	-4.83	0.896
3.9Ag/PVA	0.247	0.077	0.946	0.070	0.182	1.49	0.967	1.56	-7.45	0.846
0.25Ag/PVA/Gr	0.002	0.389	0.996	0.001	0.462	0.81	0.9983	0.61	-1.20	0.998
0.5Ag/PVA/Gr	0.010	0.276	0.971	0.002	0.419	1.72	0.986	0.72	-2.44	0.985
1.0Ag/PVA/Gr	0.137	0.120	0.976	0.053	0.199	1.08	0.986	1.45	-6.50	0.901
3.9Ag/PVA/Gr	0.316	0.064	0.970	0.118	0.146	1.17	0.983	1.69	-8.14	0.826

in Figures 2.11 and 2.12. It could be also noticed that the Higuchi model agrees better with the experimental data for hydrogels with lower AgNPs concentrations (0.25 and 0.5 mM $AgNO_3$), whereas the correlation holds only for the first two days in the case of hydrogels with 1.0 and 3.9 mM $AgNO_3$.

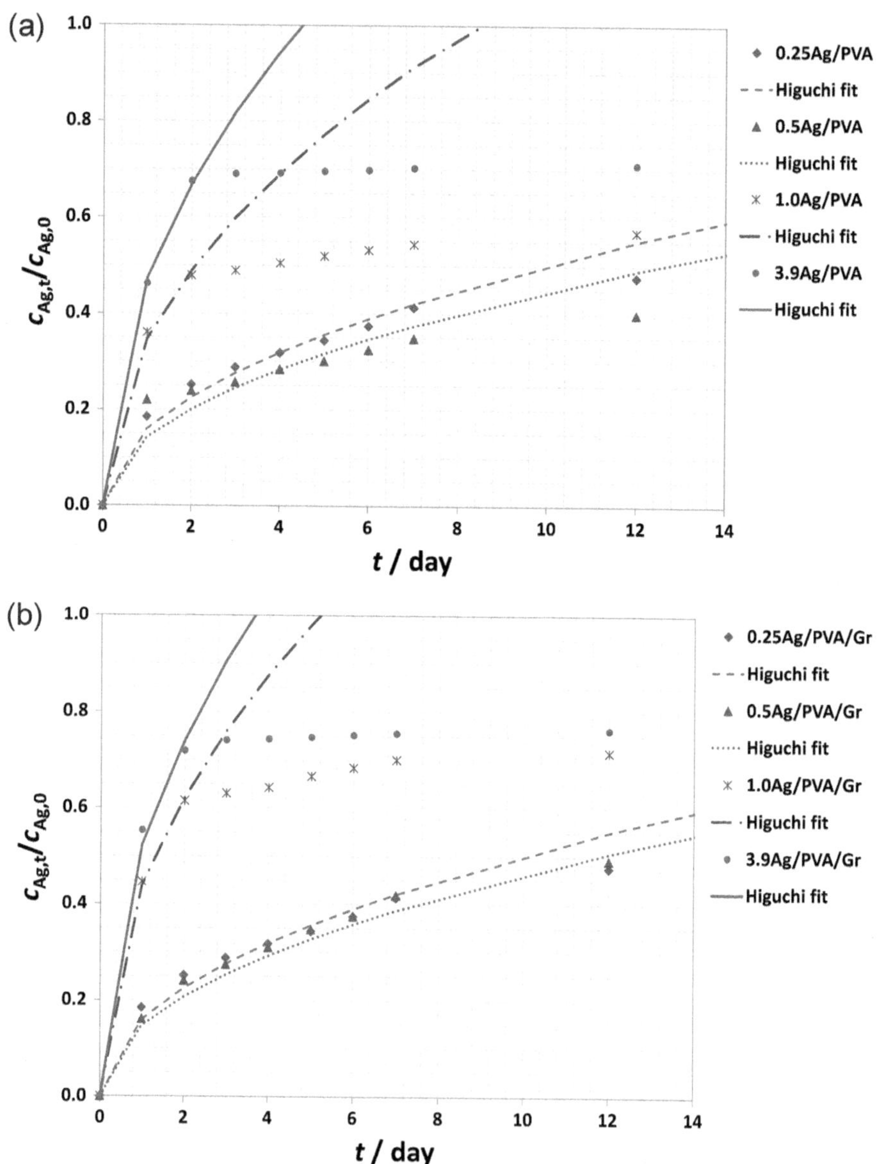

FIGURE 2.15 Higuchi model for (a) Ag/PVA and (b) Ag/PVA/Gr hydrogels with different AgNPs concentrations (reprinted from Nešović and Mišković-Stanković 2022 with permission from John Wiley & Sons)

$$\frac{c_{\mathrm{Ag,t}}}{c_{\mathrm{Ag,0}}} = k_{\mathrm{H}} \cdot t^{1/2} \tag{2.15}$$

2.1.4.5 *In Vivo* Studies

In accordance with the standard ISO-10993-1, Annex A, for implanted materials, it is mandatory to determine the physicochemical characteristics and cytotoxicity, then to include testing of tissue sensitization, tissue irritation response, systemic acute toxicity, chronic toxicity, histocompatibility, genotoxicity, carcinogenicity, and biodegradation, depending on the purpose in clinical trials (Ratner 2016). Finally, the most important step is to evaluate the tissue response *in vivo*, after implanting biomaterials in various animal models prior to clinical use in human or veterinary medicine. The evaluations include the foreign body reaction (FBR), inflammation, encapsulation, and the accumulation of macrophages in the periimplantzone (Trindade et al. 2016). The type of tissue response to biomaterials depends on the nature, structure, size, and form of the implanted biomaterials (Chen et al. 2019; Ward et al. 2002), the tissue area of implantation and period of observation after implantation (J. Sharma et al. 2015). The FBR is followed by local inflammatory tissue response provoked by both the surgical incision and the presence of the biomaterial in the body, after which wound regeneration processes and fibrous encapsulation of the implanted materials begins (Trindade et al. 2016; S. Han et al. 2019; Sheikh et al. 2015). The FBR includes a complex cascade of space-depended, interconnected processes, such as triggering signals (soluble mediators – growth factors, cytokines, chemokines, and matrix metalloproteinases and their inhibitors), followed by cellular activation involving inflammatory cells, angiogenesis, extravasation, cell migration, phagocytosis, and changes that occur in the biomaterial itself (Luttikhuizen, Harmsen, and Luyn 2006). Neutrophils are one of the first inflammatory cells that arrive at the implant site and they have a crucial role thath is reflected in the production of chemokines, which attract other inflammatory cells, including monocytes (James M. Anderson, Rodriguez, and Chang 2008). The presence of neutrophils is followed by the expression of monocyte attractant chemokines MCP1 and MIP1α that act as proinflammatory regulators and through mediation with other proinflammatory factors (IL6 and IFN-γ) promote macrophage activation and their phagocytic behavior (Ye et al. 2010).

The macrophage is an indicator of increased host protection against foreign bodies, acting as a phagocyte, engulfs small particles of foreign substances. In the case of implants, macrophages cannot absorb them, so they fuse together and form foreign body giant cells (FBGC) (Dadsetan et al. 2004). In order for the material-cell interface to act optimally, specific performance of the FBR is required (Ye et al. 2010). The biomaterial should provide a biomimetic environment to ensure cell survival and directed cell migration to ensure that relevant cells migrate to, and adhere to, the implant (James M. Anderson, Rodriguez, and Chang 2008; Hench and Thompson 2010). Nanotechnology and biomaterials science can greatly contribute to the design of devices for specific clinical needs, and the introduction of Gr has been showed to have various applications in medicine (J. Sharma et al. 2015). For example, Gr or carbon nanotubes, owing to their specific properties, have enormous potential as wound dressing fillers (Wujcik and Monty 2013; Thompson, Murray, and Wallace 2015). Graphene has even been used for the synthesis of antibacterial nanomaterials; however, the specific mechanistic aspects of its antibacterial activity are still generally unknown and debatable (Ji, Sun, and Qu 2016). Therefore, there is absolutely a great need for *in vivo* studies and extensive testing for all new graphene-based biomaterials intended for medical practice in order to investigate the connection of these implantable biomaterials with the cellular components of the tissue reaction. The *in vivo* data should provide the necessary evidence and enable development of better technologies for developing novel and biocompatible devices for clinical use (Hench and Thompson 2010; Hotaling et al. 2015).

Cell-surface interactions stimulate adhesion and activation of macrophages whose acquaintance can assist in designing Ag/PVA and Ag/PVA/Gr hydrogels that promote favorable macrophage-biomaterial surface interactions for clinical application. The distribution and number of macrophages were determined as a means of biocompatibility evaluation of Ag/PVA and Ag/PVA/Gr hydrogels *in vivo*. Sixteen rats (Albino strain, Wistar breed), female, three months old, were used for subcutaneous implantation of the hydrogels. Macrophages and giant cells were analyzed in tissue sections stained by routine (H&E) and immunohistochemical methods (CD68+) (Lužajić Božinovski, Todorović, Milošević, Prokić et al. 2021). The presence of giant cells around the foreign body localized around the subcutaneously implanted Ag/PVA and Ag/PVA/Gr hydrogels and Suprasorb©, a commercial calcium-alginate dressing (Lohmann & Rauscher GmbH & Co. KG, Neuwied, Germany) during post-operation follow-up (7, 15, 30, and 60 p.o.d.) is shown in Figure 2.16. The results of the giant cells number study, localized around the implant, showed that the number of these cells was highest on day 7 in the group implanted with Ag/PVA and Suprasorb©. With the Ag/PVA/Gr hydrogel, a gradual increase of giant formations was observed from day 7 to day 30. On the 60th p.o.d. the number of giant cells drops by 45 % compared to day 30. In the group implanted with Ag/PVA, the periimplant connective tissue analysis showed that giant cells number reached a maximum on day 7 and then declined, maintaining similar values on day 15 and day 30 and then statistically significantly decreasing on day 60. In the case of Suprasorb©, the giant cells number was the highest on day 7 and successively and uniformly decreased towar day 60, although it should be noted that the total values in this category are three and four times lower compared to the values gained for the Ag/PVA and Ag/PVA/Gr hydrogels. In contrast, in the case of Ag/PVA/Gr implants, the number of giant cells increased linearly until day 30, to be significantly reduced on day 60 (Figure 2.16a, d, e). However, the number of giant cells around Ag/PVA/Gr implants at the end of the follow-up period, on day 60, was significantly higher (9.9360 ± 1.9030) compared to Ag/PVA (3.8835 ± 0.7822) and Suprasorb© (1.9030 ± 0.7054).

The number of macrophages in the connective tissue capsule and pericapsular connective tissue after subcutaneous implantation during the postoperative period is shown in Figures 2.17a and b. The structure of the poly(vinyl alcohol) hydrogels enriched with silver and graphene particles stimulate capsule formation and collagenation, increasing leukocyte infiltration. Thus, the increased number of macrophages in the periimplant connective tissue surrounding the Ag/PVA and Ag/PVA/

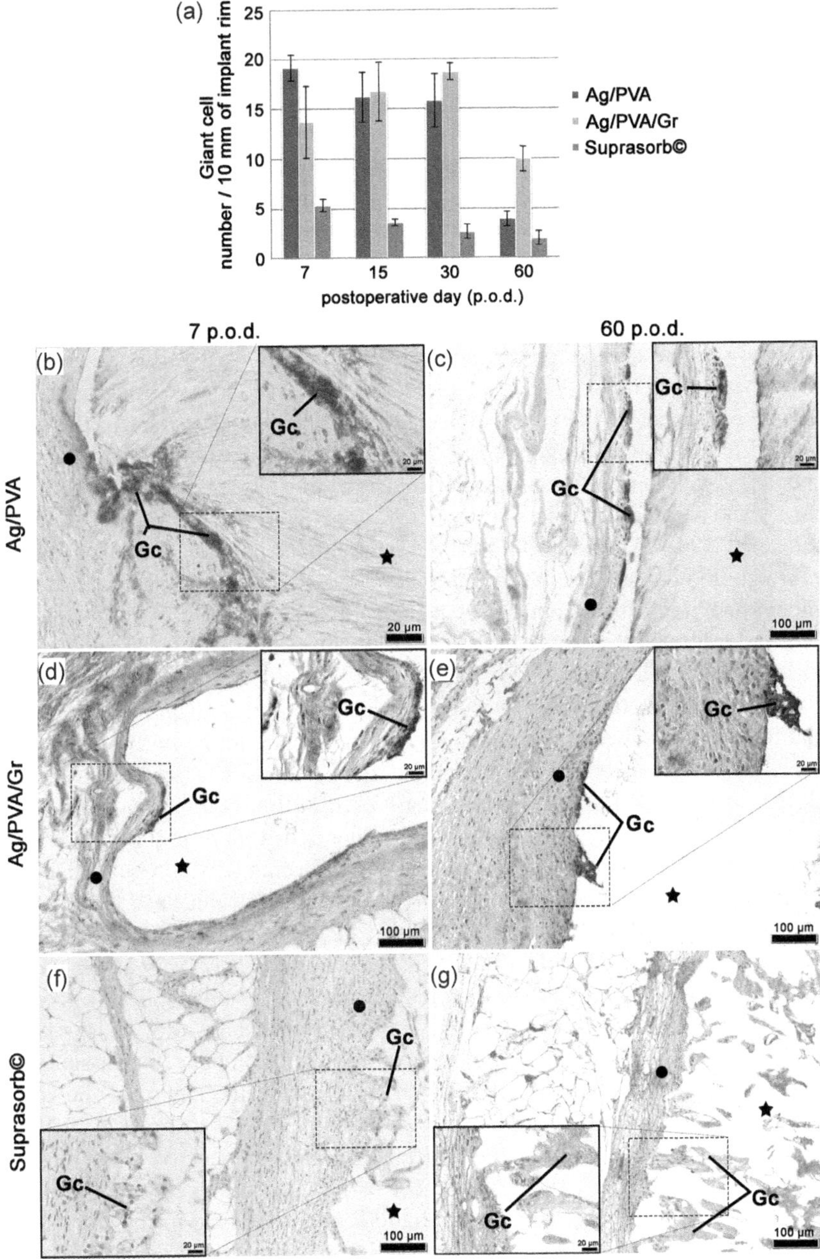

FIGURE 2.16 Giant cells number after 7, 15, 30, and 60 p.o.d. (a), giant cells around the foreign body (dot – capsule, star – implant location, Gc – giant cells) after 7 and 60 p.o.d. for: Ag/PVA (b, c), Ag/PVA/Gr (d, e) and Suprasorb© (f, g). Bar: 100 µm, insets: bar: 20 µm (reprinted from Lužajić Božinovski, Todorović, Milošević, Prokić et al. 2021 with permission from SAGE Publications)

Gr hydrogels is a part of the physiological skin healing process during the chronic stage of wound inflammation, followed by phagocytosis, which is desirable tissue reaction to a foreign body. Recently, immunohistochemistry was used to analyze and visualize skin regenerative processes after subcutaneous implantation of Ag/PVA and Ag/PVA/Gr hydrogels in an animal model (Lužajić Božinovski, Todorović, Milošević, Gajdov et al. 2021). Biocompatibility markers' *in vivo* evaluation demonstrated tissue remodeling processes. The cellular and extracellular components such as laminins, vessel density, and angiogenesis in the wound bed, collagenization, capsulation, fibroblast, and keratinocyte migration and proliferation on the 7th, 15th, 30th, and 60th p.o.d. have been observed. Screening tests deal with results comparison of semi-quantitative data and morphometric and immunohistochemical methods that adhere to the criteria prescribed by the standards used in the assessment of the tissue irritation index (TIrI), i.e., the degree of tissue damage. Macrophages are the basic parameter of these tissue changes, and their number rises in the chronic phases of the wound healing process. Collagenation, encapsulation, and magnification of tissue macrophages are indicators of a receding tissue reaction and its gradual recovery and healing (Lužajić Božinovski, Todorović, Milošević, Gajdov et al. 2021; DeFife et al. 1999). The renewal of the matrix components (collagen), the restraint of the foreign body by encapsulation, and the increase in macrophages and giant cells number are an indicator of normal tissue defect regeneration.

It is believed that the increased number of macrophages and giant cells is associated with the increase in surface area of more voluminous implants, depending on the size, shape, structure, and binding surface at the point of contact. Proper interpretation of the number of macrophages and giant cells in the periimplant zone is especially important today, when nanomaterials that have larger contact surfaces with the surrounding tissue are increasingly used in tissue engineering for scaffold construction (Hench and Thompson 2010; Collier and Anderson 2002). In line with this opinion is Ratner's proposal (Ratner 2016) according to which biocompatibility is directly proportional to the number of macrophages (Martinez and Gordon 2014). The increasing number of macrophages and giant cells in the periimplant zone of the Ag/PVA and Ag/PVA/Gr hydrogels (Figures 2.16 and 2.17) is in agreement with the findings of other authors (Ratner 2016; Collier and Anderson 2002; Gordon, Plüddemann, and Martinez Estrada 2014; Kzhyshkowska et al. 2015; Ohashi, Hattori, and Hattori 2015). High numbers of macrophages in the connective tissue around the commercial Suprasorb© were expected, considering the nature of the calcium alginate, which is easily decomposed in the dermis. The structure of Ag/PVA and Ag/PVA/Gr hydrogels should make a difference in the connective tissue response, so a well-formed capsule, signs of connective collagen production and infiltration of leukocytes are expected here, according to Ratner's formula for biocompatibility assessment (Ratner 2016; Sood, Granick, and Tomaselli 2013; Lužajić Božinovski, Todorović, Milošević, Gajdov et al. 2021). An increased number of macrophages in the periimplantation connective tissue corresponds to the processes of proper skin recovery (G. Han and Ceilley 2017), where phagocytosis is expected and is a desirable host reaction to a foreign body.

One of the constant issues that appear around some implants is the inability of macrophages to eliminate inflammation and their tendency to be in a state of

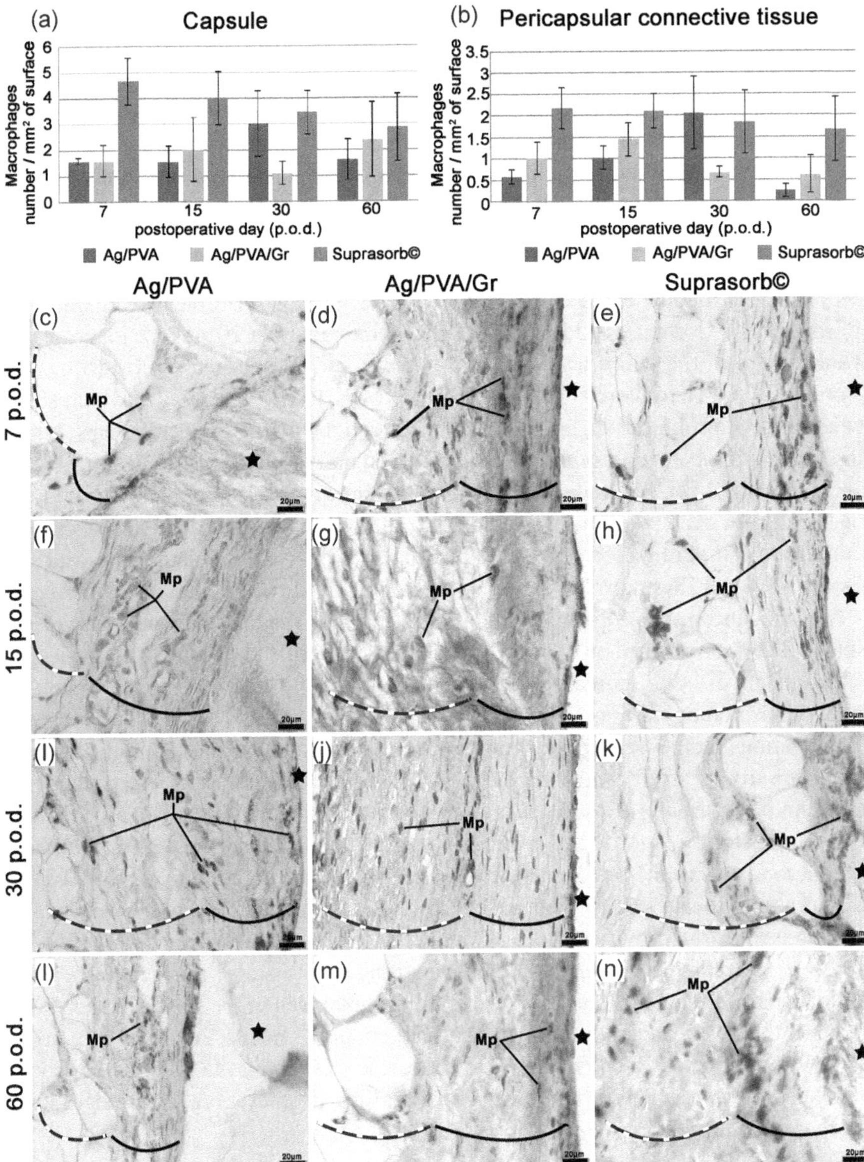

FIGURE 2.17 (a, b) CD68+ positive macrophages in the connective tissue capsule and pericapsular connective tissue (Mp – macrophages, star – implant location, solid curved line – capsule, dashed curved line – pericapsular connective tissue) after 7, 15, 30, and 60 p.o.d. for: Ag/PVA, (c, f, i, l), Ag/PVA/Gr (d, g, j, m) and Suprasorb© (e, h, k, n). Bar: 20 μm (reprinted from (Lužajić Božinovski, Todorović, Milošević, Prokić et al. 2021 with permission from SAGE Publications)

so-called frustrated phagocytosis. During the initial phase of inflammation, proinflammatory macrophages (M1-polarized) induce an acute reaction to trauma and foreign material, while tolerogenic anti-inflammatory macrophages (M2-polarized) control the withdrawal of inflammation and induce the next phase, which is healing (Gordon, Plüddemann, and Martinez Estrada 2014). However, implanted materials can induce a mixed pro- and anti-inflammatory phenotype and, thus, support the maintenance of chronic inflammation followed by microorganism infection and implantation failure (Kzhyshkowska et al. 2015). Therefore, the immunomodulatory properties of implant coating materials in the future should become part of personalized medicine (so-called personalized implant therapies) (Martinez and Gordon 2014; Gordon, Plüddemann, and Martinez Estrada 2014). M2-macrophages are involved in the withdrawal of inflammation and wound healing (Martinez and Gordon 2014). They secrete TGF-β, PDGF, MMPs, CCL7, and CCL8, which stimulate fibroblast proliferation, migration, and activation and increase collagen synthesis in myofibroblasts, thus promoting fibrosis (Shen and Horbett 2001; Ohashi, Hattori, and Hattori 2015; J. M. Anderson et al. 1999). Some authors note that certain factors released from M2 macrophages, such as CCL18 (CC chemokine ligand 18), can sustain chronic inflammation and delay healing (Gordon, Plüddemann, and Martinez Estrada 2014; Kzhyshkowska et al. 2015; Ohashi, Hattori, and Hattori 2015).

As conclusion, macrophages were present in both the capsular and pericapsular space. The numerical density of macrophages in both the capsule and pericapsular connective tissue increased significantly on the 7th and 15th p.o.d. around all implanted biomaterials as expected for the chronic phase of the tissue response. Observations on the 30th p.o.d. showed a significant increase in the number of macrophages around Ag/PVA compared to Ag/PVA/Gr. The number of macrophages on the 60th p.o.d. around Ag/PVA declined significantly, but in the area of Ag/PVA/Gr it lowered slightly. A striking finding in this period (60th) was the higher abundance of macrophages in the tissue surrounding Ag/PVA/Gr compared to Ag/PVA. These differences indicate that in the case of Ag/PVA/Gr a thicker capsule is formed, significantly infiltrated by macrophages and with a larger number of giant cells. The addition of graphene to Ag/PVA achieved strong and effective binding to the extracellular matrix elements and affects signaling molecules in the tissue in such a way that stimulates the activation of physical and chemical bonds. As a result, a microenvironment is created, which plays a major role in shaping the biological response in a specific way which modulates wound healing, regeneration, and integration of biomaterials into the tissue.

2.1.5 Polyvinyl Alcohol/Chitosan-Based Hydrogels with Silver Nanoparticles

2.1.5.1 Electrochemical Synthesis and Characterization of Silver/Poly(Vinyl Alcohol)/Chitosan Hydrogels

Poly(vinyl alcohol)/chitosan blend hydrogels can be obtained by simple freezing-thawing method, forming strong inter- and intramolecular hydrogen bonds to achieve reversibly cross-linked matrices without the use of aldehyde-based cross linkers, rendering the final product non-toxic – an important feature from safety standpoint in medical applications. AgNPs-incorporated poly(vinyl alcohol) and chitosan hydrogels have been investigated for wound dressing and other biomaterials applications (Abdelgawad, Hudson, and Rojas 2014; N.-T. Nguyen and Liu 2014; Elbarbary and El-Sawy 2017; Mishra, Ferreira, and Kannan 2015), and silver nanoparticles were usually synthesized via chemical reduction (Ghasemzadeh and Ghanaat 2014) or gamma irradiation (Uttayarat et al. 2015; Jovanović et al. 2011). Alternative route for AgNPs synthesis is in an electrochemical setup, where the silver nanoparticles were obtained by reduction with electrical current and hydrogen gas that evolves on the cathode surface during the synthesis. This simple and environment-friendly method allowed obtaining small-sized AgNPs directly inside the physically cross-linked PVA/CHI hydrogel matrices. The effect of chitosan content on AgNPs characteristics, swelling, silver release, and biological properties of hydrogels was investigated by varying the amount of chitosan (0.1 wt.% and 0.5 wt.%) in the PVA/0.1CHI and PVA/0.5CHI hydrogels, respectively, while concentration of PVA was 10 wt.% (Nešović, Janković, Radetić et al. 2019).

The cross-linked PVA/0.1CHI and PVA/0.5CHI hydrogels were obtained following a simple and green freezing-thawing method in five cycles (one cycle involved freezing for 16 hours at -18 °C and thawing for 8 hours at 4 °C). The physicochemical properties of such physically obtained hydrogels strongly depend on the duration, number of cycles, and temperatures of freezing and thawing (Fukumori and Nakaoki 2014). It is widely considered that the polymer chains inside the hydrogel are mainly bound by inter- and intramolecular hydrogen bonds, which makes the hydrogel reversible so that it can be returned to the sol phase without breaking of chemical bonds and without destruction of the polymer structure (Maitra and Shukla 2014). As both PVA and CHI contain many functional groups (–OH and $–NH_2$) that participate in hydrogen bonding, freezing-thawing is a viable method for obtaining their hydrogels, allowing us to avoid the use of conventional, difficult to remove and often toxic cross linkers (e.g., aldehyde-based substances). The cross-linking mechanism is a combination of several parallel and/or consecutive processes. These processes include liquid-solid and liquid-liquid phase separation (Peppas and Stauffer 1991; Yokoyama et al. 1986) during which hydrogen bonding takes place among the functional groups (–OH, $–NH_2$) on polymer chains, thus forming hydrogel matrix. Besides hydrogen bonding, there is also a possibility for formation of microcrystalline, ordered regions in the bulk polymer phase, as well as the formation of semi-permanent entanglements, which enable the strengthening of the polymer matrix in the hydrogel (Peppas and Stauffer 1991). The gelation degree, W_g, was calculated to be 94.0 ± 2.0 % for PVA/0.1CHI and 95.6 ± 0.84 % for PVA/0.5CHI (Nešović, Janković, Radetić et al. 2019), indicating high cross-linking degree achieved using the freezing-thawing technique. The FE-SEM micrographs of PVA/0.1CHI and PVA/0.5CHI hydrogels highlighted the microporous structure of the hydrogels, which is highly favorable for wound dressing materials and provides excellent porous matrix for better incorporation of AgNPs.

Prior to electrochemical synthesis of AgNPs at constant voltage of 90 V for 4 minutes, swelling of the PVA/0.1CHI and PVA/0.5CHI hydrogels was achieved during 48 hours in 0.25 mM and 3.9 mM $AgNO_3$ and 0.1 M KNO_3 (which was added as a base electrolyte to increase the electrical conductivity). During the synthesis, some amount of Ag^+ ions diffuses to the cathode and is deposited on the Pt surface (Eq. 2.4), lowering the yield of the AgNPs synthesis. For this reason, the polarity of the electrodes is switched periodically (every 1 minute) during the synthesis, which allows the dissolution of the deposited bulk Ag layer, oxidizing the silver back to Ag^+ and increasing the yield of AgNPs. As already mentioned, the primary reaction is the water electrolysis; therefore, the hydrogen evolution at the cathode surface (Eq. 2.1) is intensive. Thus, it is likely that the formation of AgNPs inside the hydrogel matrix is achieved via the reduction of Ag^+ ions by H_2 gas molecules. It is well known that the silver nanoparticles could be obtained by reduction reactions in H_2 atmosphere (T. C. Wang, Rubner, and Cohen 2002; X. Xu et al. 2006; Evanoff and Chumanov 2004). The reduction of Ag^+ by H_2 and the nucleation of AgNPs can be described by Eq. 2.5 (Merga et al. 2007).

The formation of silver nanoparticles inside the PVA/0.1CHI and PVA/0.5CHI hydrogels was confirmed by FE-SEM and UV-visible spectroscopy (Figure 2.18), by appearance of surface plasmon resonant (SPR) peaks at ~400 nm. The absorbance maxima for both 3.9Ag/PVA/0.5CHI (Figure 2.18a) and 0.25Ag/PVA/0.5CHI (Figure 2.18b) exhibited higher values compared to 3.9Ag/PVA/0.1CHI and 0.25Ag/PVA/0.1CHI, respectively, indicating the greater synthesis yield and higher AgNPs concentration in the presence of higher chitosan amount in the hydrogel, which could be due to the ability of CHI to act as a mild reducent (Kozicki et al. 2016), contributing to the quicker formation of AgNPs.

The incorporation of AgNPs was additionally confirmed by energy-dispersive X-ray spectroscopy (EDS), and the measured silver content in 3.9Ag/PVA/0.1CHI and 3.9Ag/PVA/0.5CHI was 0.17 and 0.25 at%, respectively, further verifying the UV-Vis conclusions about higher concentration of AgNPs in 3.9Ag/PVA/0.5CHI hydrogels (Nešović, Janković, Radetić et al. 2019).

The stabilization of the obtained AgNPs inside the hydrogel matrix is generally achieved through ion-dipole interactions with polymer chain functional groups, especially with electron-donor atoms such as oxygen and nitrogen of hydroxyl and amino groups of PVA and CHI chains (H. Huang, Yuan, and Yang 2004). There is also a possibility to form coordination bonds and polymer-metal complexes between AgNPs, and PVA and CHI, which could be denoted as $[PVA\text{-}Ag_n]^{n+}$ and $[CHI\text{-}Ag_m]^{m+}$, where *n* and *m* are the numbers of Ag^+ interacting with PVA and CHI, respectively (M M Abudabbus et al. 2016). If silver ions that are part of this sort of complex are reduced, the process results with nucleation and further growth of AgNPs, which remain bound and stabilized through the interactions with polymer chains (Mohamed M Abudabbus et al. 2018; M M Abudabbus et al. 2016). Many studies have shown that chitosan, as a polycation with many–NH_2 and –OH groups, has the ability to interact with silver ions and nanoparticles, facilitating their immobilization and stabilization in a colloid dispersion, film, or a hydrogel (Hang, Tae, and Park 2010; Twu, Chen, and Shih 2008; Reicha et al. 2012; Regiel et al. 2013).

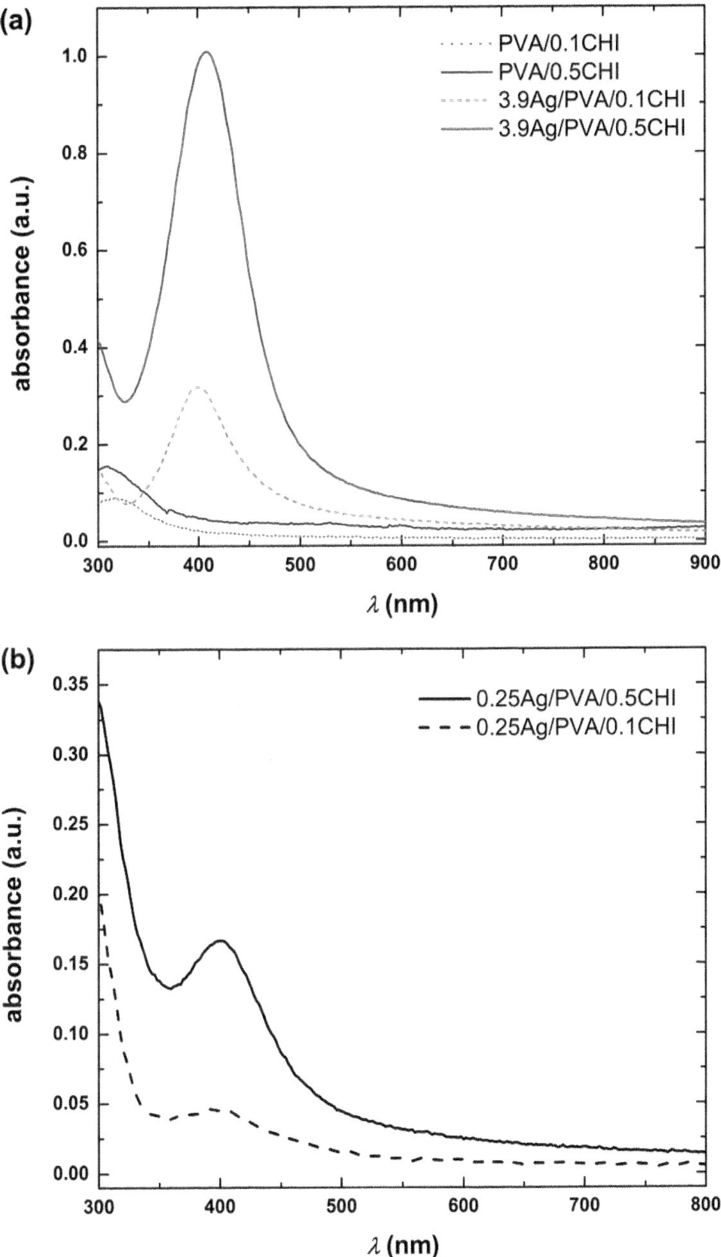

FIGURE 2.18 UV-Vis spectra of (a) PVA/0.1CHI, PVA/0.5CHI, 3.9Ag/PVA/0.1CHI and 3.9AgPVA/0.5CHI; (b) 0.25Ag/PVA/0.1CHI and 0.25AgPVA/0.5CHI hydrogels (reprinted from Nešović, Janković, Radetić et al. 2019) with permission from Elsevier)

Furthermore, it was shown that chitosan also possesses reducing properties, so that it is possible to obtain chitosan/Ag nanocomposites via direct reduction of Ag^+ with chitosan (Kozicki et al. 2016; Tran et al. 2010; Biswas et al. 2018). This method, however, can be very slow and time consuming, so the electrochemical AgNP synthesis presents substantial improvement with an implementation time of only 4 minutes, and the yield of the synthesis can be even further improved with increased chitosan content, as shown by UV-Vis spectroscopy (Figure 2.18).

A dynamic light scattering (DLS) technique enabled determination of the statistically averaged particle size and size distributions (PSD). The obtained PSD results, which are presented in Figure 2.19, confirmed fairly narrow distributions of particle diameters, with intensity- and volume-weighted PSD curves for both samples adopting lognormal monomodal shape. For 3.9Ag/PVA/0.1CHI (Figure 2.19a), the majority of AgNPs (99.3 % by intensity) were in the 9.09 nm group, although another small peak was observed at ~3000 nm, possibly originating from light scattering off the polymer chains in the solution. The volume-weighted PSD (Figure 2.19b), however, revealed that effectively 100 % of AgNPs were in the small-sized group (5.92 nm diameter by volume). Similarly, the PSD for 3.9AgPVA/0.5CHI hydrogel indicated that the overwhelming majority of AgNPs was sub-10 nm in size – 98.6 % by intensity was in the 8.14 nm group (Figure 2.19a), which translated to 100 % of nanoparticles in 4.78 nm group by volume (Figure 2.19b). The obtained Z-average hydrodynamic diameters, D_Z, and polydispersity indices (PDI) were 7.33 ± 0.088 nm (PDI = 0.211 ± 0.013) for 3.9Ag/PVA/0.1CHI and 6.11 ± 0.10 nm (PDI = 0.269 ± 0.009) for 3.9Ag/PVA/0.5CHI. The D_Z values were in good accordance with the nanoparticle diameters estimated from the UV-Vis spectra. These results also indicated that the AgNPs were slightly smaller in size in the hydrogels with higher chitosan content, corroborating the assumption of their better stabilization by interactions with hydroxyl and amino groups of CHI chains.

The incorporation of spherical silver nanoparticles in both 3.9Ag/PVA/0.1CHI and 3.9AgPVA/0.5CHI hydrogels was further characterized by high-resolution transmission electron microscopy (HRTEM) (Figure 2.20). Agglomerates in the range of several hundred nanometers were observed for 3.9Ag/PVA/0.1CHI, although agglomeration might be an artifact of sample preparation and drying of the suspensions on the Cu grids. The example of agglomerate shown in Figure 2.20a consists of several sharply faceted nanoparticles with facets parallel to {111} and {100} planes. The FFT pattern (inset in Figure 2.20a) of one of the nanoparticles confirmed face-centered cubic (fcc) crystal structure. Smaller (5–10 nm sized) polycrystalline particles were also observed, as in Figure 2.20b. These polycrystalline AgNPs were mainly decahedral, with irregular fivefold twinned structure (such as the circled nanoparticle in Figure 2.20b), which is typical morphology for smaller-sized (< 20 nm) nanoparticles due to their tendency to reduce surface energy (Z. L. Wang 2000). While the nanoparticles greater than 5–10 nm tended to be polycrystalline and heavily twinned, the smallest ones (≈5 nm and smaller) were single crystals, e.g., the nanoparticle in Figure 2.20c has cuboctahedral shape. The single crystal nature of smallest AgNPs is possibly indicative of favorable interactions with polymer chains, which could help stabilize the nanoparticles and reduce their surface energy, thus enabling the formation of high-energy structures.

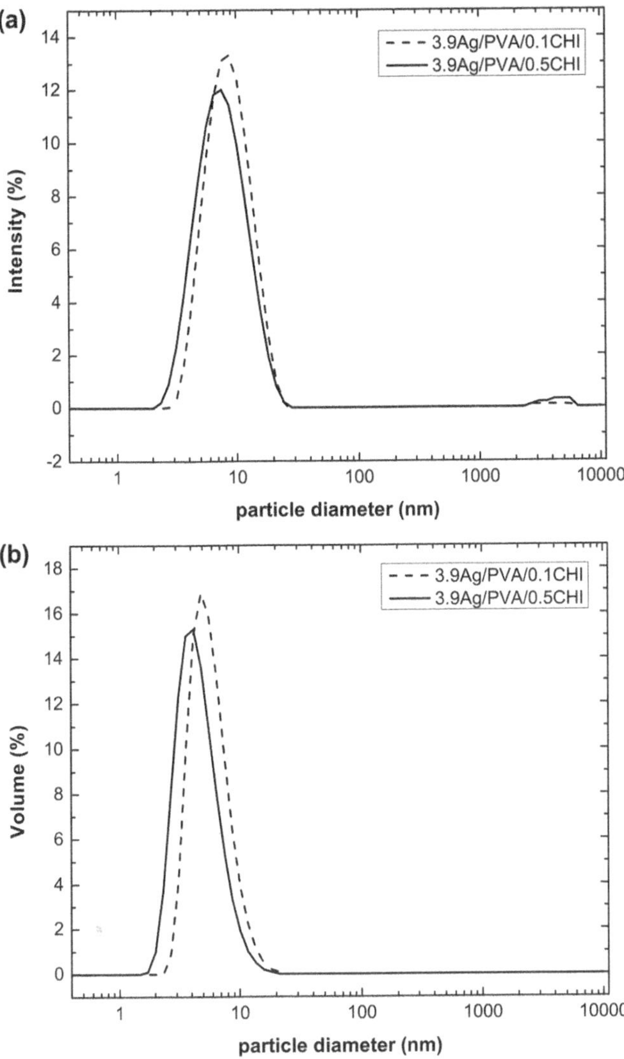

FIGURE 2.19 (a) Intensity-weighted and (b) volume-weighted AgNP size distributions of 3.9Ag/PVA/0.1CHI and 3.9AgPVA/0.5CHI hydrogels measured by DLS (reprinted from Nešović, Janković, Radetić et al. 2019 with permission from Elsevier)

The 3.9AgPVA/0.5CHI hydrogels (Figures 2.20d, e, and f) contained many small-sized AgNPs (Figure 2.20d), and less of large agglomerates, which might be due to better stabilization provided by the increased chitosan content. Larger nanoparticles ($\geq$ 5–10 nm) were polycrystalline, consisting of a number of crystallites without regular polyhedral structure (Figure 2.20e). Some of the nanoparticles appear to have rough surfaces with many defects (as indicated by arrows in Figure 2.20f). It has been shown that the nanoparticles with surface defects exhibited stronger cytotoxicity effect toward the fish gill cell line compared to the regular NPs (George

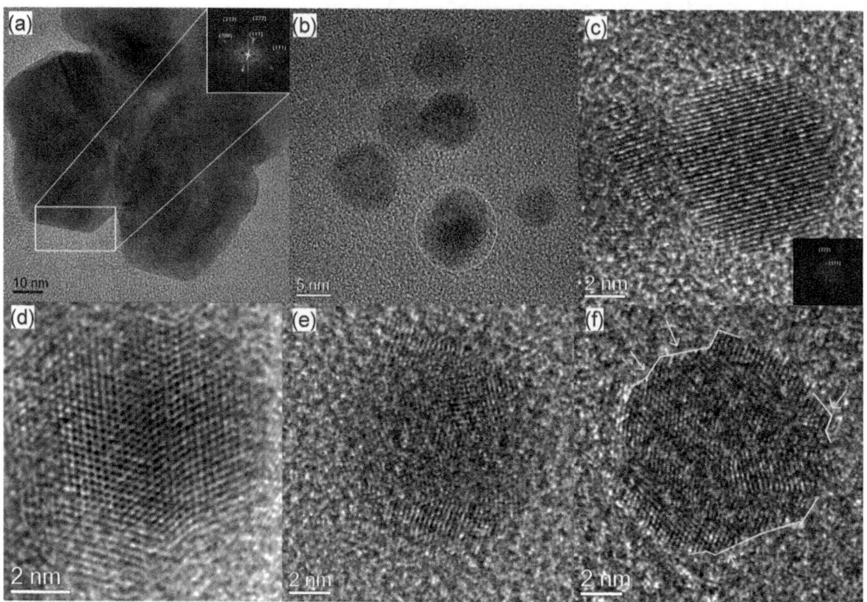

FIGURE 2.20 HRTEM images of selected nanoparticles incorporated in (a-c) 3.9Ag/PVA/0.1CHI and (d-f) 3.9AgPVA/0.5CHI hydrogels (reprinted from Nešović, Janković, Radetić et al. 2019 with permission from Elsevier)

et al. 2012), so the irregularity of AgNPs in 3.9AgPVA/0.5CHI could affect both cytotoxicity and antibacterial activity of these hydrogels. Moreover, surface defects, such as edges, corners, and surface charges, were shown to play a major role in the antibacterial activity of ZnO nanoparticles (Sirelkhatim et al. 2015), e.g., through the formation of reactive oxygen species (ROS). The ROS generation has been mentioned before in the literature as one of the possible antibacterial mechanisms of AgNPs (Banerjee et al. 2010; H. Xu et al. 2012), so the existence of surface defects could lead to enhanced ROS production and thus to improved antibacterial activity. Smaller nanoparticles were also found to exhibit significantly stronger antibacterial activity.

Using FT-IR spectroscopy, the most prominent peaks were observed at 3251 cm^{-1} (PVA/0.1CHI), 3257 cm^{-1} (PVA/0.5CHI), 3271 cm^{-1} (3.9Ag/PVA/0.1CHI), and 3268 cm^{-1} (3.9Ag/PVA/0.5CHI) and ascribed to the valence vibrations (stretching) of O–H bonds from hydroxyl groups. The O–H stretching band positions indicated that the –OH groups strongly participated in hydrogen bonding, as this vibration was observed at lower wavenumbers, rather than in the usual 3700–3600 cm^{-1} region. The hydrogen bonding between polymer chains plays an important role in the hydrogel matrix formation, as explained earlier. Additionally, the N–H stretching vibrations bands (from $-NH_2$ groups of chitosan) usually appear in the same region (P. Sharma et al. 2016), so some overlapping is also possible. The absorption maxima were slightly blue-shifted in the case of hydrogels with AgNPs, namely, 3.9Ag/PVA/0.1CHI and

3.9Ag/PVA/0.5CHI, compared to PVA/0.1CHI and PVA/0.5CHI, possibly indicating AgNPs binding to the –OH groups, which was assumed to be responsible for their stabilization in the hydrogel matrices. Several characteristic bands were also observed in the lower wavenumber ("fingerprint") region of the FT-IR spectra, i.e., the bands corresponding to C=O stretching from 2° amides (amide I band ~1654 cm^{-1}), in-plane bending of C–H bonds from vinyl groups (~1415 cm^{-1}), in-plane bending of O–H bonds from 2° alcohol (~1322–1325 cm^{-1}), stretching of the C–OH bonds (~1236–1240 cm^{-1}), symmetric stretching of the C–C bonds from the polymers' aliphatic chains (~1140 cm^{-1}). The C–O stretching band from 2° alcohol (PVA) was observed at 1083 cm^{-1} (PVA/0.1CHI), 1076 cm^{-1} (PVA/0.5CHI), 1087 cm^{-1} (3.9Ag/PVA/0.1CHI), and 1083 cm^{-1} (3.9Ag/PVA/0.5CHI). These peaks were shifted toward slightly higher wavenumbers (blue shift) in hydrogels with AgNPs, indicating some possible interactions of AgNPs with –OH groups, which caused change in the frequencies of C–O bond vibrations.

Using X-ray photoelectron spectroscopy (XPS), the high-resolution C1s, O1s, and N1s spectra of PVA/0.1CHI, PVA/0.5CHI, 3.9Ag/PVA/0.1CHI, and 3.9AgPVA/0.5CHI hydrogels were fitted with Voigt profiles in order to determine types of bonds (Nešović, Janković, Radetić et al. 2019). Four modes were present in C1s spectra and the peak maxima were positioned at binding energies (BE) of 284.7 eV, 286.2 eV, 287.5 eV, and 288.6 eV (PVA/0.1CHI); 284.8 eV, 286.2 eV, 287.7 eV, and 288.7 eV (PVA/0.5CHI); 284.8 eV, 286.2 eV, 287.1 eV, and 288.9 eV (3.9Ag/PVA/0.1CHI); and 284.7 eV, 286.1 eV, 287.1 eV, and 288.2 eV (3.9Ag/PVA/0.5CHI). Evidently, there were no significant variations among the different samples, and the peaks could be assigned to C-C/C-H, C-O/C-OH, C-N and C=O (R. Liu et al. 2014), originating from the polymer backbone and functional groups. Similarly, the O1s spectra could be fitted into three different peaks, positioned at BE of 531.2 eV, 532.3 eV, and 533.3 eV (PVA/0.1CHI); 531.4 eV, 532.4 eV, and 533.4 eV (PVA/0.5CHI); 531.2 eV, 532.3 eV, and 533.2 eV (3.9Ag/PVA/0.1CHI); and 531.3 eV, 532.3 eV, and 533.5 eV (3.9Ag/PVA/0.5CHI), and assigned to C-O, C-OH, and C=O bonds, respectively. The BE of N1s peaks were positioned at 399.9 eV (PVA/0.1CHI) and 399.7 eV for (PVA/0.5CHI), and were ascribed to the N-H single bonds from primary amino groups in chitosan (Lawrie et al. 2007). In the case of 3.9Ag/PVA/0.1CHI and 3.9AgPVA/0.5CHI hydrogels, however, another peak appeared at higher BE (406.9 eV for 3.9Ag/PVA/0.1CHI and 406.5 eV for 3.9AgPVA/0.5CHI hydrogels), which apparently originated from nitrogen bonding in nitrate groups. The presence of the $-NO_3$ groups could be explained by remnants of the $AgNO_3/KNO_3$ solution in which the hydrogels had swollen before the electrochemical synthesis of AgNPs. The high-resolution Ag3d spectra for 3.9Ag/PVA/0.1CHI and 3.9AgPVA/0.5CHI hydrogels exhibited typical appearance of the metallic silver with spin-orbit splitting doublet separated by 6 eV and positioned at 368.2 eV ($Ag3d_{5/2}$) and 374.2 eV ($Ag3d_{3/2}$) (Joshi, Markad, and Haram 2015; Song and Kim 2009; Larrude, Maia da Costa, and Freire 2014), indicating the presence of AgNPs in both 3.9Ag/PVA/0.1CHI and 3.9AgPVA/0.5CHI hydrogels.

Thermogravimetric analysis of PVA/0.1CHI, PVA/0.5CHI, 3.9Ag/PVA/0.1CHI, and 3.9Ag/PVA/0.5CHI was performed in order to elucidate the hydrogels thermal stability (Nešović, Janković, Radetić et al. 2019). The TG and DTG curves indicated three-step weight loss. The first step is water evaporation from the hydrogel matrix and occurred over a wider temperature range, including several sub-steps. Three sub-steps of mass loss for PVA/0.1CHI hydrogel covered the temperature regions 42 °C–95 °C, 95 °C–107 °C, and 107 °C–141.5 °C, with DTG peaks positioned at 89.6 °C, 105 °C, and 126.3 °C, respectively. The total weight loss in this region covered almost 80 wt.%, indicating that hydrogel contained a large amount of water. The DTG peaks and different sub-steps indicated that the water inside the hydrogel network exists in different states. The evaporation of free water, absorbed in the hydrogel pores, occurs at lower temperatures (T. Wang and Gunasekaran 2006), whereas the other types (evaporating at higher temperature of 126.3 °C) are bound to the polymer chains (e.g., by hydrogen bonding to –OH and $–NH_2$ of PVA and CHI) and, therefore, are more difficult to remove from the network (T. Wang and Gunasekaran 2006; Koosha and Mirzadeh 2015). For PVA/0.5CHI, the water evaporation step occurred in the temperature range 40 °C –98 °C and 98 °C –127.2 °C (DTG peaks at 76 °C and 103 °C, respectively). In the case of hydrogels with silver nanoparticles, this step is found in the range 34 °C–75.3 °C and 75.3 °C–110 °C with DTG peaks positioned at 66.7 °C and 103.7 °C (for 3.9Ag/PVA/0.1CHI) and 34.2 °C –76 °C and 76 °C –118.8 °C with DTG peaks positioned at 66.1 °C and 101.2 °C (for 3.9Ag/PVA/0.5CHI). After the first weight loss step, the TG curves for all the samples exhibited a plateau with no mass change up to about 250 °C -280 °C, followed by second weight loss step, which covered the onset of decomposition of the polymer matrix and further thermal degradation of polymer components. This second step occurred at 260°C–373.2 °C (DTG peaks at 274.6 °C and 355.8 °C) for PVA/0.1CHI, 257 °C–379 °C (DTG peaks at 280.4 °C and 361.5 °C) for PVA/0.5CHI, 282 °C–334 °C (DTG peak at 309 °C) for 3.9Ag/PVA/0.1CHI and 128.8 °C–280.4 °C (DTG peak at 314.7 °C) for 3.9Ag/PVA/0.5CHI. Endothermic thermal decomposition of PVA occurs through direct backbone degradation, whereas chitosan degradation involves amino groups destruction, followed by destruction of glycosidic bonds, depolymerization of macromolecular chains and pyranose rings destruction at higher temperatures (Koosha and Mirzadeh 2015; An, Beh, and Xiao 2014). The third, final thermal degradation steps occurred at temperatures higher than 400 °C, probably involving thermal decomposition of the remaining polymer components.

2.1.5.2 Swelling and Silver Release Kinetics

Swelling ability is one of the most important properties of hydrogels aimed for wound dressings. Hydrogels will optimally have a high swelling ratio in order to allow efficient absorbing of wound exudates and to ensure that the wound environment is kept moist in order to prevent drying of the wound and sticking of the dressing. The swelling degree, q_t, was calculated as the ratio of the absorbed solution, determined as the difference between hydrogel masses after, m_t, and before, m_0, swelling, and hydrogel mass before swelling, m_0

$$q_t = \frac{m_t - m_0}{m_0} \tag{2.16}$$

TABLE 2.4
Equilibrium Swelling Degrees and Diffusion Coefficients of Swelling Medium for PVA/0.1CHI, PVA/0.5CHI, 0.25Ag/PVA/0.1CHI, 0.25Ag/PVA/0.5CHI, 3.9Ag/PVA/0.1CHI and 3.9Ag/PVA/0.5CHI Hydrogels (Reprinted from Nešović, Janković, Radetić et al. 2019 with Permission from Elsevier)

Hydrogel	q_{eq}	D_{ETA} / 10^{-8} cm^2 s^{-1} (ETA)	D_{LTA} / 10^{-8} cm^2 s^{-1} (LTA)	D / 10^{-8} cm^2 s^{-1} (Etters)
PVA/0.1CHI	2.34 ± 0.06	1.22	2.15	1.80
PVA/0.5CHI	2.58 ± 0.04	2.50	4.65	3.53
0.25Ag/PVA/0.1CHI	2.90 ± 0.21	0.446	0.772	0.828
0.25Ag/PVA/0.5CHI	3.28 ± 0.14	0.350	0.641	0.738
3.9Ag/PVA/0.1CHI	3.96 ± 0.87	0.334	0.513	1.42
3.9Ag/PVA/0.5CHI	4.13 ± 0.20	0.626	1.03	2.20

The values of equilibrium swelling degree, q_{eq}, of Ag/PVA/CHI hydrogels are presented in Table 2.4. From the presented data, it was evident that the incorporation of AgNPs improved the swelling ability of hydrogels (higher equilibrium swelling degrees). This could be caused by stretching of the polymer matrix due to the presence and interactions of AgNPs with polymer chains, or could be caused by solvation of nanoparticles, inducing the absorption of more water molecules which would bind to AgNPs and form a solvation shell around them. Additionally, the hydrogels with higher chitosan content exhibited higher q_{eq}, indicating improved swelling of gels with more chitosan.

Other than calculating the equilibrium swelling degrees, the obtained swelling data were fitted with three different models from the literature, in order to calculate the diffusion coefficients of PB through hydrogel matrix during swelling, and to discern the predominant swelling mechanism. The sorption of convenient medium into the polymer network and swelling of the hydrogel usually occurs in several steps, involving initial fast absorption of the solvent into the pores of the hydrogel, followed by diffusion of the solvent inside the hydrogel matrix, governed by the concentration gradient, which causes formation of a moving boundary between the swollen and the unsolvated inner region of the hydrogel. During the latter phase of swelling, the sorption mechanism is generally governed by polymer chains plasticizing and relaxation (Xiaomin Yang et al. 2008).

The experimental swelling profiles (Figure 2.21) were fitted with several theoretical models, in order to investigate the kinetics of swelling. The chosen models were early time approximation (ETA), late time approximation (LTA), and Etters model. For ETA, a widely used standard ETA (Eq. 2.17) and a modified ETA (Eq. 2.18) proposed by Ritger and Peppas (Ritger and Peppas 1987) were applied

$$\frac{q_t}{q_{eq}} = 4\left(\frac{D_{ETA}t}{\pi\delta^2}\right)^{1/2} \tag{2.17}$$

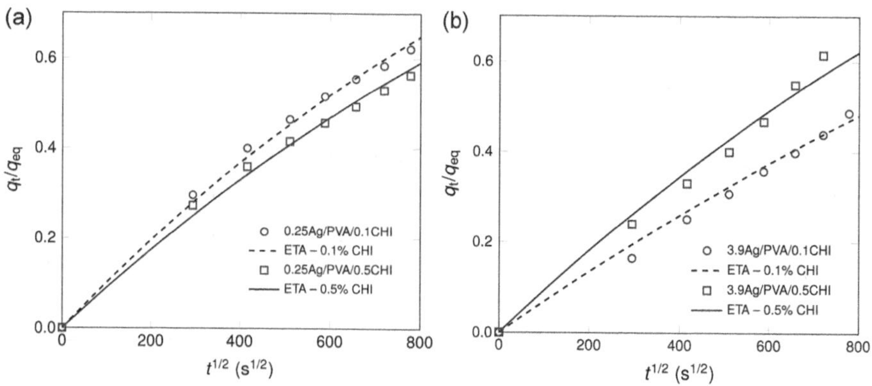

FIGURE 2.21 Swelling properties of (a) 0.25Ag/PVA/0.1CHI and 0.25Ag/PVA/0.5CHI, and (b) 3.9Ag/PVA/0.1CHI and 3.9Ag/PVA/0.5CHI hydrogels (experimental – points, ETA model – line) (reprinted from Nešović, Janković, Radetić et al. 2019)with permission from Elsevier)

$$\frac{q_t}{q_{eq}} = 4\left(\frac{D_{ETA}\,t}{\pi r^2}\right)^{\frac{1}{2}} - \pi\left(\frac{D_{ETA}\,t}{\pi r^2}\right) - \frac{\pi}{3}\left(\frac{D_{ETA}\,t}{\pi r^2}\right)^{\frac{3}{2}} + 4\left(\frac{D_{ETA}\,t}{\pi \delta^2}\right)^{\frac{1}{2}} - \frac{2r}{\delta}\left[8\left(\frac{D_{ETA}\,t}{\pi r^2}\right) - 2\pi\left(\frac{D_{ETA}\,t}{\pi r^2}\right)^{3/2} - \frac{2\pi}{3}\left(\frac{D_{ETA}\,t}{\pi r^2}\right)^{2}\right] \tag{2.18}$$

where D_{ETA} is swelling medium diffusion coefficient (subscript "ETA" indicates ETA model), t is the time of swelling, q_t is swelling degree, and δ is hydrogel thickness. The LTA model (Eq. 2.19) was used to fit the latter 40 % of swelling and the Etters model (Eq. 2.20) is supposed to be valid for the entire swelling period. D_{LTA} is swelling medium diffusion coefficient (subscript "LTA" indicates LTA model), D is swelling medium diffusion coefficient obtained using Etters model, a, b, k are Etters constants, q_t is swelling degree.

$$\frac{q_t}{q_{eq}} = 1 - \frac{8}{\pi^2}\exp\left(-\frac{D_{LTA}\,\pi^2 t}{\delta^2}\right) \tag{2.19}$$

$$\frac{q_t}{q_{eq}} = 1 - \exp\left[-k\left(\frac{Dt}{\delta^2}\right)^{a}\right]^{1/b} \tag{2.20}$$

According to Ritger and Peppas, the standard ETA is frequently misused, even though it only applies to very specific cases of swelling, and for specific geometries of thin films with very high aspect ratio (diameter divided by thickness; a thin film will typically have aspect ratio of the order of ~100, whereas for thick hydrogel disks it is closer to unity) (Ritger and Peppas 1987). Since hydrogels were thick disks with an aspect ratio of ~2 the modified ETA model was applied (Figure 2.21). The obtained diffusion coefficients, D_{ETA}, are presented in Table 2.4. The LTA model is generally thought to be valid for the last 40 % of swelling, and the diffusion coefficients, D_{LTA}, calculated using Eq. (2.19) were slightly higher than those calculated using ETA model (Eq. 2.17). The Etters model (Eq. 2.20) provided good correlation with experimental data over the entire swelling period, and the obtained diffusion coefficients, D, are presented in Table 2.4. The largest values of Etters diffusion coefficients, D, were calculated for PVA/0.1CHI (1.80×10^{-8} cm^2 s^{-1}) and PVA/0.5CHI (3.53×10^{-8} cm^2 s^{-1}), indicating that hydrogels without silver nanoparticles exhibited faster swelling; however, their equilibrium swelling degrees were lower (2.34 ± 0.06 and 2.58 ± 0.04, respectively), compared to AgNP-containing hydrogels.

Silver release from a hydrophilic hydrogel matrix is usually diffusion controlled; however, it can also be controlled by other effects, such as hydrogel swelling, polymer chains relaxation, carrier erosion, or, of course, by any combination of the aforementioned processes (Ritger and Peppas 1987). The experimental silver release profiles for 0.25Ag/PVA/0.1CHI, 0.25Ag/PVA/0.5CHI, 3.9Ag/PVA/0.1CHI, and 3.9Ag/PVA/0.5CHI hydrogels are presented in Figure 2.22. The release profiles indicated that chitosan concentration does not affect the silver release kinetics, while higher amount of silver loaded in the hydrogel matrix could have a pronounced effect on the release behavior, i.e., faster initial release and shorter time needed to reach the plateau. The Makoid-Banakar, Korsmeyer-Peppas, and Kopcha models (described by Eqs. 2.12, 2.13 and 2.14, respectively) are depicted along in Figure 2.22, while the calculated parameters and the fit quality using both R^2 and adjusted R^2_{adj} coefficients are listed in Table 2.5. The Makoid-Banakar model provided better correlation with experimental data (higher values of R^2 and R^2_{adj}) in respect to other models. The values of $n<0.5$ from Korsmeyer-Peppas model for all the samples confirmed that the silver release is predominantly governed by Fickian diffusion, which is additionally supported by the values of $|A/B|>1$ from the Kopcha model. To calculate the diffusion coefficient of silver release, the release of silver during the initial period was fitted with the modified ETA model (Figure 2.22). The greater values of diffusion coefficients of silver through the polymer matrix, D_{Ag}, calculated from this model (Table 2.5), confirmed the faster release from hydrogel with higher silver concentration.

2.1.5.3 Antibacterial Activity and Cytotoxicity

The antibacterial properties of PVA/0.1CHI, PVA/0.5CHI, 0.25Ag/PVA/0.1CHI, and 0.25AgPVA/0.5CHI hydrogels were evaluated by monitoring bacterial viability in their presence for 24 hours (Figures 2.23a and b). In the case of both bacterial strains, the hydrogels with AgNPs caused complete reduction in bacterial cell numbers even after 1 hour of incubation, indicating exceptionally powerful antibacterial activity of these hydrogels. In the case of *S. aureus*, there was a visible reduction of ~4 logarithmic units even after 15 minutes. The hydrogels without AgNPs, however, proved to be slightly less effective, but nonetheless caused 100 % reduction in *S. aureus* cell count after 1 hour. In the case of *E. coli*, on the other hand, the PVA/0.1CHI and PVA/0.5CHI hydrogels did not exhibit significant inhibitory effect, and only after 24 hours incubation were the cell counts reduced by a notable

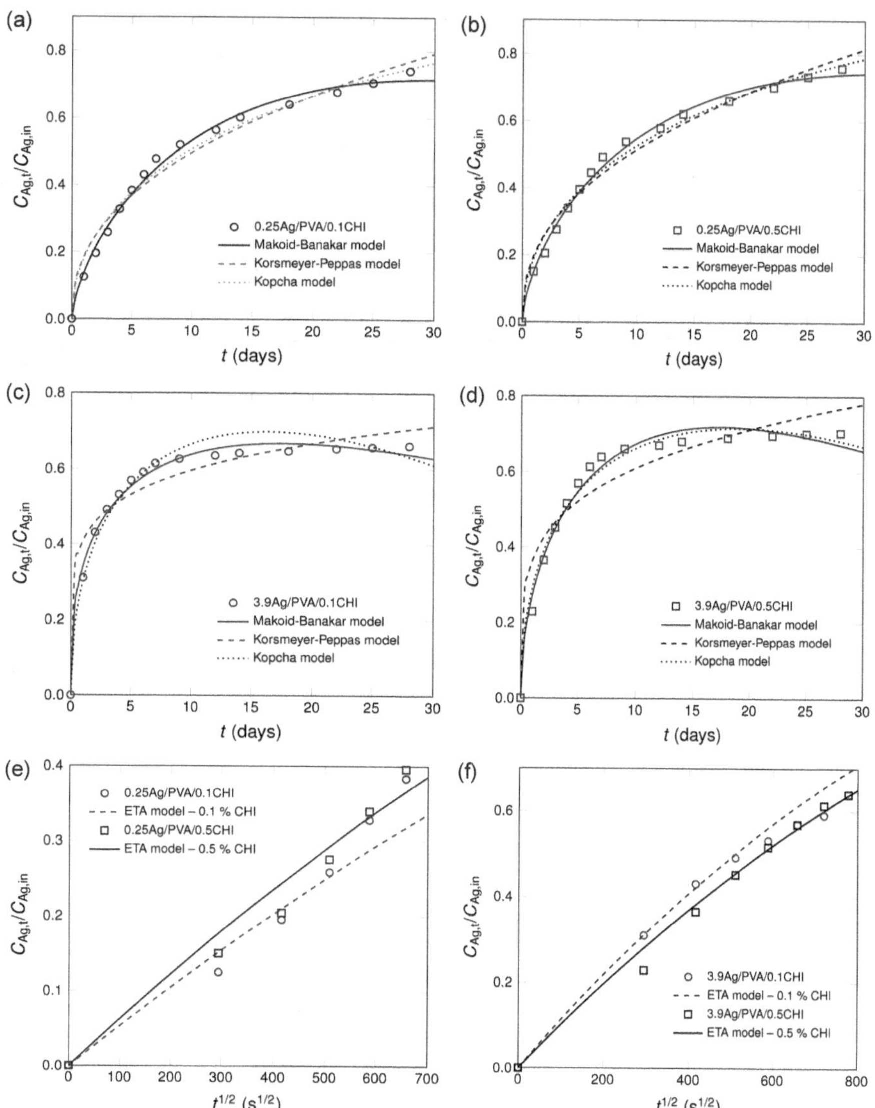

FIGURE 2.22 Makoid-Banakar, Korsmeyer-Peppas and Kopcha release models for (a) 0.25Ag/PVA/0.1CHI, (b) 0.25Ag/PVA/0.5CHI, (c) 3.9Ag/PVA/0.1CHI and (d) 3.9AgPVA/0.5CHI hydrogels, and ETA model for (e) 0.25Ag/PVA/0.1CHI and 0.25Ag/PVA/0.5CHI, (f) 3.9Ag/PVA/0.1CHI and 3.9AgPVA/0.5CHI hydrogels (reprinted from Nešović, Janković, Radetić et al. 2019 with permission from Elsevier)

TABLE 2.5
Fitting Parameters for Different Models of Silver Release from 0.25Ag/PVA/0.1CHI, 0.25Ag/PVA/0.5CHI, 3.9Ag/PVA/0.1CHI and 3.9Ag/PVA/0.5CHI Hydrogels (Reprinted from Nešović, Janković, Radetić et al. 2019 with Permission from Elsevier)

Model		0.25Ag/PVA/0.1CHI	0.25Ag/PVA/0.5CHI	3.9Ag/PVA/0.1CHI	3.9Ag/PVA/0.5CHI
Korsmeyer-Peppas	k_{kp} (s^{-n})	0.186	0.196	0.409	0.363
	n	0.427	0.419	0.163	0.225
	R^2	0.975	0.979	0.949	0.918
	R^2_{adj}	0.973	0.977	0.945	0.912
Makoid-Banakar	k_{mb} (s^{-n})	0.140	0.152	0.349	0.280
	n	0.678	0.645	0.347	0.509
	c	0.0225	0.0203	0.0198	0.0292
	R^2	0.994	0.995	0.992	0.987
	R^2_{adj}	0.993	0.994	0.99	0.985
Kopcha	A ($s^{-1/2}$)	0.189	0.198	0.342	0.329
	B (s^{-1})	-0.00893	-0.00983	-0.0427	-0.0377
	R^2	0.983	0.987	0.978	0.984
	$R^2_{adj.}$	0.981	0.985	0.977	0.983
ETA	D_{Ag} / 10^{-9} cm^2 s^{-1}	2.85	3.94	14.3	11.4
	R^2	0.974	0.966	0.999	0.99
	R^2_{adj}	0.981	0.971	0.999	0.992

~4 logarithmic units in the presence of PVA/0.5CHI hydrogel. Chitosan is well known for its intrinsic antibacterial properties (Rabea et al. 2003; Kong et al. 2010); however, some studies have shown that neat chitosan films might not be effective over a longer period as their surfaces tend to saturate with dead bacteria cells and lose their favorable activity (Wei et al. 2009). Many different factors could influence the antibacterial effect of the samples against a specific strain, such as the initial number of bacteria in the suspension, the sensitivity of the particular strain, the type of media used for culture, etc. It has been shown that the antibacterial activity of silver nanoparticles is significantly strain-specific, and even different strains of the same species exhibited varying sensitivity. It has been shown that chitosan indeed differently affects *S. aureus* and *E. coli*, specifically, that CHI of higher molecular weight (MW) possesses stronger activity against *S. aureus* than against *E. coli*. The mechanism of action could be different, i.e., the interaction of positively charged CHI with negatively charged bacteria surfaces and the adsorption of macromolecules, disrupting respiration and preventing nutrients to enter the cell is possibly a dominant mechanism in the case of *S. aureus*, whereas CHI acts on *E. coli* by pervading the membrane and entering the cell. Additionally, chitosan could cause the rupture of the cell membrane. Thus, for CHI of higher MW, it is difficult to penetrate the bacterial cells, leading to lower antibacterial activity against *E. coli*. Probably, only in the case of the sample with higher CHI content (PVA/0.5CHI), a sufficient amount of chitosan was released after 24 hours into the suspension, which could explain the lag of CHI bacteriostatic effect against *E. coli*.

The MTT cytotoxicity tests confirmed non-toxicity of all tested hydrogels toward both cell lines, MRC-5 (human fibroblast line), and L929 (mice fibroblast cell line). The MTT results (Figure 2.23c) showed high survival rate for both cell lines in the presence of all hydrogel samples, and in some cases, viabilities higher than 100 % were observed, indicating that the investigated hydrogels could even induce proliferation and growth in the observed assay period (48 h + 48 h). The results were similar for both cell lines used; however, the viability of MRC-5 cell line was slightly lower compared to L929, in the case of AgNP-containing hydrogels. The statistical analysis showed that the cell viabilities in the presence of hydrogels without silver were significantly different ($p < 0.01$), compared to silver-containing hydrogels, as well as compared to each other. These results indicated that, as the chitosan as well as AgNPs content increased, the viability of the MRC-5 and L929 cells decreased. Research has shown that chitosan could cause mild reduction in cell viability of the MRC-5 line (Je, Cho, and Kim 2006), although the effect cannot be considered cytotoxic. The TEM results indicated that the AgNPs in the hydrogel with 0.5 wt.% CHI had some surface defects in the crystalline structure, which was also shown to be a cause of cytotoxicity for fish gill cell line (George et al. 2012). All of this could be the reason for the reduced viability of cells in the presence of hydrogels with AgNPs, as well as lower viability of both cell lines in the presence of PVA/0.5CHI, compared to PVA/0.1CHI. However, cell viability was always higher than 90 %, even in the case of 3.9Ag/PVA/0.1CHI and 3.9Ag/PVA/0.5CHI hydrogels, so all the hydrogel samples can be considered non-cytotoxic and therefore safe for biomedical applications.

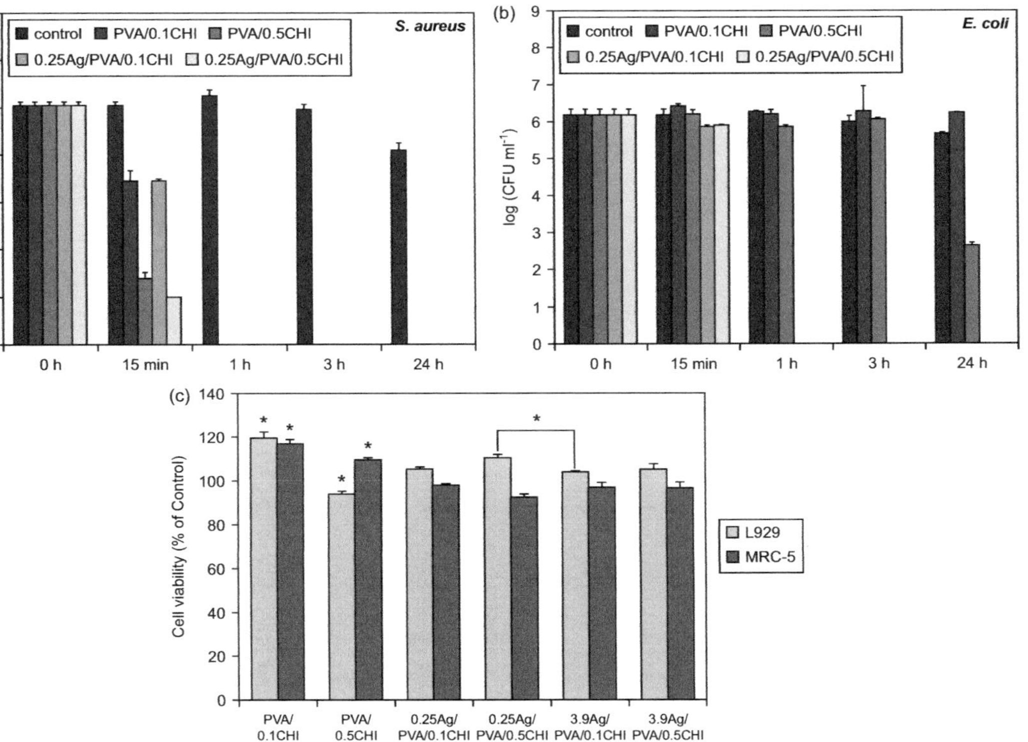

FIGURE 2.23 The number of surviving bacteria cells: (a) *S. aureus* and (b) *E. coli*, for PVA/0.1CHI, PVA/0.5CHI, 0.25Ag/PVA/0.1CHI, and 0.25AgPVA/0.5CHI hydrogels, and (c) cell viability of L929 and MRC-5 cell lines in the presence of PVA/0.1CHI, PVA/0.5CHI, 0.25Ag/PVA/0.1CHI, 0.25Ag/PVA/0.5CHI, 3.9Ag/PVA/0.1CHI, and 3.9Ag/PVA/0.5CHI hydrogels. *-$p < 0.01$ (reprinted from Nešović, Janković, Radetić et al. 2019 with permission from Elsevier)

Even though the hydrogels with both higher and lower AgNP concentrations have proved to be non-cytotoxic in this MTT test, when choosing a material for bio-applications, it is always advisable to be on the safe side regarding the concentrations of active components. The risks of potential harmful effects of AgNPs during prolonged use are well known, as they have been shown to accumulate in brain cells in a time- and dose-dependent manner (Luther et al. 2011) as well as to induce *in vivo* repeated-dose toxicity in mice (Park, Bae et al. 2010). Therefore, even if the material did not exhibit cytotoxicity upon single-time exposure, it is still best to opt for the lowest possible AgNPs concentration that provides satisfactory antibacterial effect.

2.1.6 Polyvinyl Alcohol/Chitosan/Graphene-Based Hydrogels with Silver Nanoparticles

2.1.6.1 Electrochemical Synthesis and Characterization of Silver/Poly(Vinyl Alcohol)/Chitosan/Graphene Hydrogels

PVA/CHI/Gr hydrogels consisting of 10 wt.% PVA, 0.01 wt.% Gr and 0.1 wt.% and 0.5 wt.% CHI (PVA/0.1CHI/Gr and PVA/0.5CHI/Gr, respectively) were obtained by freezing-thawing in five cycles, where one cycle was 16 hours at –18°C and 8 hours at +4°C. Prior to electrochemical synthesis of AgNPs at constant voltage of 90 V for 4 minutes, swelling of PVA/0.1CHI/Gr and PVA/0.5CHI/Gr hydrogels was achieved during 48 hours in 0.25 mM and 3.9 mM AgNO3 (Nešović et al. 2018).

In UV-Vis spectra, silver nanoparticles exhibited absorbance peak at 397 nm for 0.25Ag/PVA/0.1CHI/Gr and at 401 nm for 0.25Ag/PVA/0.5CHI/Gr, confirming the presence of spherical AgNPs with supposed diameters of a few tens of nanometers. Similarly, in previous work (Yenier et al. 2016), UV-Vis spectra of 3.9Ag/PVA/0.1CHI/Gr and 3.9Ag/PVA/0.5CHI/Gr hydrogels exhibited peaks at 401 nm and 405 nm, respectively. In addition, 3.9Ag/PVA/0.1CHI/Gr and 3.9Ag/PVA/0.5CHI/Gr showed higher absorbance than 3.9Ag/PVA/Gr. Finally, the 3.9Ag/PVA/0.1CHI/Gr and 3.9Ag/PVA/0.5CHI/Gr hydrogels with 3.9 mM $AgNO_3$ exhibited higher absorbance than 0.25Ag/PVA/0.1CHI/Gr and 0.25Ag/PVA/0.5CHI/Gr hydrogels with 0.25 mM $AgNO_3$, proving higher amount of AgNPs synthesized in hydrogels from more concentrated $AgNO_3$ swelling solution as expected.

FE-SEM micrographs of PVA/0.1CHI/Gr, PVA/0.5CHI/Gr, 3.9Ag/PVA/0.1CHI/Gr and 3.9Ag/PVA/0.5CHI/Gr showed that with an increase in chitosan content to 0.5 wt.%, the hydrogel surface structure becomes more porous, which is desirable for the effective immobilization of silver nanoparticles in the hydrogel matrix. In addition, higher chitosan content decreases AgNPs dimensions, due to stronger interactions of AgNPs with amino and hydroxyl groups on the CHI chains. Finally, AgNPs content, as determined from EDS analysis, in 3.9Ag/PVA/0.5CHI/Gr (0.49 at%) is more than two times higher than in 3.9Ag/PVA/0.1CHI/Gr (0.21 at% (Yenier et al. 2016)), which is in agreement with UV-Vis spectroscopy results.

Raman spectra of PVA/0.5CHI/Gr and 3.9Ag/PVA/0.5CHI/Gr hydrogels confirmed the incorporation of graphene by the presence of characteristic bands – the D-band, which is known to indicate presence of imperfections, defects, and rough edges in graphene layers, and the G-band, originating from sp^2-bonded C-atom in-plane vibrations. The positions of the D-band for PVA/0.5CHI/Gr and 3.9Ag/PVA/0.5CHI/Gr were at 1350 cm^{-1} and 1346 cm^{-1}, respectively, and G-bands were observed at 1585 cm^{-1} and 1582 cm^{-1}, respectively. Similarly, in the case of PVA/0.1CHI/Gr and 3.9Ag/PVA/0.1CHI/Gr hydrogels (Yenier et al. 2016), the D-band was observed at 1345 cm^{-1} and 1351 cm^{-1}, respectively, whereas the G-bands were positioned at 1591 cm^{-1} and 1586 cm^{-1}, respectively. The graphene G-band also overlaps with in-plane bending vibrations of bonds in $–NH_2$ groups on chitosan chain. The intensity of band corresponding to $-NH_2$ groups on chitosan chain in 3.9Ag/PVA/0.5CHI/Gr is obviously increased in respect to PVA/0.5CHI/Gr and its position is shifted from 1585 cm^{-1} to 1582 cm^{-1}, which may indicate interactions of AgNPs with $-NH_2$ groups of chitosan. Other bands in the Raman spectra originate from the bond vibrations in the polymer matrix. The most prominent band in the PVA/0.5CHI/Gr spectrum was at 2915 cm^{-1}, which corresponds to the symmetrical stretching of the C-H bond from the CH_2 group in the polymer backbone. This was also found at the same wavenumber in the PVA/0.1CHI/Gr spectrum. In the case of 3.9Ag/PVA/0.5CHI/Gr hydrogel, this peak is wider, split into two maxima, and with several overlapping bands. The range of 2900–3100 cm^{-1} contains peaks at 2937, 2968, and a smaller one at 3038 cm^{-1}. This region usually reflects the CH and CH_2 stretching, so these bands can be ascribed to C-H stretching modes from the PVA and CHI structure. Similarly, for 3.9Ag/PVA/0.1CHI/Gr hydrogel (Yenier et al. 2016), there is also a split of the largest band into peaks at 2915 and 2970 cm^{-1}, with the appearance of another one at 3034 cm^{-1}. The bands at 1440 cm^{-1} for PVA/0.5CHI/Gr (as well as both PVA/0.1CHI/Gr and 3.9Ag/PVA/0.1CHI/Gr (Yenier et al. 2016)) and at 1437 cm^{-1} for 3.9Ag/PVA/0.5CHI/Gr originate from the in-plane bending of CH_2 and OH bonds. The only red shift of this band position occurs for 3.9Ag/PVA/0.5CHI/Gr, indicating interactions of AgNPs with -OH groups, which are stronger in the hydrogel with higher CHI content that also contains more AgNPs as confirmed by UV-vis. A prominent feature in the 3.9Ag/PVA/0.5CHI/Gr spectrum is the band at 236 cm^{-1}, also found in the 3.9Ag/PVA/0.1CHI/Gr spectrum at 235 cm^{-1} (Yenier et al. 2016), that pointed to AgNPs in the hydrogel.

The XPS C1s peaks for PVA/0.5CHI/Gr and 3.9Ag/PVA/0.5CHI/Gr were fitted into four different modes with binding energy (BE) values of 284.8, 286.2, 287.5, 289.1 eV and 284.8, 286.2, 287.7, 289.1 eV, respectively. These peaks were assigned to the C-C/C-H, C-O/C-OH, C-N, and C=O bonds, respectively. Similar BE for C1s peaks were also found for hydrogels with 0.1 wt.% CHI (Yenier et al. 2016), where the C-C/C-H, C-O/C-OH, C-N, and C=O responses were positioned at 284.8, 286.2, 287.7, 289.1 eV, respectively, for PVA/0.1CHI/Gr and at 284.8, 286.2, 287.5, 289.1 eV for 3.9Ag/PVA/0.1CHI/Gr. As shown, there is good agreement in the BE of deconvoluted peaks for all samples, and no significant change was observed upon introduction of AgNPs. The O1s peak was fitted by three peaks corresponding to the C-O, C-OH, and C=O bonds, positioned at 530.0, 531.5, and 532.3 eV, respectively, for PVA/0.1CHI/Gr and at 530.0, 531.6 and 532.4 eV for Ag/PVA/0.1CHI/Gr (Yenier et al. 2016). For PVA/0.5CHI/Gr, these peaks were positioned at 530.0, 531.4, and 532.2 eV, and for 3.9Ag/PVA/0.5CHI/Gr they were at 530.1, 531.4, and

532.4 eV, respectively. The presence of C-O, C-OH, and C=O bonds was confirmed by both C1s and O1s peaks analyses. The much smaller area of the C=O peak can be explained by this peak originating from carbonyl groups in the chitosan structure, where the amount of chitosan was very low in the hydrogel, whereas the C-OH bond can be found in both PVA and CHI. The BE of N1s peaks were found at 399.4 eV for PVA/0.1CHI/Gr, 399.5 eV for 3.9Ag/PVA/0.1CHI/Gr 399.6 eV for PVA/0.5CHI/Gr, and at 399.8 eV for 3.9Ag/PVA/0.5CHI/Gr. These were ascribed to single-bonded nitrogen from primary amines in the chitosan structure. Finally, the core level Ag3d peak of 3.9Ag/PVA/0.5CHI/Gr consisted of two well-separated distinct peaks at 368 and 374 eV, corresponding to the $3d_{5/2}$ and $3d_{3/2}$ modes, respectively. The position of these peaks and their separation by 6 eV is an indication of metallic silver (Ma et al. 2007), confirming the incorporation of AgNPs in the hydrogels.

The dynamic light scattering (DLS) method was employed in order to determine hydrodynamic size (diameter) and size distributions of silver nanoparticles incorporated in the hydrogels (Nešović, Janković, Perić-Grujić et al. 2019). The averaged intensity- and volume-weighted distributions were determined for 3.9Ag/PVA/0.1CHI/Gr and 3.9Ag/PVA/0.5CHI/Gr, indicating relatively narrow distributions with particle size in nm range. A rather small portion of large-sized fraction was also detected. The hydrogel with lower chitosan content (0.1 wt.%) exhibited a monomodal distribution. Based on intensity data, the most abundant was the 9.97 nm-sized particle population (96.7 % share in the scattered light). The hydrogel with higher chitosan content (0.5 wt.%) contained even smaller-sized AgNPs, which could be due to better stabilization of nanoparticles by interactions with functional groups on chitosan chains. Additionally, the particle size distribution (PSD) for 3.9Ag/PVA/0.5CHI/Gr hydrogel exhibited a bimodal distribution of particle sizes, with two peaks at 8.22 nm and 1.76 nm, respectively. Upon transformation to volume-weighted distribution, it was observed that the nanoparticles were predominantly (87.0 % by volume) in the smaller-sized group (peak at ~1.57 nm), further corroborating the assumption that chitosan highly influenced the stabilization and growth of AgNPs in the hydrogel. The related Z-average hydrodynamic diameters, D_Z, of AgNPs were 8.06 ± 0.098 nm (PDI = 0.265 ± 0.032) for 3.9Ag/PVA/0.1CHI/Gr and 6.38 ± 0.12 nm (PDI = 0.387 ± 0.079) for 3.9Ag/PVA/0.5CHI/Gr. The polydispersity indices were relatively large, however, and larger in the case of 3.9Ag/PVA/0.5CHI/Gr (0.387 ± 0.079), suggesting that the nanoparticles incorporated in both hydrogel samples were not monodisperse.

TEM characterization confirmed the results of DLS analysis. The low-magnification micrographs revealed the presence of some larger agglomerates, hundreds of nm in size, surrounded by numerous, finer AgNPs. Similarly to DLS results, characterization showed an almost bimodal distribution of AgNPs. Larger particles, ~10-20 nm in size, are heavily twinned and polycrystalline with faceted morphology. Smaller AgNPs, ~5 nm in size, tend to be single crystals with cuboctahedral shape. In the case of 3.9Ag/PVA/0.5CHI/Gr hydrogel, there are many very small nanoparticles with sizes ~2 nm surrounding some larger particles between 10 and 20 nm in size. The presence of very small AgNPs in 3.9Ag/PVA/0.5CHI/Gr hydrogel could be due to the contribution of higher chitosan content, as chitosan could influence both growth and stabilization of nanoparticles It is known that smaller-sized AgNPs possess much better antibacterial activity than larger nanoparticles, so the presence of AgNPs in a size range of <10 nm could prove invaluable for antibacterial applications of the prepared hydrogels. That the observed nanoparticles are indeed AgNPs has been unquestionably confirmed by the FFT patterns typical for fcc crystal structure and lattice fringe spacing of 0.24 nm and 0.20 nm corresponding to (111) and (200) crystal planes of fcc Ag (Nešović, Janković, Perić-Grujić et al. 2019).

FT-IR spectra of PVA/0.1CHI/Gr and 3.9Ag/PVA/0.1CHI/Gr hydrogels exhibited a broad, well-defined absorption band ascribed to the stretching vibrations of hydrogen-bonded –OH groups positioned at 3295 cm^{-1} for PVA/0.1CHI/Gr and at 3294 cm^{-1} for 3.9Ag/PVA/0.1CHI/Gr, with a possible overlap of $–NH_2$ stretching from chitosan. A slight red shift in the absorption maximum in the sample with silver suggested the interactions of silver nanoparticles with –OH groups in the polymer. The red shift of this band is also prominent, with the –OH stretching band shifting from 3275 cm^{-1} for PVA/0.5CHI/Gr to 3274 cm^{-1} for 3.9Ag/PVA/0.5CHI/Gr. This indicates stronger interactions between AgNPs and chitosan. The –OH valence vibration band is also very sensitive to hydrogen bonding; therefore, it is obvious that increases in CHI concentration led to the formation of stronger and more numerous inter- and intramolecular hydrogen bonds, as evidenced by the significant shift of this band from 3295 cm^{-1} (PVA/0.1CHI/Gr) to 3275 cm^{-1} (PVA/0.5CHI/Gr). Bands corresponding to C–O stretching vibrations in secondary alcohols (PVA) were located at 1087 cm^{-1} (PVA/0.1CHI/Gr), 1086 cm^{-1} (3.9A PVA/0.1CHI/Gr), 1088 cm^{-1} (PVA/0.5CHI/Gr) and 1080 cm^{-1} (3.9Ag/PVA/0.5CHI/Gr). The shift in the absorption maxima to lower wavenumbers in hydrogels containing silver indicated interactions of AgNPs with PVA chains and the formation of complex bonds with –OH groups, leading to changes in C–O bond vibrations and IR absorption at lower wavenumbers. A sharp weak band originating from C–C symmetric stretching in PVA, is located at 1143 cm^{-1} (for both PVA/0.1CHI/Gr and PVA/0.5CHI/Gr), 1142 cm^{-1} (3.9A PVA/0.1CHI/Gr) and 1141 cm^{-1} (3.9AgPVA/0.5CHI/Gr). As this band's location and intensity are sensitive to polymer crystallinity, it can be assumed that the presence of AgNPs influenced the crystalline structure of the PVA chain. Stretching of the carbonyl (C=O) bond of secondary amides (R–CO–NH–R') is present as a broad, but sharp band around 1650 cm^{-1} (the so-called amide I absorption band). A slight shift of this band to higher wavenumbers was observed in the spectra of nanocomposite hydrogels with AgNPs (1652 cm^{-1} for 3.9Ag/PVA/0.1CHI/Gr and 1654 cm^{-1} for 3.9Ag/PVA/0.5CHI/Gr). Additionally, an increase in CHI content in the hydrogel increased the wavenumber as well as the intensity of the band. This occurs due to hydrogen bonding of acetamide groups on the chitosan chain with OH and NH_2 groups on PVA and CHI. Bands at around 830 cm^{-1} correspond to out-of-plane wagging and twisting of the primary amino ($–NH_2$) group in the chitosan macromolecule. A significant increase in intensity and a slight red shift of this band in the FT-IR spectra of samples with silver nanoparticles also indicated AgNP-CHI complex formation, contributing to the stabilization of AgNPs in the silver-doped hydrogels (Nešović, Janković, Perić-Grujić et al. 2019).

TABLE 2.6
Mechanical Properties of PVA/0.1CHI, PVA/0.5CHI and PVA/0.5CHI/Gr: σ_R – Tensile Yield Strength, ε_R – Yield Elongation, E_J – Young's Elasticity Modulus, σ_U – Ultimate Strength, ε_U – Ultimate Elongation (Reprinted from Nešović, Janković, Perić-Grujić et al. 2019 with Permission from Elsevier)

	σ_R (MPa)	ε_R (%)	E_J (MPa)	σ_U (MPa)	ε_U (%)
PVA/0.1CHI	30.7	2.7	21.4	38.5	28.1
PVA/0.5CHI	22.6	3.8	14.0	24.4	38.0
PVA/0.5CHI/Gr	78.0	1.3	121.7	63.1	23.2

2.1.6.2 Biomechanical Properties

The influence of graphene on the hydrogels mechanical properties was evaluated by tensile testing (Nešović, Janković, Perić-Grujić et al. 2019). The stress-strain curves of reference PVA/0.1CHI and PVA/0.5CHI samples without graphene exhibited fairly similar behavior, whereas the PVA/0.5CHI/Gr exhibited much higher tensile yield, indicating improved mechanical properties with the addition of graphene. The quantitative tensile data, namely, tensile yield strength, σ_R, yield elongation, ε_R, Young's elasticity modulus, E_J, ultimate strength, σ_U, ultimate elongation, ε_U, were calculated from stress-strain curves and presented in Table 2.6. The PVA/0.5CHI/Gr sample exhibited much higher yield and ultimate strengths (78.0 MPa and 63.1 MPa, respectively), as well as higher elasticity modulus (121.7 MPa), compared to both PVA/0.1CHI and PVA/0.5CHI, confirming that the incorporation of graphene significantly improved hydrogels' tensile strength and elasticity. On the other hand, the elongation at break for PVA/0.5CHI/Gr (23.2 %) was slightly lower than for PVA/0.1CHI (28.1 %) and PVA/0.5CHI (38.0 %), indicating that graphene-containing gels and films could be slightly more brittle. Chitosan is known to possess poor mechanical properties; therefore, PVA/0.5CHI exhibited lower tensile strength, ultimate strength, and elastic modulus than PVA/0.1CHI.

2.1.6.3 Thermal Stability

The DSC curves of all hydrogels revealed apparently endothermic peaks (Nešović, Janković, Perić-Grujić et al. 2019). The first peak, depicted by a large endothermic peak with two maxima, was ascribed to the evaporation and loss of water in different states in the hydrogel. Water in a hydrogel can adopt different states due to different interactions and dipole orientations. Freezable or free water inside the pores of the gel accounts for the largest proportion in the hydrogel, and it evaporates at lower temperatures. The bound or intermediate forms of water consist of dipoles polarized and oriented around charged and hydrogen-bonded groups and/or structured into a solvent cage around hydrophobic segments. The first step of free water evaporation was observed at 74 °C for PVA/0.1CHI/Gr, 97 °C for 3.9Ag/PVA/0.1CHI/Gr, 88 °C for PVA/0.5CHI/Gr and at 80 °C for 3.9Ag/PVA/0.5CHI/Gr. The bound water evaporated in the range of approximately 130 °C–160 °C, with DSC peaks positioned at 137 °C for PVA/0.1CHI/Gr, 156 °C for 3.9Ag/PVA/0.1CHI/Gr, 147 °C for PVA/0.5CHI/Gr, and 150 °C for 3.9Ag/PVA/0.5CHI/Gr. The first observation is a change in the areas of the first two peaks with a change in chitosan content; namely, the area of the second peak increased in the hydrogels with 0.5 wt.% CHI compared to those with 0.1 wt.% CHI. This means that the ratio of bound-to-free water is higher in hydrogels with higher chitosan content, which can be explained by the increase in the amount of polar hydrophilic groups (i.e., $-NH_2$, –OH) that are able to interact with water dipoles and cause orientation and ordering, subsequently lowering the free water content in favor of bound water. This conclusion is also corroborated by the increase in evaporation temperatures for both peaks in PVA/0.5CHI/Gr (88 °C and 147 °C) in comparison to PVA/0.1CHI/Gr (74 °C and 137 °C). Some further changes can be observed in the DSC curves with the addition of AgNPs. Water evaporation occurred at higher temperatures for 3.9Ag/PVA/0.1CHI/Gr in comparison to PVA/0.1CHI/Gr, and the peaks exhibited a larger area, indicating that the hydrogel with AgNPs contained a higher amount of both bound and free water. This could be due to interactions of water dipoles with AgNPs, which result in a solvent cage around them as well as separation of macromolecule chains due to the incorporation of AgNPs. However, the peak areas are significantly lower for the 3.9Ag/PVA/0.5CHI/Gr as compared to the PVA/0.5CHI/Gr, and the peak of free water evaporation is much wider, with a maximum at lower temperature (80 °C as compared to 88 °C for PVA/0.5CHI/Gr). Neto et al. (Neto et al. 2005) hypothesized that the interactions of water dipoles with polar groups differ in strength. Specifically, the binding of water to amino groups in chitosan is weaker than binding to hydroxyl groups, and consequently this type of water bound to $-NH_2$ can be removed at lower temperatures. This may be an explanation for the higher bound water content in hydrogels with AgNPs, as AgNPs readily interact with $-NH_2$, which is an important factor in their stabilization and was explained previously. For that reason, $-NH_2$ groups are less available for interactions with water, and the dipoles are tightly bound (mainly to –OH groups), leading to an increase in bound water content. UV-Vis showed that the hydrogel with higher chitosan content contained a higher amount of AgNPs than the hydrogel with lower chitosan content as a consequence of more interactions with both $-NH_2$ groups of CHI and –OH groups of CHI and PVA. This reduces the number of polar groups available for orientation and binding of water dipoles. Additionally, a high amount of AgNPs can contribute to the rigidity of a polymer network, thus reducing its water uptake capability. Those effects collectively lowered the amounts of both free and bound water in the 3.9Ag/PVA/0.5CHI/Gr hydrogel and resulted in a lower temperature of evaporation.

The second and third peaks in the DSC curves are related to the melting and onset of polymer matrix degradation, respectively. The peaks for these events were positioned at 220 °C and 272 °C for PVA/0.1CHI/Gr, 215 °C and 282 °C for 3.9Ag/PVA/0.1CHI/Gr, 218 °C and 276 °C for PVA/0.5CHI/Gr and at 219 °C and 293 °C for 3.9Ag/PVA/0.5CHI/Gr. The melting point, T_m, for pure PVA is usually found in the range of 202 °C–218 °C, depending on the degree of crystallinity, cross-linking density, and preparation conditions. The degradation of both PVA and CHI begins close to 300 °C, but their degradation behavior is different. Due to the much higher amount of PVA, the degradation peaks mainly represent the endothermic decomposition of PVA chains through scission reactions (Tanpichai and Oksman 2016; An, Beh, and Xiao 2014). The increase in degradation temperature of PVA/0.5CHI/Gr (276 °C) compared to PVA/0.1CHI/Gr (272 °C) agrees with the literature (Guo et al. 2011) and can be ascribed to the influence of chitosan. The thermal degradation of chitosan occurs via free radical-induced cross-linking of the chains and the destruction of amino groups (Koosha and Mirzadeh 2015; Zawadzki and Kaczmarek 2010). Depolymerization of the CHI chains continues up to 400 C through dehydration, deamination, and destruction of pyranose rings (Zawadzki and Kaczmarek 2010), also seen as slight peaks and shoulders at higher temperatures. The onset of degradation is clearly shifted toward higher temperatures in both 3.9Ag/PVA/0.1CHI/Gr (282 °C) and 3.9Ag/PVA/0.5CHI/Gr (293 °C) hydrogels, indicating that the thermal stability is improved with the addition of AgNPs. A higher peak area for 3.9Ag/PVA/0.5CHI/Gr could be due to additional breakage of coordination bonds between AgNPs and polymer functional groups. Finally, at temperatures higher than 400 °C, the DSC curves exhibited mainly stable baselines, with few changes, indicating a thermally stable graphene-containing residue. At even higher temperatures, there is the possibility of some thermal oxidation of the residual graphene structure.

2.1.6.4 Swelling

The swelling of hydrophilic polymer gels is a complex process, especially in the case of polymers containing ionizable functional groups, such as amino groups on chitosan chain. The process of swelling is generally understood to take place via the formation of a moving front, with a sharp boundary between the solvated region (i.e., the swollen hydrogel phase) and the unsolvated polymer chains. Initially, the concentration gradient of the swelling medium governs the swelling, as the dynamic sorption takes place by the mass transport of the solvent into the unsolvated region, moving the mentioned boundary inwards. Inside the swollen region, the disassociation of hydrogen bonds occurs, and just before the moving front, the presence of swelling medium causes the plasticizing of polymer chains, thus initiating the relaxation of polymer chains (Yao et al. 1994). This complex mechanism of gel swelling is thus governed by the three main processes – initial fast uptake of the medium through the pores of the gel, followed by longer, diffusion-controlled period of solvent penetration due to the concentration gradient inside the gel, and the last, usually short, phase where increase in swelling is achieved due to the polymer chain relaxation (Xiaomin Yang et al. 2008).

It was shown that the equilibrium swelling degree, q_{eq}, for PVA/0.5CHI/Gr (212 ± 14 %) was higher than for PVA/0.1CHI/Gr (182 ± 33 %) (Nešović et al. 2018), indicating higher uptake capability of hydrogels with higher CHI content. This is a consequence of larger number of -OH and -NH_2 groups on the CHI chain capable of hydrogen bonding. The hydrogen bonding of water molecules is much stronger with amino groups than with hydroxyl, which explains the higher water uptake capability of hydrogels with more chitosan. The presence of AgNPs slightly increased the swelling degree of 0.25Ag/PVA/0.1CHI/Gr hydrogel (187 ± 11 %), compared to

PVA/0.1CHI/Gr hydrogel (182 ± 33 %), as the AgNPs could contribute to the stretching of polymer network and increase in the bound water content. On the other hand, the equilibrium swelling degree of 0.25Ag/PVA/0.5CHI/Gr hydrogel (199 ± 16 %) decreased compared to PVA/0.5CHI/Gr hydrogel (212 ± 14 %). As hypothesized earlier, the AgNPs are stabilized in the hydrogel matrix by forming coordination bonds with side groups on polymer chains and interactions with $-NH_2$ groups of chitosan, which are especially strong and actively contribute to the immobilization of AgNPs inside the hydrogel. Consequently, for the hydrogel with higher CHI content, it is assumed more interactions of AgNPs and $-NH_2$, which would prevent the amino groups from taking part in hydrogen bonding with water molecules and subsequently cause a decrease in the swelling degree. Moreover, the 0.25Ag/PVA/0.5CHI/Gr hydrogel contains higher concentration of AgNPs than the 0.25Ag/PVA/0.1CHI/Gr, which explains the stronger effect of AgNPs on the swelling behavior of 0.25Ag/PVA/0.5CHI/Gr hydrogel. However, upon statistical analysis for the equilibrium swelling degree data, none of the differences have proved to be statistically significant ($p>0.05$).

The diffusion coefficients determined from the ETA (D_{ETA}), LTA (D_{LTA}) and Etters (D) models are presented in Table 2.7. All the diffusion coefficients of PB swelling medium through the hydrogel matrices were of the order of 10^{-8}. Generally, the D_{ETA} had the lowest and D_{LTA} the highest values, while D was always between these two values for all the samples. This means that the ETA model underestimates, while the LTA slightly overestimates the value of diffusion coefficient with regard to the Etters model, which provides the best fit for the entire time period. The highest values of Etters diffusion coefficient, D, were observed for PVA/0.1CHI/Gr (3.12×10^{-8} cm^2 s^{-1}) and PVA/0.5CHI/Gr (3.53×10^{-8} cm^2 s^{-1}) and the lowest for 3.9Ag/PVA/0.1CHI/Gr (0.940×10^{-8} cm^2 s^{-1}) and 3.9Ag/PVA/0.5CHI/Gr (0.983×10^{-8} cm^2 s^{-1}), indicating that the hydrogels without the AgNPs exhibit the higher swelling rate and

TABLE 2.7
Diffusion Coefficients of the Swelling Medium, Calculated from Different Sorption Models, for PVA/0.1CHI/Gr, PVA/0.5CHI/Gr, 0.25Ag/PVA/0.1CHI/Gr, 0.25Ag/PVA/0.5CHI/Gr, 3.9Ag/PVA/0.1CHI/Gr and 3.9Ag/PVA/0.5CHI/Gr Hydrogels (Reprinted from (Nešović, Janković, Perić-Grujić et al. 2019) with Permission of Elsevier)

Hydrogel	D_{ETA} /10^{-8} cm^2 s^{-1} (ETA)	D_{LTA} /10^{-8} cm^2 s^{-1} (LTA)	D /10^{-8} cm^2 s^{-1} (Etters)
PVA/0.1CHI/Gr	1.87	3.62	3.12
PVA/0.5CHI/Gr	2.40	4.65	3.53
0.25Ag/PVA/0.1CHI/Gr	1.41	2.39	1.74
0.25Ag/PVA/0.5CHI/Gr	2.22	3.70	2.36
3.9Ag/PVA/0.1CHI/Gr	0.610	1.04	0.940
3.9Ag/PVA/0.5CHI/Gr	0.876	1.50	0.983

reach the equilibrium faster, whereas the hydrogels with AgNPs have a slower swelling rate, but their equilibrium swelling degree is higher (273 ± 40 % and 261 ± 21 % for 3.9Ag/PVA/0.1CHI/Gr and 3.9Ag/PVA/0.5CHI/Gr, respectively, in comparison with 182 ± 33 % and 212 ± 14 % for PVA/0.1CHI/Gr and PVA/0.5CHI/Gr, respectively (Nešović et al. 2018)).

2.1.6.5 Cytotoxicity and Antibacterial Activity

The MTT test was done on PVA/0.1CHI/Gr, PVA/0.5CHI/Gr, 0.25Ag/PVA/0.1CHI/Gr, and 0.25Ag/PVA/0.5CHI/Gr prepared from 0.25 mM $AgNO_3$ swelling solutions. According to the cytotoxicity scale, there is no evidence of toxicity for any of the samples (Figure 2.24a). MTT assays even showed that PVA/0.1CHI/Gr, PVA/0.5CHI/Gr, and 0.25Ag/PVA/0.1CHI/Gr samples promote differentiation and growth of MRC-5 (human fibroblasts), as evidenced by cell viability values higher than 100%, and the 0.25Ag/PVA/0.1CHI/Gr sample exhibits a statistically significant increase in cell viability ($p < 0.05$). The MRC-5 exhibits slightly decreased viability in the presence of 0.25Ag/PVA/0.5CHI/Gr. However, in the case of L929 cells, the viability is clearly decreased for all samples in comparison with PVA/0.1CHI/Gr due to the enhanced sensitivity of the mice cell line toward hydrogels.

Figures 2.24b and c represent the quantification of surviving bacterial cells in the presence of PVA/0.1CHI/Gr, PVA/0.5CHI/Gr, 0.25Ag/PVA/0.1CHI/Gr, and 0.25Ag/PVA/0.5CHI/Gr hydrogels. A visible reduction of the cell number occurred even after 15 minutes of incubation, especially in the case of 0.25Ag/PVA/0.5CHI/Gr sample. After 1 hour, 0.25Ag/PVA/0.1CHI/Gr and 0.25Ag/PVA/0.5CHI/Gr hydrogels caused complete reduction of bacterial cells for both *S. aureus* and *E. coli*. Against *S. aureus*, all the samples exhibited strong bactericidal activity even after 1 hour of incubation; however, the effect of PVA/0.1CHI/Gr and PVA/0.5CHI/Gr against *E. coli* was much less pronounced. The number of *E. coli* bacteria was progressively reduced, however, only after 24 hours PVA/0.5CHI/Gr caused ~5 logarithmic units reduction. Toward the end of monitoring, PVA/0.1CHI/Gr lost its antibacterial effect against *E. coli*, as observed by the slow bacterial growth (Figure 24b). Those results indicated that the hydrogels with higher CHI content possessed stronger antibacterial activity, and moreover, the 0.25Ag/PVA/0.5CHI/Gr hydrogels exhibited synergistic antibacterial effect of CHI and AgNPs. Based on the results obtained for a strong antibacterial activity of 0.25Ag/PVA/0.1CHI/Gr and 0.25Ag/PVA/0.5CHI/Gr hydrogels, and considering the fact that they are non-cytotoxic toward both MRC-5 and L929 fibroblast cell lines, it can be concluded that the 0.25Ag/PVA/0.1CHI/Gr and 0.25Ag/PVA/0.5CHI/Gr hydrogels are potentially good materials for topical wound dressing applications.

2.1.6.6 Silver Release

The experimental silver release profiles of hydrogels with 0.25 mM $AgNO_3$ were fitted with Makoid-Banakar, Korsmeyer-Peppas, and Kopcha models (Figure 2.25) described by equations (2.12), (2.13), and (2.14), while Table 2.8 presents the values of parameters obtained by these fits. According to the Korsmeyer-Peppas model, the values of exponent n were calculated to be 0.313 and 0.380 for 0.25Ag/PVA/0.1CHI/

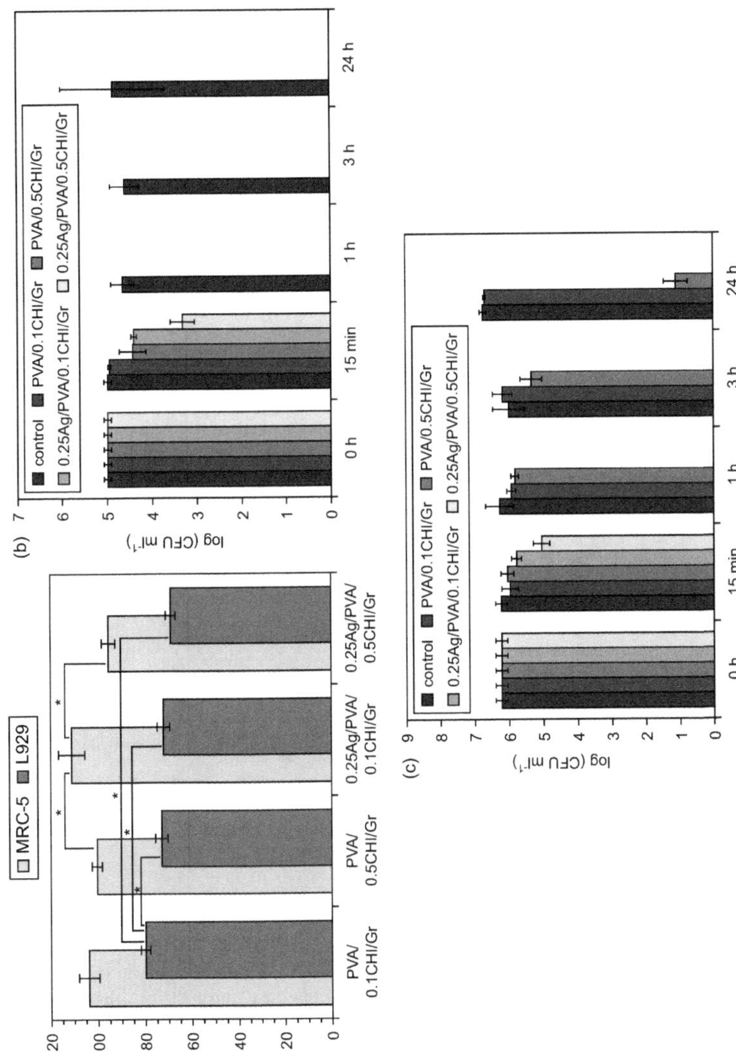

FIGURE 2.24 (a) Average viability of MRC-5 and L929 cell cultures (* - $p < 0.05$) (reprinted from Nešović et al. 2018 with permission from Elsevier), and reduction of viable cells of (b) *S. aureus* and (c) *E. coli* before and after incubation in PB at 37 °C with PVA/0.1CHI/Gr, PVA/0.5CHI/Gr, 0.25Ag/PVA/0.1CHI/Gr, and 0.25Ag/PVA/0.5CHI/Gr hydrogels (reprinted from Nešović, Janković, Perić-Grujić et al. 2019 with permission from Elsevier)

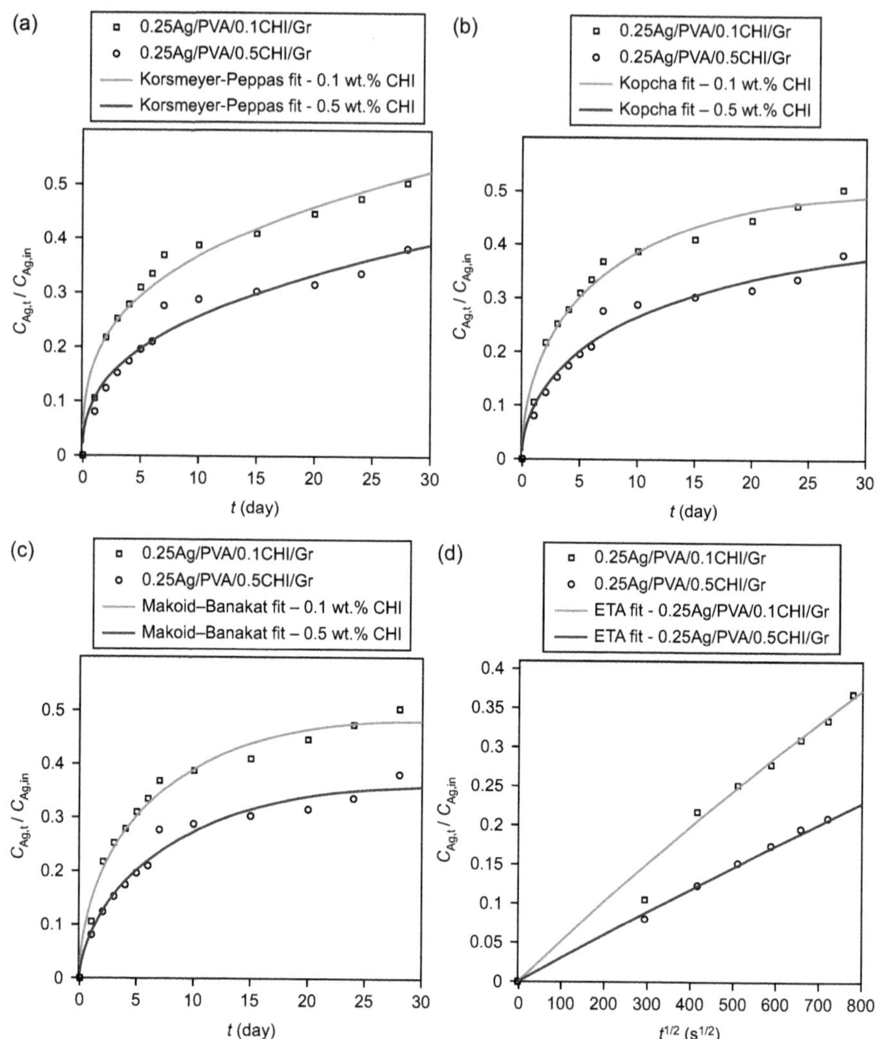

FIGURE 2.25 Release profiles from 0.25Ag/PVA/0.1CHI/Gr and 0.25Ag/PVA/0.5CHI/Gr hydrogels; (a) Korsmeyer-Peppas, (b) Kopcha, (c) Makoid-Banakar, and (d) ETA models of silver release from 0.25Ag/PVA/0.1CHI/Gr and 0.25Ag/PVA/0.5CHI/Gr hydrogels. Release conditions: 37 °C in PB (pH 7.42), 28 days (reprinted from Nešović et al. 2018 with permission from Elsevier)

Gr and 0.25Ag/PVA/0.5CHI/Gr, respectively. As the value of this parameter indicates transport mechanism of active substance, and for both samples $n < 0.5$, it was confirmed that the release of silver from PVA/CHI/Gr hydrogel matrices follows Fick's diffusion law, i.e., it is influenced by the concentration gradient of Ag^{+} ions in the polymer matrix. This conclusion is supported by the fact that the ratio of

TABLE 2.8
Fitting Parameters of Silver Release Profiles from 0.25Ag/PVA/0.1CHI/Gr and 0.25Ag/PVA/0.5CHI/Gr Hydrogels, Models Korsmeyer-Peppas, Kopcha, and Makoid-Banakar (Reprinted from Nešović et al. 2018 with Permission from Elsevier)

Hydrogel	Korsmeyer-Peppas			Kopcha		
	k_{KP} ($^{-n}$)	n	R^2	A ($s^{-1/2}$)	B (s^{-1})	R^2
0.25Ag/PVA/0.1CHI/Gr	0.176	0.313	0.968	0.167	-0.0142	0.983
0.25Ag/PVA/0.5CHI/Gr	0.107	0.380	0.962	0.106	-0.00685	0.972
	Makoid-Banakar					
	c	n	k_{MB} (s^{-n})	R^2		
0.25Ag/PVA/0.1CHI/Gr	0.0163	0.487	0.150	0.983		
0.25Ag/PVA/0.5CHI/Gr	0.0178	0.569	0.0882	0.975		

Kopcha parameters is A > |B|, which points to greater influence of diffusion processes on the silver release, compared to the polymer network relaxation effects, as well as by the values of exponent n in the Makoid-Banakar model, which are always close to 0.5, indicating diffusion-controlled release. The parameter c of the Makoid-Banakar model was close to zero for both samples, which is in agreement with the Korsmeyer-Peppas model, as when c → 0, the Makoid-Banakar model equates to Korsmeyer-Peppas. Thus, it can be considered that AgNPs are released from both 0.25Ag/PVA/0.1CHI/Gr and 0.25Ag/PVA/0.5CHI/Gr polymer matrix via a diffusion-controlled mechanism, with mass transport in compliance with Fick's law of diffusion.

The diffusion coefficient of Ag^+ ions from the polymer matrix was determined by modified ETA (Eq. 2.11), which is valid for shorter times in the initial 60 % of release. The ETA fits for 0.25Ag/PVA/0.1CHI/Gr and 0.25Ag/PVA/0.5CHI/Gr hydrogels are presented in Figure 2.25d. The average diffusion coefficient of silver, D_{Ag}, for 0.25Ag/PVA/0.5CHI/Gr (1.22 x 10^{-9} cm^2 s^{-1}) is smaller than for 0.25Ag/PVA/0.1CHI/Gr (3.63 x10^{-9} cm^2 s^{-1}), proving slower release from hydrogel with higher CHI content. This is due to the higher stability and stronger bonding of AgNPs in hydrogels with -OH and -NH_2 groups in chitosan chains, as shown by UV and Raman analyses.

2.1.6.7 *In Vivo* Studies

Sterilized Ag/PVA, Ag/PVA/Gr, Ag/PVA/CHI, and Ag/PVA/CHI/Gr hydrogel disks, as well as commercial Suprasorb©, a calcium-alginate dressing (Lohmann & Rauscher GmbH & Co. KG, Neuwied, Germany), were implanted in subcutaneous tissues of 16 anesthetized adult female rats. A small skin incision on the rat back, at the level of the midline of the thoracic spinal column, was made to create five pockets in the subcutis of back lateral sides, which was 3 cm distanced from back midline. The implants were introduced through pockets. Surgical incision made on the right lateral side opposite of the Suprasorb© implantation as a control area. The experiment lasted 60 days. Surgical implantation of hydrogels was done according to the permeation of the Ethical Committee of the Faculty of Veterinary Medicine, University of Belgrade (Lužajić Božinovski et al. 2018).

To estimate the processes of tissue response, regeneration and the tissue-implant interface, the obtained slides were examined semiquantitatively by histological reactions: epithelial alterations, relative number of inflammatory cells, vascular congestion, edema and connective tissue capsule thickness. These parameters were presented as the tissue irritation index (TIrI) score, according to the ISO 10993-6, 2007. The TIrI values of 1 to 5, 6 to 10, 11 to 15, and 16 to 20 indicates minimal, mild, moderate, and severe tissue responses, respectively. Morphometric methods included the counting of number of inflammatory cells per mm^2 of peri-implanted area and measuring the capsule thickness. The time dependences of TIrI score, leukocyte number around the implanted materials, and connective tissue capsule thickness for subcutaneously implanted Ag/PVA, Ag/PVA/Gr, Ag/PVA/CHI, Ag/PVA/CHI/Gr hydrogels, and Suprasorb©, as well as pseudooperated regions (incision skin) is shown in Figures 2.26a, b, and c, respectively.

The results of study *in vivo* biocompatibility of novel PVA-based hydrogels with AgNPs have shown that TIrI scores, leukocyte number around the implanted materials, and capsule thickness were gradually decreased during the 60 days follow-up. At the endpoint of follow-up, Ag/PVA/CHI/Gr implant was surrounded with a thinner capsule, while the both TIrI score and number of leukocytes of periimplant zone were greater compared to Ag/PVA/Gr implant. Despite the observed differences, it can be considered that novel hydrogels were biocompatible and potentially suitable for medical use.

2.2 HYDROGELS WITH GENTAMICIN AIMED FOR WOUND DRESSINGS AND SOFT TISSUE IMPLANTS

Simultaneous with the development of modern chemistry, pharmacy, and medicine, a significant increase in treating soft and hard tissues, as well as bones and joints diseases, injuries, and wounds, has been achieved. However, application of soft and hard tissue implants also brings a risk of infection by various microorganisms. Traditionally, antibiotics have been used to treat bacterial infections. The most common route for their application is oral administration. In the case of severe infections, antibiotics are usually administered intramuscularly or, more often, intravenously. The choice of antibacterial agent is an important one, and different antibiotics are often used. However, prolonged systemic application of antibiotics may lead to an increase in their side and toxic effects as well as development of resistance. Today, a large area of interest in nanomedicine is the application of antibiotics-loaded soft tissue implants, wound dressings, or hard tissue implants. Many advantages accrue from their application since they can significantly reduce side and toxic effects of

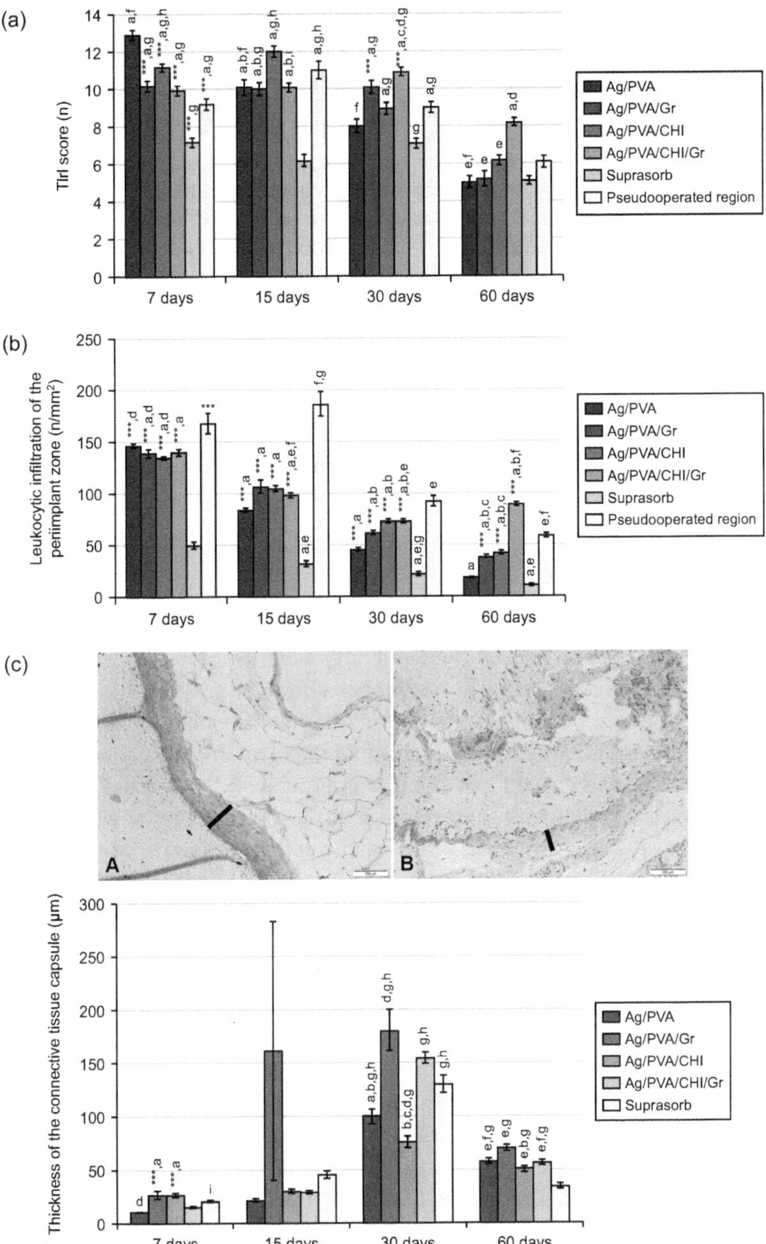

FIGURE 2.26 Time dependences of: (a) TIrI score and control area of skin incision. Legend: ***p < 0.001 relative to Ag/PVA; a - p < 0.001 relative to Suprasorb; b - p < 0.01 relative to Ag/PVA/CHI; c - p < 0.001 relative to Ag/PVA/CHI; d - p < 0.001 relative to Pseudooperated region; e - p < 0.001 relative to Ag/PVA/CHI/Gr; f - p < 0.001 relative to all other observed period; g - p < 0.001 relative to 60 days; h - p < 0.001 relative to 30 days; i - p < 0.01 relative to

FIGURE 2.26 CONTINUED 60 days; (b) leukocytic infiltration of the periimplant zone and control area of skin incision. Legend: ***$p < 0.001$ relative to Suprasorb; a - $p < 0.001$ relative to pseudooperated region; b - $p < 0.001$ relative to Ag/PVA; c - $p < 0.001$ relative to Ag/PVA/CHI/Gr; d - $p < 0.001$ relative to all other observed period; e - $p < 0.001$ relative to 7 days; f - $p < 0.001$ relative to 30 days; g - $p < 0.05$ relative to 60 days; (c) connective tissue capsule thickness around implanted A – Ag/PVA/Gr and B – AG/PVA/CHI/Gr hydrogels at postimplantation day 60, C – connective tissue capsule thickness for all implanted biomaterials. Legend: ***$p < 0.001$ relative to Ag/PVA; a - $p < 0.01$ relative to Ag/PVA/CHI/Gr; b - $p < 0.001$ relative to Ag/PVA/Gr; c - $p < 0.001$ relative to Ag/PVA/CHI/Gr; d - $p < 0.05$ relative to Suprasorb; e - $p < 0.001$ relative to Suprasorb; f - $p < 0.01$ relative to Ag/PVA/Gr; g - $p < 0.001$ relative to 7 days; h - $p < 0.001$ relative to 60 days; i - $p < 0.01$ relative to 60 days (reprinted from Lužajić Božinovski et al. 2018 with permission from the Faculty of Veterinary Medicine, University of Belgrade, Serbia)

incorporated antibiotics or bacteria resistance in comparison to systemic application of antibiotics.

2.2.1 Soft Tissue Infections

Human skin as a physical barrier serves as the first line of defense against microbial infection by secreting sebaceous fluid and fatty acids to inhibit growth of pathogens and by possessing its own normal flora, thus deterring colonization by other pathogenic organisms. However, human skin is an environment for many microbes. Infecting microorganisms may cause tissue damage and incite an inflammation process. Also, different skin and tissue damages break this protective barrier and enable activity of pathogens. The organisms characteristic of the skin above the waist are usually Gram-positive species such as *Staphylococcus epidermidis*, *Corynebacterium* species, *Staphylococcus aureus*, and *Streptococcus pyogenes* while both Gram-positive and Gram-negative species are microorganisms that inhabit the skin below the waist. The infection agents *Enterobacteriaceae* and *Enterococcus* species (enteric species) mainly colonize this area of the skin and they may originate from the colon and faeces (Jadranka Odović and Vesna Mišković Stanković 2023; Eron et al. 2003).

Different factors such as chronic diseases, age, or trauma as well as injuries of the soft tissue represent specific risk factors that may increase the growth of skin and soft tissue infections. Potential risk factors may be divided into two types. There are patient-related factors, including critical illness, elderly age, immunocompromised state, liver and kidney disease, and vascular (especially lymphatic or venous) insufficiency. Certain risk factors (chronic renal or liver failure, immunocompromised state, vascular insufficiency, or neuropathy) should be considered in the determination of disease severity. The second category is etiological risk factors. The mechanism of injury (trauma or others) or specific exposures to some infection agents can increase the incidence of skin and soft tissue infections. The overlap between risk different factors in this grouping can be noticed (Ki and Rotstein 2008). Many different risk factors and their bacterial causes are presented in Table 2.9, as well as antibiotics for different infection agents and degrees.

TABLE 2.9
Risk Elements for Soft Tissue Infections and Antimicrobial Agents for Skin and Soft Tissue Infections

Risk Element	**Pathogen**
Diabetes mellitus	*Staphylococcus aureus*, anaerobes, Gram-negative bacilli
Cat or dog bite wounds	*Pasteurella multocida, C canimorsus*
Rat bite wounds	*Streptobacillus moniliformis*

Infection	**Etiology**	**Antibiotic(s)**
Mild infections (above waist)	*Staphylococcus aureus* *Streptococcus pyogenes*	Cloxacillin, cephalexin, or clindamycin
Severe infections (above waist)	*Staphylococcus aureus* *Streptococcus pyogenes*	Cefazolin, cloxacillin, cephalexin
Mild infections (below waist)	*Staphylococcus aureus* *Streptococcus pyogenes*	Cloxacillin or cephalexin, clindamycin or metronidazole (anaerobes), second-generation cephalosporin or fluoroquinolone
Severe infections (below waist)	*Escherichia coli* *Enterococcus species* *Staphylococcus aureus* *Streptococcus pyogenes*	Second-, third- or fourth-generation cephalosporin, fluoroquinolones or piperacillin-tazobactam

However, prolonged antibiotic or exposure hospitalization promotes a risk for infections with resistant organisms. In the first place it can be *Methicillin-resistant Staphylococcus aureus* (MRSA) as well as *Pseudomonas aeruginosa*, *Enterococcus* species, *Streptococcus pyogenes*, or *Clostridium* species. In such cases, guidelines recommend second- or third-generation cephalosporin (mild to moderate), beta-lactam plus a fluoroquinolone or aminoglycoside with the addition of vancomycin if MRSA is suspected (Cohen and Kurzrock 2004). The infections caused by MRSA bacteria are especially challenging since it is resistant to a number of commonly used drugs. Antibiotics commonly recommended for treatment of MRSA infections are mupirocin, clindamycin, trimethoprim-sulfamethoxazole, doxycycline, cephalexin, amoxicillin, and vancomycin (Rajan 2012).

Different drugs can be locally administered through the skin due its possibility to absorb by application of adhesive transdermal patch or wound dressings. Application of antibiotics-loaded wound dressing can importantly improve soft tissue infections healing and today is of considerable interest in nanomedicine. The local antibiotics application reduces side, toxic effects or bacteria resistance on applied antibiotics. For soft tissue implants the most frequently used antibiotics according to the available literature are gentamicin, ciprofloxacin, clindamycin, ampicillin, tetracycline, and vancomycin. Hwang et al. (Hwang et al. 2010) investigated application of gentamicin in wound dressing. For that purpose, polyvinyl alcohol (PVA) and dextran were used for preparation of cross-linked hydrogel films by application of the freezing-thawing method. Two wound dressings with different compositions were prepared. The first was composed of PVA (2.5%), dextran (1.13%) with gentamicin (0.1%) addition, while no drug was added into the second wound dressings. The gentamicin-loaded wound dressing (rat model) enhanced the reepithelialization rate, which was higher for hydrogel with gentamicin (98±2%) then hydrogel without drug (91±2%). Also, hydrogels with gentamicin significantly decreased the possible granulation tissue area. Therefore, gentamicin-loaded wound dressing can be recommended as a potential wound dressing with improved healing effect in wound care. Another material with natural characteristics suitable for applications in wound dressing, chitosan (CHI) and nanofiber mesh (NFM), was proposed by Monteiro et al. (Monteiro et al. 2015). The gentamicin-loaded liposomes were immobilized at the surface of Ch/NFM. For *Staphylococcus aureus, Escherichia coli, and Pseudomonas aeruginosa* reduction was more than 99.9%. The bactericidal activity of released gentamicin and developed system has promising performance for wound dressing applications, avoiding infections caused by these common pathogens. The new hydrogels with gentamicin addition for infected wound treatment were proposed by Pãunicã-Panea et al. (Păunică-Panea et al. 2015). Two proteins, fibrous, type I collagen and globula, albumin, were the main components of proposed hydrogels. The hydrogels provided good antimicrobial properties for a maximum of 20% albumin and 0.2% gentamicin. Further, improved topical hydrogels were produced using three commercial polymeric agents with addition of gentamicin (0.03, 0.06, and .09 w/w) in order to achieve predictable permeation of gentamicin in skin. The gentamicin-loaded hydrogels with a higher percentage of drug offered better permeation and possible treatment of skin infections caused by gentamicin-susceptible bacteria (Nnamani et al. 2013). Lukáč et al. (Lukáč et al. 2019) proposed a novel collagen wound dressing sponge prepared from freshwater fish (*Cyprinus Carpio*) skin collagen type I. Half of the sponges were cross-linked with carbodiimide. Both cross-linked and non-cross-linked collagen sponges were impregnated with gentamicin. The sponges were tested through a rat model for activity on *Pseudomonas aeruginosa* infected wound and compared with a reference commercial product. The obtained results indicate that gentamicin released from the sponges had good clinical properties and was active against investigated infective agents. Fibers composed of poly(lactic acid) (PLA), poly(ε-caprolactone) (PCL), and the copolymer poly(D,L,lactic-co-glycolide) (PLGA, L/G 50:50, ester terminated) as materials for immobilization of the antibiotic gentamicin sulfate (in concentration of 10% of the polymer weight) have been produced by an electrospinning method. The antibacterial activity of the gentamicin sulfate-loaded fibers was proved against *Staphylococcus aureus* (Coimbra et al. 2019).

Puoci et al. (Puoci et al. 2012) proposed application of ciprofloxacin-collagen conjugate (CFX-T1C) for successful wound healing with reducing side effects usually recorded in systematic patients' therapy. The antibacterial activity of CFX-T1C with the addition of gentamicin has been proved against *Staphylococcus aureus* and *Escherichia coli* at 37 °C. The bilayer dressing was prepared from succinylated collagen with incorporated ciprofloxacin in final concentration 0.2 mg/cm^2. *In vitro* investigation of ciprofloxacin-incorporating dressings antimicrobial properties made on agar plates inoculated with a mixed culture of *Staphylococcus aureus* and *Pseudomonas aeruginosa* showed an important zone of inhibition. *In vivo* investigations of prepared ciprofloxacin-loaded wound dressing showed significant higher wound closure and confirmed possibility of its application in proper wound healing (Sripriya et al. 2007). Roy et al. (Roy et al. 2014) investigated ciprofloxacin-loaded keratose hydrogels using a porcine wound model, infected with *Pseudomonas aeruginosa*. Prepared hydrogels contained from 0 to 20 mg/mL of ciprofloxacin. *In vivo* investigations (pig model) were performed to determine if ciprofloxacin-loaded keratose hydrogels inhibit *Pseudomonas aeruginosa*. Treatment with keratose hydrogels loaded with 5 mg/mL or 10 mg/mL ciprofloxacin significantly reduced the amount of *Pseudomonas aeruginosa* in the wound by > 99.9% and displayed wound contraction and reepithelialization.

The poly(vinyl alcohol) and sodium alginate (SA) were used to develop clindamycin wound dressing (J. O. Kim et al. 2008). The hydrogel films were prepared using the freeze-thawing method from solutions consisting of different proportions of poly(vinyl alcohol) and sodium alginate and 3%w/v clindamycin. The healing effect of prepared hydrogels was investigated on male rats. Their wounds infected with *Pseudomonas aeruginosa* were covered with PVA/SA wound dressings containing antibiotic clindamycin. Hydrogel with clindamycin led to a significant decrease of inflammation and inflammatory cells in wound. The obtained results could recommend application of clindamycin-loaded wound dressing for efficient hilling of wounds infected with *Pseudomonas aeruginosa*. The polymeric nanofiber patch for topical treatment were prepared using several different concentrations of poly(vinyl alcohol) and tamarind seed gum with clindamycin (in concentration 1.0% to 2.5%) as antibacterial agent. The antimicrobial activity of the drug-loaded poly(vinyl alcohol)/gum polymeric nanofiber patch was evaluated against *Staphylococcus aureus* and *Propionibacterium* and compared to that of a commercially available clindamycin gel for acne treatment. The antibacterial activities of the clindamycin-loaded wound dressing were significantly higher in comparison to commercial 1% clindamycin gel, indicating that the investigated clindamycin-loaded wound dressing has good antibacterial activity and can be applied as wound dressings in acne healing (Sangnim et al. 2018).

Ampicillin-loaded wound dressing was prepared from hydrophobic polyurethane and hydrophilic ampicillin, which were mixed together in the same solvent and electrospun into a fibrous scaffold (Sabitha and Rajiv 2015). The various ratios of ampicillin: polyurethane were prepared (1:10 wt.%, 1.5:10 wt.%, 2:10 wt.%). *In vitro* study of cytotoxicity of the examined nanofibrous scaffolds was performed with human keratinocyte showing that prepared scaffolds can be used as an appropriate biocompatible wound dressing material. Ampicillin polyurethane fibers exhibited antibacterial activity against *Staphylococcus aureus* and *Klebsiella pneumonia*.

For preparation, tetracycline-loaded wound dressing poly(vinyl alcohol) and chitosan were used with the addition of tetracycline hydrochloride to the polymer solution before the electrospinning process. The 5 mg/mL of tetracycline were mixed to the polymer solution, which correspond to 5% of the polymer weight in the nanofibers (Alavarse et al. 2017). Antibacterial activity was proved against *Escherichia coli*, *Staphylococci epidermidis*, and *Staphylococcus aureus*.

Vancomycin-loaded wound dressings were prepared by application of alginate or gelatin/alginate hydrogel with the addition of vancomycin in a concentration 10 mg per gram of the dried gel. The strong antimicrobial activity against various *Staphylococcus* and *Streptococcus* bacteria was obtained (Kurczewska et al. 2015).

2.2.2 Polyvinyl Alcohol-Based Hydrogels with Gentamicin

2.2.2.1 Synthesis and Characterization

The PVA/Gent hydrogel was prepared by physical cross-linking of poly (vinyl alcohol) dispersion (10 wt.% PVA) using the freezing-thawing method in five cycles. One cycle consisted of freezing for 16 hours at 18 °C, followed by thawing for 8 hours at 4 °C. Then, the hydrogel was swollen in 5.0 mg/ml gentamicin solution at 37 C° for 48 hours (Miskovic-Stankovic, Janev, and Atanackovic 2023). The PVA/CHI/Gent hydrogel was prepared by the physical cross-linking of poly(vinyl alcohol)/chitosan dispersion (10 wt.% PVA and 0.5 wt.% CHI) using the freezing-thawing method and then was swollen in 5.0 mg/ml gentamicin solution at 37°C for 48 hours (Miskovic-Stankovic and Atanackovic 2023).

FE-SEM microphotographs (Figures 2.27a and b) revealed hydrogels porosity (Mišković-Stanković et al. 2024) as a desirable property of biomaterials that allows better incorporation of antimicrobial and antibacterial agents (Greene et al. 2023; Fathollahipour et al. 2020) along with the ability to stabilize penetration of nutrients and oxygen (Hu et al. 2022; Ferreira et al. 2020). FT-IR spectra showed characteristics bands at 3250 cm^{-1} (O–H stretching), 2935 cm^{-1} (asymmetric CH_2 stretching), 2910 cm^{-1} (C–H symmetric stretching), 2850 cm^{-1} (C–H stretching in chitosan), 1650 cm^{-1} (C=O stretching), 1415 cm^{-1} (-OH in-plane coupling with C–H wagging in CH_2), 1375 cm^{-1} (–CH_2 wagging), 1142 cm^{-1} (symmetric C–O stretching), 1086 cm^{-1} (C–O stretching of secondary alcohols), 916 cm^{-1} (CH_2 rocking), 832 cm^{-1} (C–C stretching) indicating established bonds between PVA, CHI and gemtamicin (Figures 2.27c and d).

2.2.2.2 Biomechanical Properties

The results of a tensile test have been obtained from stress-strain curves for PVA, PVA/CHI, and PVA/CHI/Gent films, while tensile strength, σ , and modulus of elasticity, E are listed in Table 2.10. Instead of breaking strain, the strain corresponding to tensile strength (maximum of curve, when geometrical weakening of material starts), ε_{m}, is presented in Table 2.10.

It can be seen that the tensile strength of PVA/CHI film increased by 13.1%, from 47.25 to 53.43 MPa, Young's modulus by 18.0%, from 1880.87 to 2223.67 MPa, and elongation ε_{m} by 83.1%, from 7.27 to 13.31%, compared to pure PVA films. This improvement of mechanical properties is due to the strong physical interactions and establishment of hydrogen bonds between PVA and CHI molecules (Chopra et al. 2022; Olewnik-Kruszkowska et al. 2019). By comparing the mechanical properties of the PVA/CHI and PVA/CHI/Gent hydrogels, a decrease in tensile strength with the addition of gentamicin is observed by 46.4%, from 53.43 to 36.50 MPa, Young's

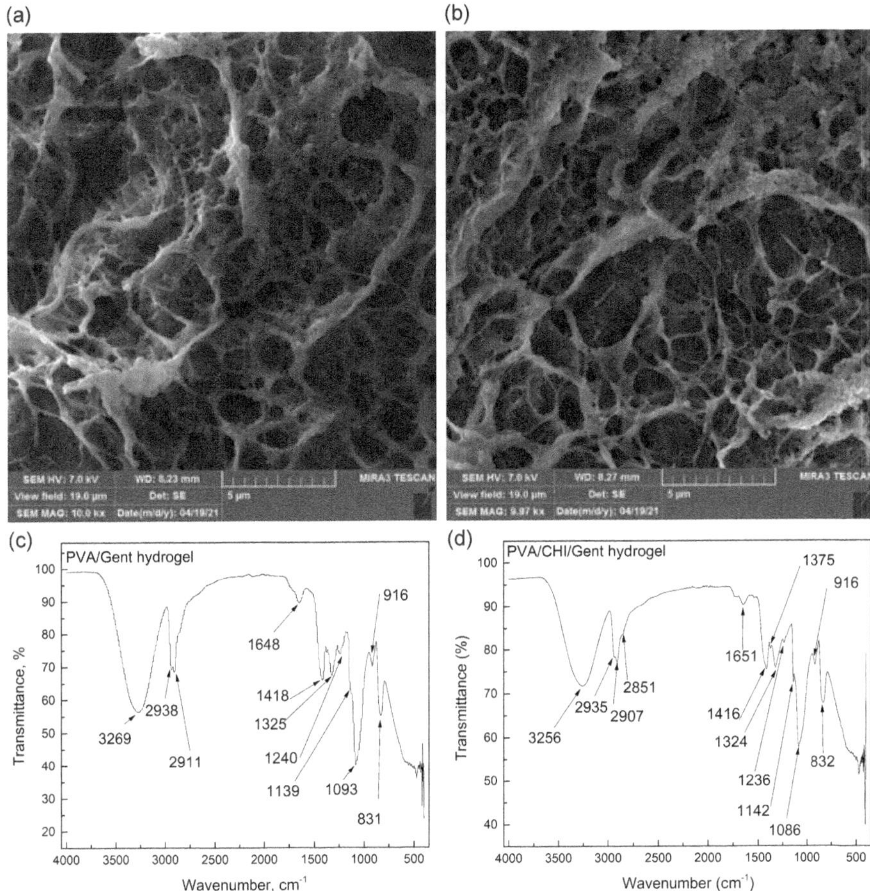

FIGURE 2.27 FE-SEM micrographs (a), (b) and FT-IR spectra (c), (d) of PVA/Gent and PVA/CHI/Gent hydrogels, respectively (reprinted from Mišković-Stanković et al. 2024 with permission from the Serbian Chemical Society)

modulus of elasticity by 13% , from 2223.67 to 1969.73 MPa, and ε_m even five times, which means that the addition of gentamicin leads to an increase in the brittleness of the films.

2.2.2.3 Cytotoxicity and Antibacterial Activity

Cytotoxicity against MRC-5 and l929 cells was determined using MTT (Figure 2.28a). Based on cytotoxicity scale, it was confirmed that both PVA/Gent and PVA/CHI/Gent hydrogels are non-cytotoxic. Strong antibacterial activity against *Escherichia coli* (Figure 2.28b) and *Staphylococcus aureus* (Figure 2.28c) was observed for both hydrogels after 15 minutes (Mišković-Stanković et al. 2024).

TABLE 2.10
Tensile Strength, σ, Modulus of Elasticity, *E*, and Tensile Strain in Maximum of Tensile Curve, ε_m (Adapted from Mišković-Stanković et al. 2024 with Permission from the Serbian Chemical Society)

Hydrogel	σ, MPa	E, MPa	ε_m, %
PVA	47.25	1886.87	7.27
PVA/CHI	53.43	2223.67	13.31
PVA/CHI/Gent	36.50	1969.73	2.61

2.2.2.4 Gentamicin Release

The concentration of released gentamicin from PVA/Gent and PVA/CHI/Gent hydrogels was determined using a high-performance liquid chromatography (HPLC) coupled with an ion trap as a mass spectrometer (MS), according to a procedure published earlier (Stevanović et al. 2021). Briefly, gentamicin release studies were carried out during a 14-day immersion in deionized water, at 37 °C, as a model system. All the measurements were done in triplicate. High-performance liquid chromatography (HPLC) was utilized for gentamicin components separation and the detection and quantitative analysis was done in an ion trap mass spectrometer (MS) with an electrospray ionizer. Methanol (A), deionized water (B), and 10 % acetic acid (C) comprised the mobile phase. The optimized HPLC and MS operating parameters (mobile-phase gradient, analytes' precursor ions, fragmentation reactions used for quantification, and optimal collision energies) for the determination of gentamicin compounds were published previously (Stevanović et al. 2020). The gentamicin mass spectra were collected in the *m/z* range of 50–1000. As expected, the MS spectrum revealed the three most abundant ions since gentamicin are composed of three compounds – gentamicin C1a, C2, and C1. These ions were further chosen as the precursor ions for each compound. Their most sensitive transitions were selected for quantification purposes. The presented gentamicin concentrations represent sums of the three determined gentamicin compounds.

The experimental cumulative gentamicin release profiles for PVA/Gent and PVA/CHI/Gent hydrogels are represented in Figure 2.29 as an average of three samples, where c_t is the concentration of released gentamicin after certain time t, $c_{gel,t}$ is the concentration of gentamicin remained in hydrogel after certain time, t, and c_0 is the initial concentration of gentamicin inside the hydrogel. Release profiles verified the initial burst release effect of gentamicin from the hydrogel (60% from PVA/Gent and 70% from PVA/CHI/Gent within first 48 hours), which could be very useful in preventing biofilm formation, followed by the slow release of gentamicin in a later time period. This behavior favors both application requirements; namely, for effective wound dressing with antibacterial properties, initial burst release can be favorable to quickly suppress the bacterial adhesion and biofilm formation in the wound environment, whereas sustained release over a longer period would ensure maintaining

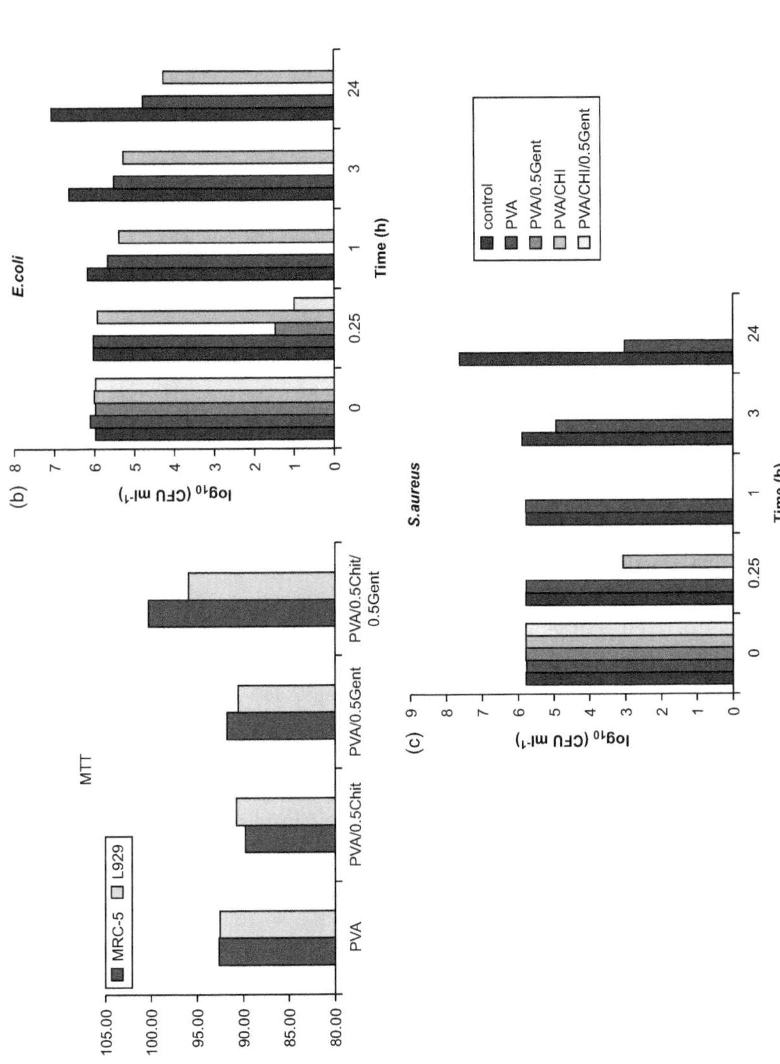

FIGURE 2.28 Cytotoxicity of PVA, PVA/Gent, PVA/CHI and PVA/CHI/Gent hydrogels (a) MTT test and antibacterial activity against (b) *Escherichia coli* and (c) *Staphylococcus aureus* (reprinted from Mišković-Stanković et al. 2024 with permission from the Serbian Chemical Society)

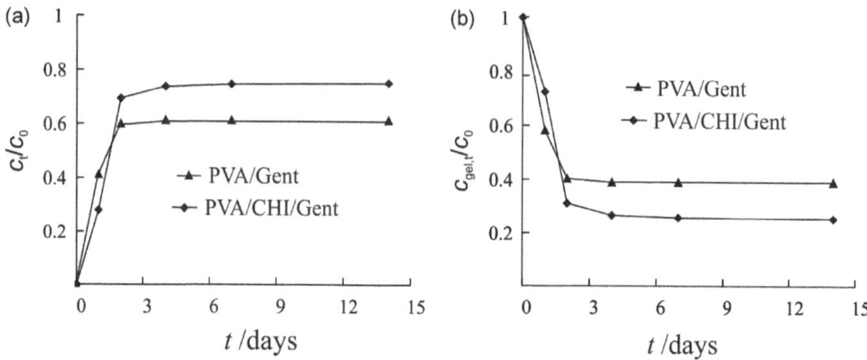

FIGURE 2.29 (a) Increase in concentration of released gentamicin, c_t, and (b) decrease in concentration of gentamicin remained in PVA/Gent and PVA/CHI/Gent hydrogel, $c_{gel,t}$, with time during 14 days in deionized water at 37 °C

the sterility of the wound and lowering of the dressing replacement frequency. This behavior is a consequence of gentamicin molecules entrapped in the cross-linked polymer matrix.

The gentamicin release profiles were fitted with the Korsmeyer-Peppas model described by Eq. 2.13. According to the Korsmeyer-Peppas model, exponent n had a mean value of 0.1030 and 0.2137 for PVA/Gent and PVA/CHI/Gent hydrogels, respectively. As the value of parameter n for both hydrogels was lower than 0.5, it pointed out that the release of gentamicin from both hydrogel matrices followed the Fick's diffusion law. Then, diffusion coefficients of gentamicin through the hydrogel network, *D*, were calculated using modified ETA (Eq. 2.11). The *D* value for PVA/CHI/Gent (4.29×10^{-8} cm^2 s^{-1}) was lower in comparison to PVA/Gent (7.16×10^{-8} cm^2 s^{-1}), meaning that the release of gentamicin is slower from the hydrogel with chitosan due to a greater number of bonds and consequently a more cross-linked polymer matrix. The detailed pharmacokinetics analysis of gentamicin release profiles using Makoid-Banakar, Korsmeyer-Peppas, and Kopcha models in comparison with the novel general fractional derivative (GFD) model is presented in Sections 4.4.1 and 4.4.2.

REFERENCES

Abdelgawad, Abdelrahman M, Samuel M Hudson, and Orlando J Rojas. 2014. "Antimicrobial Wound Dressing Nanofiber Mats from Multicomponent (Chitosan/Silver-NPs/Polyvinyl Alcohol) Systems." *Carbohydrate Polymers* 100: 166–78. https://doi.org/10.1016/j.carbpol.2012.12.043.

Abudabbus, MM, I Jevremović, A Janković, A Perić-Grujić, I Matić, M Vukašinović-Sekulić, D Hui, KY Rhee, and V Mišković-Stanković. 2016. "Biological Activity of Electrochemically Synthesized Silver Doped Polyvinyl Alcohol/Graphene Composite Hydrogel Discs for Biomedical Applications." *Composites Part B: Engineering* 104: 26–34. https://doi.org/10.1016/j.compositesb.2016.08.024.

Abudabbus, MM, Ivana Jevremović, Katarina Nešović, Aleksandra Perić-Grujić, Kyong Yop Rhee, and Vesna Mišković-Stanković. 2018. "In Situ Electrochemical Synthesis of Silver-Doped Poly(Vinyl Alcohol)/Graphene Composite Hydrogels and Their Physico-Chemical and Thermal Properties." *Composites Part B: Engineering* 140: 99–107. https://doi.org/10.1016/j.compositesb.2017.12.017.

Agnihotri, Shekhar, Soumyo Mukherji, and Suparna Mukherji. 2012. "Antimicrobial Chitosan–PVA Hydrogel as a Nanoreactor and Immobilizing Matrix for Silver Nanoparticles." *Applied Nanoscience* 2 (3): 179–88. https://doi.org/10.1007/s13204-012-0080-1.

Ahmad, AL, NM Yusuf, and BS Ooi. 2012. "Preparation and Modification of Poly (Vinyl) Alcohol Membrane: Effect of Crosslinking Time towards Its Morphology." *Desalination* 287: 35–40. https://doi.org/10.1016/j.desal.2011.12.003.

Alavarse, Alex Carvalho, Fernanda Waitman de Oliveira Silva, Jandir Telleria Colque, Viviam Moura da Silva, Tatiane Prieto, Everaldo Carlos Venancio, and Jean-Jacques Bonvent. 2017. "Tetracycline Hydrochloride-Loaded Electrospun Nanofibers Mats Based on PVA and Chitosan for Wound Dressing." *Materials Science and Engineering: C* 77: 271–81. https://doi.org/10.1016/j.msec.2017.03.199.

Alexandre, Nuno, Irina Amorim, Ana Rita Caseiro, Tiago Pereira, Rui Alvites, Alexandra Rêma, Ana Gonçalves, et al. 2017. "Long Term Performance Evaluation of Small-Diameter Vascular Grafts Based on Polyvinyl Alcohol Hydrogel and Dextran and MSCs-Based Therapies Using the Ovine Pre-Clinical Animal Model." *International Journal of Pharmaceutics* 523 (2): 515–30. https://doi.org/10.1016/j.ijpharm.2017.02.043.

Alipour, Reza, Alireza Khorshidi, Abdollah Fallah Shojaei, Farhad Mashayekhi, and Mohammad Javad Mehdipour Moghaddam. 2019. "Skin Wound Healing Acceleration by Ag Nanoparticles Embedded in PVA/PVP/Pectin/Mafenide Acetate Composite Nanofibers." *Polymer Testing* 79: 106022. https://doi.org/10.1016/j.polymertesting.2019.106022.

An, Qiaozhi, Catherine Beh, and Huining Xiao. 2014. "Preparation and Characterization of Thermo-Sensitive Poly(Vinyl Alcohol)-Based Hydrogel as Drug Carrier." *Journal of Applied Polymer Science* 131 (1). https://doi.org/10.1002/app.39720.

Anderson, JM, K Defife, A Mcnally, T Collier, and C Jenney. 1999. "Monocyte, Macrophage and Foreign Body Giant Cell Interactions with Molecularly Engineered Surfaces." *Journal of Materials Science: Materials in Medicine* 10 (10): 579–88. https://doi.org/10.1023/A:1008976531592.

Anderson, James M, Analiz Rodriguez, and David T Chang. 2008. "Foreign Body Reaction to Biomaterials." *Seminars in Immunology* 20 (2): 86–100. https://doi.org/10.1016/j.smim.2007.11.004.

Angelescu, Daniel G, Marilena Vasilescu, Raluca Somoghi, Dan Donescu, and Valentin S Teodorescu. 2010. "Kinetics and Optical Properties of the Silver Nanoparticles in Aqueous L64 Block Copolymer Solutions." *Colloids and Surfaces A: Physicochemical and Engineering Aspects* 366 (1): 155–62. https://doi.org/10.1016/j.colsurfa.2010.06.001.

Augustine, Robin, Anwarul Hasan, VK Yadu Nath, Jince Thomas, Anitha Augustine, Nandakumar Kalarikkal, Ala-Eddin Al Moustafa, and Sabu Thomas. 2018. "Electrospun Polyvinyl Alcohol Membranes Incorporated with Green Synthesized Silver Nanoparticles for Wound Dressing Applications." *Journal of Materials Science: Materials in Medicine* 29 (11): 163. https://doi.org/10.1007/s10856-018-6169-7.

Bajpai, SK, Navin Chand, and Manika Mahendra. 2013. "In Situ Formation of Silver Nanoparticles in Poly(Methacrylic Acid) Hydrogel for Antibacterial Applications." *Polymer Engineering & Science* 53 (8): 1751–59. https://doi.org/10.1002/pen.23424.

Baker, Maribel I, Steven P Walsh, Zvi Schwartz, and Barbara D Boyan. 2012. "A Review of Polyvinyl Alcohol and Its Uses in Cartilage and Orthopedic Applications." *Journal of Biomedical Materials Research Part B: Applied Biomaterials* 100B (5): 1451–57. https://doi.org/10.1002/jbm.b.32694.

Bal, A, FE Çepni, Ö Çakir, I Acar, and G Güçlü. 2015. "Synthesis and Characterization of Copolymeric and Terpolymeric Hydrogel-Silver Nanocomposites Based on Acrylic Acid, Acrylamide and Itaconic Acid: Investigation of Their Antibacterial Activity Against Gram-Negative Bacteria." *Brazilian Journal of Chemical Engineering* 32 (2): 509–18. https://doi.org/10.1590/0104-6632.20150322s00003066.

Banerjee, Madhuchanda, Sadhucharan Mallick, Anumita Paul, Arun Chattopadhyay, and Siddhartha Sankar Ghosh. 2010. "Heightened Reactive Oxygen Species Generation in the Antimicrobial Activity of a Three Component Iodinated Chitosan–Silver Nanoparticle Composite." *Langmuir* 26 (8): 5901–8. https://doi.org/10.1021/la9038528.

Bhowmick, Sirsendu, and Veena Koul. 2016. "Assessment of PVA/Silver Nanocomposite Hydrogel Patch as Antimicrobial Dressing Scaffold: Synthesis, Characterization and Biological Evaluation." *Materials Science and Engineering: C* 59: 109–19. https://doi.org/10.1016/j.msec.2015.10.003.

Bianchera, Annalisa, Ovidio Catanzano, Joshua Boateng, and Lisa Elviri. 2020. "The Place of Biomaterials in Wound Healing." In *Therapeutic Dressings and Wound Healing Applications*, 337–66. https://doi.org/10.1002/9781119433316.ch15.

Biswas, Dhee P, Neil M O'Brien-Simpson, Eric C Reynolds, Andrea J O'Connor, and Phong A Tran. 2018. "Comparative Study of Novel in Situ Decorated Porous Chitosan-Selenium Scaffolds and Porous Chitosan-Silver Scaffolds towards Antimicrobial Wound Dressing Application." *Journal of Colloid and Interface Science* 515: 78–91. https://doi.org/10.1016/j.jcis.2018.01.007.

Blair, Jessica MA, Mark A Webber, Alison J Baylay, David O Ogbolu, and Laura JV Piddock. 2015. "Molecular Mechanisms of Antibiotic Resistance." *Nature Reviews Microbiology* 13 (1): 42–51. https://doi.org/10.1038/nrmicro3380.

Boateng, Joshua S, Kerr H Matthews, Howard NE Stevens, and Gillian M Eccleston. 2008. "Wound Healing Dressings and Drug Delivery Systems: A Review." *Journal of Pharmaceutical Sciences* 97 (8): 2892–923. https://doi.org/10.1002/jps.21210.

Bon, Silvia Bittolo, Luca Valentini, Raquel Verdejo, Jose L Garcia Fierro, Laura Peponi, Miguel A Lopez-Manchado, and Jose M Kenny. 2009. "Plasma Fluorination of Chemically Derived Graphene Sheets and Subsequent Modification With Butylamine." *Chemistry of Materials* 21 (14): 3433–38. https://doi.org/10.1021/cm901039j.

Broussard, Karen C, and Jennifer Gloeckner Powers. 2013. "Wound Dressings: Selecting the Most Appropriate Type." *American Journal of Clinical Dermatology* 14 (6): 449–59. https://doi.org/10.1007/s40257-013-0046-4.

Bryaskova, Rayna, Daniela Pencheva, Girish M Kale, Umesh Lad, and T Kantardjiev. 2010. "Synthesis, Characterisation and Antibacterial Activity of PVA/TEOS/Ag-Np Hybrid Thin Films." *Journal of Colloid and Interface Science* 349 (1): 77–85. https://doi.org/10.1016/j.jcis.2010.04.091.

Bugarski, Branko, Qiangliang Li, Mattheus FA Goosen, Denis Poncelet, Ronald J Neufeld, and Gordana Vunjak. 1994. "Electrostatic Droplet Generation: Mechanism of Polymer Droplet Formation." *AIChE Journal* 40 (6): 1026–31. https://doi.org/10.1002/aic.690400613.

Caló, Enrica, and Vitaliy V Khutoryanskiy. 2015. "Biomedical Applications of Hydrogels: A Review of Patents and Commercial Products." *European Polymer Journal* 65: 252–67. https://doi.org/10.1016/j.eurpolymj.2014.11.024.

Chen, Hao, Ruoyu Cheng, Xin Zhao, Yuhui Zhang, Allison Tam, Yufei Yan, Haokai Shen, et al. 2019. "An Injectable Self-Healing Coordinative Hydrogel with Antibacterial and Angiogenic Properties for Diabetic Skin Wound Repair." *NPG Asia Materials* 11 (1): 3. https://doi.org/10.1038/s41427-018-0103-9.

Chitra, G, DS Franklin, S Sudarsan, M Sakthivel, and S Guhanathan. 2018. "Noncytotoxic Silver and Gold Nanocomposite Hydrogels with Enhanced Antibacterial and Wound Healing Applications." *Polymer Engineering & Science* 58 (12): 2133–42. https://doi.org/10.1002/pen.24824.

Chopra, H., Bibi, S., Kumar, S., Khan, M.S., Kumar, P., Singh, I. 2022. Preparation and evaluation of chitosan/PVA based hydrogel films loaded with honey for wound healing application. *Gels* 8: 111. https://doi.org/10.3390/ gels8020111.

Choudhury, Rupasree, Moumita Majumdar, Piyali Biswas, Shamim Khan, and Tarun K Misra. 2019. "Kinetic Study of Functionalization of Citrate Stabilized Silver Nanoparticles with Catechol and Its Anti-Biofilm Activity." *Nano-Structures & Nano-Objects* 19: 100326. https://doi.org/10.1016/j.nanoso.2019.100326.

Chung, Ying-chien, Ya-ping Su, Chiing-chang Chen, Guang Jia, Huey-lan Wang, JC Gaston Wu, and Jaung-geng Lin. 2004. "Relationship between Antibacterial Activity of Chitosan and Surface Characteristics of Cell Wall." *Acta Pharmacologica Sinica* 25 (7): 932–36.

Chuysinuan, P, N Chimnoi, N Reuk-Ngam, P Khlaychan, A Makarasen, N Wetprasit, D Dechtrirat, P Supaphol, and S Techasakul. 2019. "Development of Gelatin Hydrogel Pads Incorporated with Eupatorium Adenophorum Essential Oil as Antibacterial Wound Dressing." *Polymer Bulletin* 76 (2): 701–24. https://doi.org/10.1007/s00289-018-2395-x.

Cohen, Philip R, and Razelle Kurzrock. 2004. "Community-Acquired Methicillin-Resistant Staphylococcus Aureus Skin Infection: An Emerging Clinical Problem." *Journal of the American Academy of Dermatology* 50 (2): 277–80. https://doi.org/10.1016/j.jaad.2003.06.005.

Coimbra, Patrícia, João P Freitas, Teresa Gonçalves, Maria H Gil, and Margarida Figueiredo. 2019. "Preparation of Gentamicin Sulfate Eluting Fiber Mats by Emulsion and by Suspension Electrospinning." *Materials Science and Engineering: C* 94: 86–93. https://doi.org/10.1016/j.msec.2018.09.019.

Collier, TO, and JM Anderson. 2002. "Protein and Surface Effects on Monocyte and Macrophage Adhesion, Maturation, and Survival." *Journal of Biomedical Materials Research* 60 (3): 487–96. https://doi.org/10.1002/jbm.10043.

Crank, J. 1970. *The Mathematics of Diffusion*. Oxford: Clarendon Press.

Croisier, Florence, and Christine Jérôme. 2013. "Chitosan-Based Biomaterials for Tissue Engineering." *European Polymer Journal* 49 (4): 780–92. https://doi.org/10.1016/j.eurpolymj.2012.12.009.

Dadsetan, Mahrokh, Jacqueline A Jones, Anne Hiltner, and James M Anderson. 2004. "Surface Chemistry Mediates Adhesive Structure, Cytoskeletal Organization, and Fusion of Macrophages." *Journal of Biomedical Materials Research Part A* 71A (3): 439–48. https://doi.org/10.1002/jbm.a.30165.

Dai, Lei, Ben Nadeau, Xingye An, Dong Cheng, Zhu Long, and Yonghao Ni. 2016. "Silver Nanoparticles-Containing Dual-Function Hydrogels Based on a Guar Gum-Sodium Borohydride System." *Scientific Reports* 6 (1): 36497. https://doi.org/10.1038/srep36497.

Daniels, Timothy R, Alastair SE Younger, Murray J Penner, Kevin J Wing, Sara Lyn Miniaci-Coxhead, Ellie Pinsker, and Mark Glazebrook. 2017. "Midterm Outcomes of Polyvinyl Alcohol Hydrogel Hemiarthroplasty of the First Metatarsophalangeal Joint in Advanced Hallux Rigidus." *Foot & Ankle International* 38 (3): 243–47. https://doi.org/10.1177/1071100716679979.

Davis, Thomas P, Malcolm B Huglin, and Daniel CF Yip. 1988. "Properties of Poly(N-Vinyl-2-Pyrrolidone) Hydrogels Crosslinked with Ethyleneglycol Dimethacrylate." *Polymer* 29 (4): 701–6. https://doi.org/10.1016/0032-3861(88)90087-0.

DeFife, Kristin M, Erica Colton, Yasuhide Nakayama, Takehisa Matsuda, and James M Anderson. 1999. "Spatial Regulation and Surface Chemistry Control of Monocyte/Macrophage Adhesion and Foreign Body Giant Cell Formation by Photochemically Micropatterned Surfaces." *Journal of Biomedical Materials Research* 45 (2): 148–54. https://doi.org/10.1002/(SICI)1097-4636(199905)45:2<148::AID-JBM10>3.0.CO;2-U.

Diniz, Flavia R, Romerito Cesar AP Maia, M Lucas Rannier, Luciana N de Andrade, Marco Vinicius Chaud Andrade, Classius F da Silva, Cristiane B Corrêa, et al. 2020. "Silver Nanoparticles-Composing Alginate/Gelatine Hydrogel Improves Wound Healing In Vivo." *Nanomaterials*. https://doi.org/10.3390/nano10020390.

Du, Yan, Lin Li, Haitao Peng, Heng Zheng, Shuang Cao, Guoyu Lv, Aiping Yang, Hong Li, and Tielong Liu. 2020. "A Spray-Filming Self-Healing Hydrogel Fabricated from Modified Sodium Alginate and Gelatin as a Bacterial Barrier." *Macromolecular Bioscience* 20 (2): 1900303. https://doi.org/10.1002/mabi.201900303.

Dubas, Stephan T, and Vimolvan Pimpan. 2008. "Optical Switch from Silver Nanocomposite Thin Films." *Materials Letters* 62 (19): 3361–63. https://doi.org/10.1016/j.matlet.2008.03.036.

Durán, Nelson, Marcela Durán, Marcelo Bispo de Jesus, Amedea B Seabra, Wagner J Fávaro, and Gerson Nakazato. 2016. "Silver Nanoparticles: A New View on Mechanistic Aspects on Antimicrobial Activity." *Nanomedicine: Nanotechnology, Biology and Medicine* 12 (3): 789–99. https://doi.org/10.1016/j.nano.2015.11.016.

Duygu Sütekin, S, and Olgun Güven. 2019. "Application of Radiation for the Synthesis of Poly(n-Vinyl Pyrrolidone) Nanogels with Controlled Sizes from Aqueous Solutions." *Applied Radiation and Isotopes* 145: 161–69. https://doi.org/10.1016/j.apradiso.2018.12.028.

Elbarbary, Ahmed M, and Naeem M El-Sawy. 2017. "Radiation Synthesis and Characterization of Polyvinyl Alcohol/Chitosan/Silver Nanocomposite Membranes: Antimicrobial and Blood Compatibility Studies." *Polymer Bulletin* 74 (1): 195–212. https://doi.org/10.1007/s00289-016-1708-1.

Eron, Lawrence J, Benjamin A Lipsky, Donald E Low, Dilip Nathwani, Alan D Tice, and Gregory A Volturo. 2003. "Managing Skin and Soft Tissue Infections: Expert Panel Recommendations on Key Decision Points." *Journal of Antimicrobial Chemotherapy* 52(Supplement 1): i3–17. https://doi.org/10.1093/jac/dkg466.

Escobar-Hernández, John MA, and Juan CM Escobar-Remolina. 2019. "Silver Nanoparticles: Synthesis and Mathematical-Geometric Formulation." *Nano-Structures & Nano-Objects* 17: 259–68. https://doi.org/10.1016/j.nanoso.2019.01.005.

Evanoff, David D, and George Chumanov. 2004. "Size-Controlled Synthesis of Nanoparticles. 1. 'Silver-Only' Aqueous Suspensions via Hydrogen Reduction." *The Journal of Physical Chemistry B* 108 (37): 13948–56. https://doi.org/10.1021/jp047565s.

Fages, E, J Pascual, O Fenollar, D García-Sanoguera, and R Balart. 2011. "Study of Antibacterial Properties of Polypropylene Filled with Surfactant-Coated Silver Nanoparticles." *Polymer Engineering & Science* 51 (4): 804–11. https://doi.org/10.1002/pen.21889.

Fathollahipour, Shahrzad, Mojtaba Koosha, Javad Tavakoli, Susan Maziarfar, and Jalil Fallah Mehrabadi. 2020. "Erythromycin Releasing PVA/Sucrose and PVA/Honey Hydrogels as Wound Dressings with Antibacterial Activity and Enhanced Bio-Adhesion." *Iranian Journal of Pharmaceutical Research* 19 (1): 448–64. https://doi.org/10.22037/ijpr.2020.1101002.

Fei Liu, Xiao, Yun Lin Guan, Dong Zhi Yang, Zhi Li, and Kang De Yao. 2001. "Antibacterial Action of Chitosan and Carboxymethylated Chitosan." *Journal of Applied Polymer Science* 79 (7): 1324–35. https://doi.org/10.1002/1097-4628(20010214)79:7<1324::AID-APP210>3.0.CO;2-L.

Feng, QL, J Wu, GQ Chen, FZ Cui, TN Kim, and JO Kim. 2000. "A Mechanistic Study of the Antibacterial Effect of Silver Ions on Escherichia Coli and Staphylococcus Aureus." *Journal of Biomedical Materials Research* 52 (4): 662–68. https://doi.org/10.1002/1097-4636(20001215)52:4<662::AID-JBM10>3.0.CO;2-3.

Ferfera-Harrar, Hafida, Dalila Berdous, and Tayeb Benhalima. 2018. "Hydrogel Nanocomposites Based on Chitosan-g-Polyacrylamide and Silver Nanoparticles Synthesized Using Curcuma Longa for Antibacterial Applications." *Polymer Bulletin* 75 (7): 2819–46. https://doi.org/10.1007/s00289-017-2183-z.

Ferreira, RV, CL Cruz, GH de Castro, KM Freitas, NM de Paula, LB Nogueira, CSB Gil, and DM Freitas-Silvaa. 2020. "Reticulated PVA Foams: Preparation, Characterization and in Vitro Evaluation for Potential 3D Microbiological Culture." *Materials Research* 23 (6). https://doi.org/10.1590/1980-5373-MR-2020-0228.

Figueroa-Pizano, MD, I Vélaz, FJ Peñas, P Zavala-Rivera, AJ Rosas-Durazo, AD Maldonado-Arce, and ME Martínez-Barbosa. 2018. "Effect of Freeze-Thawing Conditions for Preparation of Chitosan-Poly (Vinyl Alcohol) Hydrogels and Drug Release Studies." *Carbohydrate Polymers* 195: 476–85. https://doi.org/10.1016/j.carbpol.2018.05.004.

Fukumori, Taishi, and Takahiko Nakaoki. 2014. "High-Tensile-Strength Polyvinyl Alcohol Films Prepared from Freeze/Thaw Cycled Gels." *Journal of Applied Polymer Science* 131 (15). https://doi.org/10.1002/app.40578.

George, Saji, Sijie Lin, Zhaoxia Ji, Courtney R Thomas, LinJiang Li, Mathew Mecklenburg, Huan Meng, et al. 2012. "Surface Defects on Plate-Shaped Silver Nanoparticles Contribute to Its Hazard Potential in a Fish Gill Cell Line and Zebrafish Embryos." *ACS Nano* 6 (5): 3745–59. https://doi.org/10.1021/nn204671v.

Georgieva, Nelly, Rayna Bryaskova, and Rumiana Tzoneva. 2012. "New Polyvinyl Alcohol-Based Hybrid Materials for Biomedical Application." *Materials Letters* 88: 19–22. https://doi.org/10.1016/j.matlet.2012.07.111.

Ghaffari-Bohlouli, Pejman, Fatemeh Hamidzadeh, Payam Zahedi, Mohsen Shahrousvand, and Mahshid Fallah-Darrehchi. 2020. "Antibacterial Nanofibers Based on Poly(l-Lactide-Co-d, l-Lactide) and Poly(Vinyl Alcohol) Used in Wound Dressings Potentially: A Comparison between Hybrid and Blend Properties." *Journal of Biomaterials Science, Polymer Edition* 31 (2): 219–43. https://doi.org/10.1080/09205063.2019.1683265.

Gharibi, Reza, Shima Kazemi, Hamid Yeganeh, and Vida Tafakori. 2019. "Utilizing Dextran to Improve Hemocompatibility of Antimicrobial Wound Dressings with Embedded Quaternary Ammonium Salts." *International Journal of Biological Macromolecules* 131 (June): 1044–56. https://doi.org/10.1016/j.ijbiomac.2019.03.185.

Ghasemzadeh, Hossein, and Fereshteh Ghanaat. 2014. "Antimicrobial Alginate/PVA Silver Nanocomposite Hydrogel, Synthesis and Characterization." *Journal of Polymer Research* 21 (3): 355. https://doi.org/10.1007/s10965-014-0355-1.

Gholamali, Iman, Manzarbanou Asnaashariisfahani, and Eskandar Alipour. 2019. "Silver Nanoparticles Incorporated in PH-Sensitive Nanocomposite Hydrogels Based on Carboxymethyl Chitosan-Poly (Vinyl Alcohol) for Use in a Drug Delivery System." *Regenerative Engineering and Translational Medicine* 6: 138–53. https://api.semanticscholar.org/CorpusID:199651520.

———. 2020. "Silver Nanoparticles Incorporated in PH-Sensitive Nanocomposite Hydrogels Based on Carboxymethyl Chitosan-Poly (Vinyl Alcohol) for Use in a Drug Delivery System." *Regenerative Engineering and Translational Medicine* 6 (2): 138–53. https://doi.org/10.1007/s40883-019-00120-7.

Gholipourmalekabadi, Mazaher, Sunaina Sapru, Ali Samadikuchaksaraei, Rui L Reis, David L Kaplan, and Subhas C Kundu. 2020. "Silk Fibroin for Skin Injury Repair: Where Do Things Stand?" *Advanced Drug Delivery Reviews* 153: 28–53. https://doi.org/10.1016/j.addr.2019.09.003.

Gómez Chabala, Luisa F, Claudia E Cuartas, and Martha E López. 2017. "Release Behavior and Antibacterial Activity of Chitosan/Alginate Blends with Aloe Vera and Silver Nanoparticles." *Marine Drugs*. https://doi.org/10.3390/md15100328.

Gong, Lei, Bo Yin, Lan-peng Li, and Ming-bo Yang. 2015. "Nylon-6/Graphene Composites Modified through Polymeric Modification of Graphene." *Composites Part B: Engineering* 73: 49–56. https://doi.org/10.1016/j.compositesb.2014.12.009.

Gonzalez, JS, AS Maiolo, CE Hoppe, and VA Alvarez. 2012. "Composite Gels Based on Poly (Vinyl Alcohol) for Biomedical Uses." *Procedia Materials Science* 1: 483–90. https://doi.org/10.1016/j.mspro.2012.06.065.

Goosen, Mattheus FA, Eltag SE Mahmud, Abdullah S Al-Ghafri, Hamad A Al-Hajri, Yousuf S Al-Sinani, and Branko Bugarski. 1997. "Immobilization of Cells Using Electrostatic Droplet Generation." In *Immobilization of Enzymes and Cells*, edited by Gordon F Bickerstaff, 167–74. Totowa, NJ: Humana Press. https://doi.org/10.1385/0-89603-386-4:167.

Gordon, Siamon, Annette Plüddemann, and Fernando Martinez Estrada. 2014. "Macrophage Heterogeneity in Tissues: Phenotypic Diversity and Functions." *Immunological Reviews* 262 (1): 36–55. https://doi.org/10.1111/imr.12223.

Greene, Caitlyn, Henry T Beaman, Darnelle Stinfort, Maryam Ramezani, and Mary Beth B Monroe. 2023. "Antimicrobial PVA Hydrogels with Tunable Mechanical Properties and Antimicrobial Release Profiles." *Journal of Functional Biomaterials*. https://doi.org/10.3390/jfb14040234.

Guo, Juan, Lulu Ren, Ruiyu Wang, Chao Zhang, Yang Yang, and Tianxi Liu. 2011. "Water Dispersible Graphene Noncovalently Functionalized with Tryptophan and Its Poly(Vinyl Alcohol) Nanocomposite." *Composites Part B: Engineering* 42 (8): 2130–35. https://doi.org/10.1016/j.compositesb.2011.05.008.

Gupta, Abhishek, Sophie M Briffa, Sam Swingler, Hazel Gibson, Vinodh Kannappan, Grazyna Adamus, Marek Kowalczuk, Claire Martin, and Iza Radecka. 2020. "Synthesis of Silver Nanoparticles Using Curcumin-Cyclodextrins Loaded into Bacterial Cellulose-Based Hydrogels for Wound Dressing Applications." *Biomacromolecules* 21 (5): 1802–11. https://doi.org/10.1021/acs.biomac.9b01724.

Hamedi, Hamid, Sara Moradi, Samuel M Hudson, and Alan E Tonelli. 2018. "Chitosan Based Hydrogels and Their Applications for Drug Delivery in Wound Dressings: A Review." *Carbohydrate Polymers* 199: 445–60. https://doi.org/10.1016/j.carbpol.2018.06.114.

Han, George, and Roger Ceilley. 2017. "Chronic Wound Healing: A Review of Current Management and Treatments." *Advances in Therapy* 34 (3): 599–610. https://doi.org/10.1007/s12325-017-0478-y.

Han, Shanying, Jie Sun, Shuangba He, Mingliang Tang, and Renjie Chai. 2019. "The Application of Graphene-Based Biomaterials in Biomedicine." *American Journal of Translational Research* 11 (6): 3246–60.

Hang, Au Thi, Beomseok Tae, and Jun Seo Park. 2010. "Non-Woven Mats of Poly(Vinyl Alcohol)/Chitosan Blends Containing Silver Nanoparticles: Fabrication and Characterization." *Carbohydrate Polymers* 82 (2): 472–79. https://doi.org/10.1016/j.carbpol.2010.05.016.

Hassan, Christie M, and Nikolaos A Peppas. 2000. "Structure and Applications of Poly(Vinyl Alcohol) Hydrogels Produced by Conventional Crosslinking or by Freezing/Thawing Methods BT - Biopolymers · PVA Hydrogels, Anionic Polymerisation Nanocomposites." In, 37–65. Berlin, Heidelberg: Springer. https://doi.org/10.1007/3-540-46414-X_2.

He, Rong, Xuefeng Qian, Jie Yin, and Zikang Zhu. 2002. "Preparation of Polychrome Silver Nanoparticles in Different Solvents." *Journal of Materials Chemistry* 12 (12): 3783–86. https://doi.org/10.1039/B205214H.

Hebeish, Ali, M Hashem, MM Abd El-Hady, and S Sharaf. 2013. "Development of CMC Hydrogels Loaded with Silver Nano-Particles for Medical Applications." *Carbohydrate Polymers* 92 (1): 407–13. https://doi.org/10.1016/j.carbpol.2012.08.094.

Hench, Larry L, and Ian Thompson. 2010. "Twenty-First Century Challenges for Biomaterials." *Journal of the Royal Society, Interface* 7 (Suppl 4): S379–91. https://doi.org/10.1098/rsif.2010.0151.focus.

Hidalgo, E, and C Domínguez. 1998. "Study of Cytotoxicity Mechanisms of Silver Nitrate in Human Dermal Fibroblasts." *Toxicology Letters* 98 (3): 169–79. https://doi.org/10.1016/S0378-4274(98)00114-3.

Hiep, Nguyen Thi, Huynh Chan Khon, Vo Van Thanh Niem, Vo Van Toi, Tran Ngoc Quyen, Nguyen Dai Hai, and Mai Ngoc Tuan Anh. 2016. "Microwave-Assisted Synthesis of Chitosan/Polyvinyl Alcohol Silver Nanoparticles Gel for Wound Dressing Applications." *International Journal of Polymer Science* 2016. https://doi.org/10.1155/2016/1584046.

Higuchi, T. 1961. "Rate of Release of Medicaments from Ointment Bases Containing Drugs in Suspension." *Journal of Pharmaceutical Sciences* 50 (October): 874–75. https://doi.org/10.1002/jps.2600501018.

———. 1963. "Mechanism of Sustained-Action Medication. Theoretical Analysis of Rate of Release of Solid Drugs Dispersed in Solid Matrices." *Journal of Pharmaceutical Sciences* 52 (12): 1145–49. https://doi.org/10.1002/jps.2600521210.

Hoffmann, B, D Seitz, A Mencke, A Kokott, and G Ziegler. 2009. "Glutaraldehyde and Oxidised Dextran as Crosslinker Reagents for Chitosan-Based Scaffolds for Cartilage Tissue Engineering." *Journal of Materials Science: Materials in Medicine* 20 (7): 1495–503. https://doi.org/10.1007/s10856-009-3707-3.

Hong, Kyung Hwa. 2007. "Preparation and Properties of Electrospun Poly(Vinyl Alcohol)/Silver Fiber Web as Wound Dressings." *Polymer Engineering & Science* 47 (1): 43–49. https://doi.org/10.1002/pen.20660.

Hotaling, Nathan A, Li Tang, Darrell J Irvine, and Julia E Babensee. 2015. "Biomaterial Strategies for Immunomodulation." *Annual Review of Biomedical Engineering* 17: 317–49. https://doi.org/10.1146/annurev-bioeng-071813-104814.

Hövel, H, S Fritz, A Hilger, U Kreibig, and M Vollmer. 1993. "Width of Cluster Plasmon Resonances: Bulk Dielectric Functions and Chemical Interface Damping." *Physical Review B* 48 (24): 18178–88. https://doi.org/10.1103/PhysRevB.48.18178.

Hu, Qingxi, Runsheng Lu, Suihong Liu, Yakui Liu, Yan Gu, and Haiguang Zhang. 2022. "3D Printing GelMA/PVA Interpenetrating Polymer Networks Scaffolds Mediated with CuO Nanoparticles for Angiogenesis." *Macromolecular Bioscience* 22 (10): e2200208. https://doi.org/10.1002/mabi.202200208.

Huang, Haizhen, Qiang Yuan, and Xiurong Yang. 2004. "Preparation and Characterization of Metal–Chitosan Nanocomposites." *Colloids and Surfaces B: Biointerfaces* 39 (1): 31–37. https://doi.org/10.1016/j.colsurfb.2004.08.014.

Huang, Mei-Hua, and Ming-Chien Yang. 2008. "Evaluation of Glucan/Poly(Vinyl Alcohol) Blend Wound Dressing Using Rat Models." *International Journal of Pharmaceutics* 346 (1): 38–46. https://doi.org/10.1016/j.ijpharm.2007.06.021.

Hussain, SM, KL Hess, JM Gearhart, KT Geiss, and JJ Schlager. 2005. "In Vitro Toxicity of Nanoparticles in BRL 3A Rat Liver Cells." *Toxicology in Vitro* 19 (7): 975–83. https://doi.org/10.1016/j.tiv.2005.06.034.

Hwang, Ma-Ro, Jong Oh Kim, Jeong Hoon Lee, Yong Il Kim, Jeong Hoon Kim, Sun Woo Chang, Sung Gju Jin, et al. 2010. "Gentamicin-Loaded Wound Dressing With Polyvinyl Alcohol/Dextran Hydrogel: Gel Characterization and In Vivo Healing Evaluation." *AAPS PharmSciTech* 11 (3): 1092–103. https://doi.org/10.1208/s12249-010-9474-0.

Innocenti Malini, Riccardo, Jessica Lesage, Claudio Toncelli, Giuseppino Fortunato, René M Rossi, and Fabrizio Spano. 2019. "Crosslinking Dextran Electrospun Nanofibers via Borate Chemistry: Proof of Concept for Wound Patches." *European Polymer Journal* 110: 276–82. https://doi.org/10.1016/j.eurpolymj.2018.11.017.

Jadranka, Odović, and Vesna Mišković Stanković. 2023. "Antibiotics Application in Biomaterials for Soft and Hard Tissue Implants." *Global Sustainability Challenges* 1 (1 SE-Articles). https://gsc.unionnikolatesla.edu.rs/index.php/gsc/article/view/15.

Jayakumar, R, M Prabaharan, PT Sudheesh Kumar, SV Nair, and H Tamura. 2011. "Biomaterials Based on Chitin and Chitosan in Wound Dressing Applications." *Biotechnology Advances* 29 (3): 322–37. https://doi.org/10.1016/j.biotechadv.2011.01.005.

Je, Jae-Young, Young-Sook Cho, and Se-Kwon Kim. 2006. "Cytotoxic Activities of Water-Soluble Chitosan Derivatives with Different Degree of Deacetylation." *Bioorganic & Medicinal Chemistry Letters* 16 (8): 2122–26. https://doi.org/10.1016/j.bmcl.2006.01.060.

Jemilugba, Olufunto T, El Hadji Mamour Sakho, Sundararajan Parani, Vuyo Mavumengwana, and Oluwatobi S Oluwafemi. 2019. "Green Synthesis of Silver Nanoparticles Using Combretum Erythrophyllum Leaves and Its Antibacterial Activities." *Colloid and Interface Science Communications* 31: 100191. https://doi.org/10.1016/j.colcom.2019.100191.

Ji, Haiwei, Hanjun Sun, and Xiaogang Qu. 2016. "Antibacterial Applications of Graphene-Based Nanomaterials: Recent Achievements and Challenges." *Advanced Drug Delivery Reviews* 105: 176–89. https://doi.org/10.1016/j.addr.2016.04.009.

Jiang, Shan, Sha Liu, and Wenhao Feng. 2011. "PVA Hydrogel Properties for Biomedical Application." *Journal of the Mechanical Behavior of Biomedical Materials* 4 (7): 1228–33. https://doi.org/10.1016/j.jmbbm.2011.04.005.

Joshi, Aditee C, Ganesh B Markad, and Santosh K Haram. 2015. "Rudimentary Simple Method for the Decoration of Graphene Oxide with Silver Nanoparticles: Their Application for the Amperometric Detection of Glucose in the Human Blood Samples." *Electrochimica Acta* 161: 108–14. https://doi.org/10.1016/j.electacta.2015.02.077.

Jovanović, Željka, Aleksandra Krklješ, Jasmina Stojkovska, Simonida Tomić, Bojana Obradović, Vesna Mišković-Stanković, and Zorica Kačarević-Popović. 2011. "Synthesis and Characterization of Silver/Poly(N-Vinyl-2-Pyrrolidone) Hydrogel Nanocomposite Obtained by in Situ Radiolytic Method." *Radiation Physics and Chemistry* 80 (11): 1208–15. https://doi.org/10.1016/j.radphyschem.2011.06.005.

Jovanović, Željka, Aleksandra Radosavljević, Zorica Kačarević-Popović, Jasmina Stojkovska, Aleksandra Perić-Grujić, Mirjana Ristić, Ivana Z Matić, Zorica D Juranić, Bojana Obradovic, and Vesna Mišković-Stanković. 2013. "Bioreactor Validation and Biocompatibility of Ag/Poly(N-Vinyl-2-Pyrrolidone) Hydrogel Nanocomposites." *Colloids and Surfaces B: Biointerfaces* 105: 230–35. https://doi.org/10.1016/j.colsurfb.2012.12.055.

Jovanović, Željka, Jasmina Stojkovska, Bojana Obradović, and Vesna Mišković-Stanković. 2012. "Alginate Hydrogel Microbeads Incorporated with Ag Nanoparticles Obtained by Electrochemical Method." *Materials Chemistry and Physics* 133 (1): 182–89. https://doi.org/10.1016/j.matchemphys.2012.01.005.

Jovanović, Željka, Aleksandra Radosavljević, Milorad Šiljegović, Nataša Bibić, Vesna Mišković-Stanković, and Zorica Kačarević-Popović. 2012. "Structural and Optical Characteristics of Silver/Poly(N-Vinyl-2-Pyrrolidone) Nanosystems Synthesized by γ-Irradiation." *Radiation Physics and Chemistry* 81 (11): 1720–28. https://doi.org/10.1016/j.radphyschem.2012.05.019.

Jovanović, Željka, Aleksandra Radosavljević, Jasmina Stojkovska, Branislav Nikolić, Bojana Obradovic, Zorica Kačarević-Popović, and Vesna Mišković-Stanković. 2014. "Silver/Poly(N-Vinyl-2-Pyrrolidone) Hydrogel Nanocomposites Obtained by Electrochemical Synthesis of Silver Nanoparticles inside the Polymer Hydrogel Aimed for Biomedical Applications." *Polymer Composites* 35 (2): 217–26. https://doi.org/10.1002/pc.22653.

Kenawy, E, AM Omer, TM Tamer, MA Elmeligy, and MS Mohy Eldin. 2019. "Fabrication of Biodegradable Gelatin/Chitosan/Cinnamaldehyde Crosslinked Membranes for Antibacterial Wound Dressing Applications." *International Journal of Biological Macromolecules* 139: 440–48. https://doi.org/10.1016/j.ijbiomac.2019.07.191.

Khampieng, Thitikan, Supisara Wongkittithavorn, Sonthaya Chaiarwut, Pongpol Ekabutr, Prasit Pavasant, and Pitt Supaphol. 2018. "Silver Nanoparticles-Based Hydrogel: Characterization of Material Parameters for Pressure Ulcer Dressing Applications." *Journal of Drug Delivery Science and Technology* 44: 91–100. https://doi.org/10.1016/j.jddst.2017.12.005.

Ki, Vincent, and Coleman Rotstein. 2008. "Bacterial Skin and Soft Tissue Infections in Adults: A Review of Their Epidemiology, Pathogenesis, Diagnosis, Treatment and Site Of Care." *Canadian Journal of Infectious Diseases and Medical Microbiology* 19: 846453. https://doi.org/10.1155/2008/846453.

Kim, Jong Oh, Jun Young Choi, Jung Kil Park, Jeong Hoon Kim, Sung Giu Jin, Sun Woo Chang, Dong Xun Li, et al. 2008. "Development of Clindamycin-Loaded Wound Dressing with Polyvinyl Alcohol and Sodium Alginate." *Biological and Pharmaceutical Bulletin* 31 (12): 2277–82. https://doi.org/10.1248/bpb.31.2277.

Kim Min-Sung, Gun-Woo Oh, Yu-Mi Jang, Seok-Chun Ko, Won-Sun Park, Il-Whan Choi, Young-Mog Kim, and Won-Kyo Jung. 2020. "Antimicrobial Hydrogels Based on PVA and Diphlorethohydroxycarmalol (DPHC) Derived from Brown Alga Ishige Okamurae: An in Vitro and in Vivo Study for Wound Dressing Application." *Materials Science and Engineering: C* 107: 110352. https://doi.org/10.1016/j.msec.2019.110352.

Koehler, Julia, Ferdinand P Brandl, and Achim M Goepferich. 2018. "Hydrogel Wound Dressings for Bioactive Treatment of Acute and Chronic Wounds." *European Polymer Journal* 100: 1–11. https://doi.org/10.1016/j.eurpolymj.2017.12.046.

Koivuniemi, Raili, Tiina Hakkarainen, Jasmi Kiiskinen, Mika Kosonen, Jyrki Vuola, Jussi Valtonen, Kari Luukko, Heli Kavola, and Marjo Yliperttula. 2020. "Clinical Study of Nanofibrillar Cellulose Hydrogel Dressing for Skin Graft Donor Site Treatment." *Advances in Wound Care* 9 (4): 199–210. https://doi.org/10.1089/wound.2019.0982.

Kong, Ming, Xi Guang Chen, Ke Xing, and Hyun Jin Park. 2010. "Antimicrobial Properties of Chitosan and Mode of Action: A State of the Art Review." *International Journal of Food Microbiology*. https://doi.org/10.1016/j.ijfoodmicro.2010.09.012.

Konop, Marek, Tatsiana Damps, Aleksandra Misicka, and Lidia Rudnicka. 2016. "Certain Aspects of Silver and Silver Nanoparticles in Wound Care: A Minireview." *Journal of Nanomaterials* 2016. https://doi.org/10.1155/2016/7614753.

Koosha, Mojtaba, and Hamid Mirzadeh. 2015. "Electrospinning, Mechanical Properties, and Cell Behavior Study of Chitosan/PVA Nanofibers." *Journal of Biomedical Materials Research Part A* 103 (9): 3081–93. https://doi.org/10.1002/jbm.a.35443.

Kopcha, M, NG Lordi, and KJ Tojo. 1991. "Evaluation of Release from Selected Thermosoftening Vehicles." *The Journal of Pharmacy and Pharmacology* 43 (6): 382–87. https://doi.org/10.1111/j.2042-7158.1991.tb03493.x.

Kora, Aruna Jyothi, RB Sashidhar, and J Arunachalam. 2010. "Gum Kondagogu (Cochlospermum Gossypium): A Template for the Green Synthesis and Stabilization of Silver Nanoparticles with Antibacterial Application." *Carbohydrate Polymers* 82 (3): 670–79. https://doi.org/10.1016/j.carbpol.2010.05.034.

———. 2012. "Aqueous Extract of Gum Olibanum (Boswellia Serrata): A Reductant and Stabilizer for the Biosynthesis of Antibacterial Silver Nanoparticles." *Process Biochemistry* 47 (10): 1516–20. https://doi.org/10.1016/j.procbio.2012.06.004.

Korsmeyer, Richard W, Robert Gurny, Eric Doelker, Pierre Buri, and Nikolaos A Peppas. 1983. "Mechanisms of Solute Release from Porous Hydrophilic Polymers." *International Journal of Pharmaceutics* 15 (1): 25–35. https://doi.org/10.1016/0378-5173(83)90064-9.

Kozicki, Marek, Marek Kołodziejczyk, Małgorzata Szynkowska, Aleksandra Pawlaczyk, Ewa Leśniewska, Aleksandra Matusiak, Agnieszka Adamus, and Aleksandra Karolczak. 2016. "Hydrogels Made from Chitosan and Silver Nitrate." *Carbohydrate Polymers* 140: 74–87. https://doi.org/10.1016/j.carbpol.2015.12.017.

Kurczewska, Joanna, Paulina Sawicka, Magdalena Ratajczak, Marzena Gajęcka, and Grzegorz Schroeder. 2015. "Will the Use of Double Barrier Result in Sustained Release of Vancomycin? Optimization of Parameters for Preparation of a New Antibacterial Alginate-Based Modern Dressing." *International Journal of Pharmaceutics* 496 (2): 526–33. https://doi.org/10.1016/j.ijpharm.2015.10.075.

Kzhyshkowska, Julia, Alexandru Gudima, Vladimir Riabov, Camille Dollinger, Philippe Lavalle, and Nihal Engin Vrana. 2015. "Macrophage Responses to Implants: Prospects for Personalized Medicine." *Journal of Leukocyte Biology* 98 (6): 953–62. https://doi.org/10.1189/jlb.5VMR0415-166R.

Larrude, Dunieskys G, Marcelo EH Maia da Costa, and Fernando L Freire. 2014. "Synthesis and Characterization of Silver Nanoparticle-Multiwalled Carbon Nanotube Composites." Edited by Claude Estournès. *Journal of Nanomaterials* 2014: 654068. https://doi.org/10.1155/2014/654068.

Lawrie, Gwen, Imelda Keen, Barry Drew, Adrienne Chandler-Temple, Llewellyn Rintoul, Peter Fredericks, and Lisbeth Grondahl. 2007. "Interactions between Alginate and Chitosan Biopolymers Characterized Using FTIR and XPS." *Biomacromolecules* 8 (8): 2533–41. https://doi.org/10.1021/bm070014y.

Levick, JR, RM Mason, PJ Coleman, and D Scott. 1999. "Physiology of Synovial Fluid and Trans-Synovial Flow." In *Biology of the Synovial Joint*, edited by CW Archer, M Benjamin, B Caterson, and JR Ralphs, 235–52. Amsterdam: Harwood Academic.

Li, Pan, Shan Jiang, Yan Yu, Jun Yang, and Zhiyong Yang. 2015. "Biomaterial Characteristics and Application of Silicone Rubber and PVA Hydrogels Mimicked in Organ Groups for Prostate Brachytherapy." *Journal of the Mechanical Behavior of Biomedical Materials* 49 (September): 220–34. https://doi.org/10.1016/j.jmbbm.2015.05.012.

Li, Wenfeng, Feiyan Gao, Jinlan Kan, Jia Deng, Bochu Wang, and Shilei Hao. 2019. "Synthesis and Fabrication of a Keratin-Conjugated Insulin Hydrogel for the Enhancement of Wound Healing." *Colloids and Surfaces B: Biointerfaces* 175: 436–44. https://doi.org/10.1016/j.colsurfb.2018.12.020.

Li, Xiaoxia, Aihua Xu, Hongguo Xie, Weiting Yu, Weiyang Xie, and Xiaojun Ma. 2010. "Preparation of Low Molecular Weight Alginate by Hydrogen Peroxide Depolymerization for Tissue Engineering." *Carbohydrate Polymers* 79 (3): 660–64. https://doi.org/10.1016/j.carbpol.2009.09.020.

Lin, Zefeng, Tingting Wu, Wanshun Wang, Binglin Li, Ming Wang, Lingling Chen, Hong Xia, and Tao Zhang. 2019. "Biofunctions of Antimicrobial Peptide-Conjugated Alginate/Hyaluronic Acid/Collagen Wound Dressings Promote Wound Healing of a Mixed-Bacteria-Infected Wound." *International Journal of Biological Macromolecules* 140: 330–42. https://doi.org/10.1016/j.ijbiomac.2019.08.087.

Liu, Hui, Yumin Du, Xiaohui Wang, and Liping Sun. 2004. "Chitosan Kills Bacteria through Cell Membrane Damage." *International Journal of Food Microbiology* 95 (2): 147–55. https://doi.org/10.1016/j.ijfoodmicro.2004.01.022.

Liu, Ruifang, Xianlin Xu, Xupin Zhuang, and Bowen Cheng. 2014. "Solution Blowing of Chitosan/PVA Hydrogel Nanofiber Mats." *Carbohydrate Polymers* 101: 1116–21. https://doi.org/10.1016/j.carbpol.2013.10.056.

Liu, Shaobin, Tingying Helen Zeng, Mario Hofmann, Ehdi Burcombe, Jun Wei, Rongrong Jiang, Jing Kong, and Yuan Chen. 2011. "Antibacterial Activity of Graphite, Graphite Oxide, Graphene Oxide, and Reduced Graphene Oxide: Membrane and Oxidative Stress." *ACS Nano* 5 (9): 6971–80. https://doi.org/10.1021/nn202451x.

Liu, Yi, Jing Huang, and Hua Li. 2013. "Synthesis of Hydroxyapatite–Reduced Graphite Oxide Nanocomposites for Biomedical Applications: Oriented Nucleation and Epitaxial Growth of Hydroxyapatite." *Journal of Materials Chemistry B* 1 (13): 1826–34. https://doi.org/10.1039/C3TB00531C.

Liu, Yusheng, Shimou Chen, Lei Zhong, and Guozhong Wu. 2009. "Preparation of High-Stable Silver Nanoparticle Dispersion by Using Sodium Alginate as a Stabilizer under Gamma Radiation." *Radiation Physics and Chemistry* 78 (4): 251–55. https://doi.org/10.1016/j.radphyschem.2009.01.003.

Lu, Bitao, Fei Lu, Yini Zou, Jiawei Liu, Bao Rong, Zhiquan Li, Fangying Dai, Dayang Wu, and Guangqian Lan. 2017. "In Situ Reduction of Silver Nanoparticles by Chitosan-l-Glutamic Acid/Hyaluronic Acid: Enhancing Antimicrobial and Wound-Healing Activity." *Carbohydrate Polymers* 173: 556–65. https://doi.org/10.1016/j.carbpol.2017.06.035.

Lu, Lehui, Atsuko Kobayashi, Keiko Tawa, and Yukihiro Ozaki. 2006. "Silver Nanoplates with Special Shapes: Controlled Synthesis and Their Surface Plasmon Resonance and Surface-Enhanced Raman Scattering Properties." *Chemistry of Materials* 18 (20): 4894–901. https://doi.org/10.1021/cm0615875.

Lukáč, Peter, Jan Miroslav Hartinger, Mikuláš Mlček, Michaela Popková, Tomáš Suchý, Monika Šupová, Jan Závora, et al. 2019. "A Novel Gentamicin-Releasing Wound Dressing Prepared from Freshwater Fish Cyprinus Carpio Collagen Cross-Linked with Carbodiimide." *Journal of Bioactive and Compatible Polymers* 34 (3): 246–62. https://doi.org/10.1177/0883911519835143.

Luther, Eva M, Yvonne Koehler, Joerg Diendorf, Matthias Epple, and Ralf Dringen. 2011. "Accumulation of Silver Nanoparticles by Cultured Primary Brain Astrocytes." *Nanotechnology* 22 (37). https://doi.org/10.1088/0957-4484/22/37/375101.

Luttikhuizen, Daniël T, Martin C Harmsen, and Marja JA Van Luyn. 2006. "Cellular and Molecular Dynamics in the Foreign Body Reaction." *Tissue Engineering* 12 (7): 1955–70. https://doi.org/10.1089/ten.2006.12.1955.

Lužajić Božinovski, Tijana, Danica Marković, Vera Todorović, Bolka Bogomir Prokić, Ivan Milošević, Neda Drndarević, Katarina Nešović, Yop Rhee Kyong, and Vesna Mišković-Stanković. 2018. "In Vivo Investigation of Soft Tissue Response of Novel Silver/Poly(Vinyl Alcohol)/Graphene and Silver/Poly(Vinyl Alcohol)/Chitosan/Graphene Hydrogels Aimed for Medical Applications – The First Experience." *Acta Veterinaria* 68 (3): 321–39. https://doi.org/10.2478/acve-2018-0027.

Lužajić Božinovski, Tijana, Vera Todorović, Ivan Milošević, Vladimir Gajdov, Bogomir Bolka Prokić, Katarina Nešović, Vesna Mišković-Stanković, and Danica Marković. 2021. "Evaluation of Soft Tissue Regenerative Processes After Subcutaneous Implantation of Silver/ Poly(Vinyl Alcohol) and Novel Silver/Poly(Vinyl Alcohol)/Graphene Hydrogels in an Animal Model." *Acta Veterinaria* 71 (3): 285–302. https://doi.org/doi:10.2478/acve-2021-0025.

Lužajić Božinovski, Tijana, Vera Todorović, Ivan Milošević, Bogomir Bolka Prokić, Vladimir Gajdov, Katarina Nešović, Vesna Mišković-Stanković, and Danica Marković. 2021. "Macrophages, the Main Marker in Biocompatibility Evaluation of New Hydrogels after Subcutaneous Implantation in Rats." *Journal of Biomaterials Applications* 36 (6): 1111–25. https://doi.org/10.1177/08853282211046119.

Ma, Xiaole, Yanlei Su, Qiang Sun, Yanqiang Wang, and Zhongyi Jiang. 2007. "Enhancing the Antifouling Property of Polyethersulfone Ultrafiltration Membranes through Surface Adsorption-Crosslinking of Poly(Vinyl Alcohol)." *Journal of Membrane Science* 300 (1): 71–78. https://doi.org/10.1016/j.memsci.2007.05.008.

Maiolo, Adolfo Sebastián, Matías Nicolás Amado, Jimena Soledad Gonzalez, and Vera Alejandra Alvarez. 2012. "Development and Characterization of Poly (Vinyl Alcohol) Based Hydrogels for Potential Use as an Articular Cartilage Replacement." *Materials Science and Engineering: C* 32 (6): 1490–95. https://doi.org/10.1016/j.msec.2012.04.030.

Maitra, Jaya, and Vivek Kumar Shukla. 2014. "Cross-Linking in Hydrogels - A Review." *American Journal of Polymer Science* 4 (2): 25–31. https://doi.org/10.5923/j.ajps.20140402.01.

Makoid, MC, A Dufour, and UV Banakar. 1993. "Modelling of Dissolution Behaviour of Controlled Release Systems." *S.T.P. Pharma Pratiques* 3 (1): 49–58.

Maleki, Homa, Sanjay Mathur, and Axel Klein. 2020. "Antibacterial Ag Containing Core-Shell Polyvinyl Alcohol-Poly (Lactic Acid) Nanofibers for Biomedical Applications." *Polymer Engineering & Science* 60 (6): 1221–30. https://doi.org/10.1002/pen.25375.

Manojlovic, Verica, Jasna Djonlagic, Bojana Obradovic, Viktor Nedovic, and Branko Bugarski. 2006. "Investigations of Cell Immobilization in Alginate: Rheological and Electrostatic Extrusion Studies." *Journal of Chemical Technology & Biotechnology* 81 (4): 505–10. https://doi.org/10.1002/jctb.1465.

Marie Arockianathan, P, S Sekar, S Sankar, B Kumaran, and TP Sastry. 2012. "Evaluation of Biocomposite Films Containing Alginate and Sago Starch Impregnated with Silver Nano Particles." *Carbohydrate Polymers* 90 (1): 717–24. https://doi.org/10.1016/j.carbpol.2012.06.003.

Martinez, Fernando O, and Siamon Gordon. 2014. "The M1 and M2 Paradigm of Macrophage Activation: Time for Reassessment." *F1000Prime Reports* 6 (March): 1–13. https://doi.org/10.12703/P6-13.

Masood, Nosheen, Rashid Ahmed, Muhammad Tariq, Zahoor Ahmed, Muhammad Shareef Masoud, Imran Ali, Rehana Asghar, Anisa Andleeb, and Anwarul Hasan. 2019. "Silver Nanoparticle Impregnated Chitosan-PEG Hydrogel Enhances Wound Healing in Diabetes Induced Rabbits." *International Journal of Pharmaceutics* 559: 23–36. https://doi.org/10.1016/j.ijpharm.2019.01.019.

Matica, Mariana Adina, Finn Lillelund Aachmann, Anne Tøndervik, Håvard Sletta, and Vasile Ostafe. 2019. "Chitosan as a Wound Dressing Starting Material: Antimicrobial Properties and Mode of Action." *International Journal of Molecular Sciences*. https://doi.org/10.3390/ijms20235889.

Matshetshe, Kabo I, Sundararajan Parani, Sarah M Manki, and Oluwatobi S Oluwafemi. 2018. "Preparation, Characterization and in Vitro Release Study of β-Cyclodextrin/Chitosan Nanoparticles Loaded Cinnamomum Zeylanicum Essential Oil." *International Journal of Biological Macromolecules* 118: 676–82. https://doi.org/10.1016/j.ijbiomac.2018.06.125.

Mbhele, ZH, MG Salemane, CGCE van Sittert, JM Nedeljković, V Djoković, and AS Luyt. 2003. "Fabrication and Characterization of Silver–Polyvinyl Alcohol Nanocomposites." *Chemistry of Materials* 15 (26): 5019–24. https://doi.org/10.1021/cm034505a.

Mekkawy, Aml I, Mohamed A El-Mokhtar, Nivien A Nafady, Naeima Yousef, Mostafa A Hamad, Sohair M El-Shanawany, Ehsan H Ibrahim, and Mahmoud Elsabahy. 2017. "In Vitro and in Vivo Evaluation of Biologically Synthesized Silver Nanoparticles for Topical Applications: Effect of Surface Coating and Loading into Hydrogels." *International Journal of Nanomedicine* 12: 759–77. https://doi.org/10.2147/IJN.S124294.

Merga, Getahun, Robert Wilson, Geoffrey Lynn, Bratoljub H Milosavljevic, and Dan Meisel. 2007. "Redox Catalysis on "Naked" Silver Nanoparticles." *The Journal of Physical Chemistry C* 111 (33): 12220–26. https://doi.org/10.1021/jp074257w.

Meriç, Gökçe, Jon E Dahl, and I Eystein Ruyter. 2008. "Cytotoxicity of Silica–Glass Fiber Reinforced Composites." *Dental Materials* 24 (9): 1201–6. https://doi.org/10.1016/j.dental.2008.01.010.

Mishra, Sandeep K, JMF Ferreira, and S Kannan. 2015. "Mechanically Stable Antimicrobial Chitosan–PVA–Silver Nanocomposite Coatings Deposited on Titanium Implants." *Carbohydrate Polymers* 121: 37–48. https://doi.org/10.1016/j.carbpol.2014.12.027.

Miskovic-Stankovic, Vesna, and Teodor M Atanackovic. 2023. "On a System of Equations with General Fractional Derivatives Arising in Diffusion Theory." *Fractal and Fractional*. https://doi.org/10.3390/fractalfract7070518.

Miskovic-Stankovic, Vesna, Marko Janev, and Teodor M Atanackovic. 2023. "Two Compartmental Fractional Derivative Model with General Fractional Derivative." *Journal of Pharmacokinetics and Pharmacodynamics* 50 (2): 79–87. https://doi.org/10.1007/s10928-022-09834-8.

Mišković-Stanković, Vesna, Ana Janković, Svetlana Grujić, Ivana Matić Bujagić, Vesna Radojević, Maja Vukašinović-Sekulić, Vesna Kojić, Marija Đošić, and Teodor M Atanacković. 2024. "Diffusion Models of Gentamicin Released in Poly(Vinyl Alcohol)/Chitosan Hydrogel." *Journal of the Serbian Chemical Society*. https://doi.org/10.2298/JSC231207010M

Mohanty, Fanismita, and Sarat K Swain. 2019. "Nano Silver Embedded Starch Hybrid Graphene Oxide Sandwiched Poly(Ethylmethacrylate) for Packaging Application." *Nano-Structures & Nano-Objects* 18: 100300. https://doi.org/10.1016/j.nanoso.2019.100300.

Monteiro, Nelson, Margarida Martins, Albino Martins, Nuno A Fonseca, João N Moreira, Rui L Reis, and Nuno M Neves. 2015. "Antibacterial Activity of Chitosan Nanofiber Meshes with Liposomes Immobilized Releasing Gentamicin." *Acta Biomaterialia* 18: 196–205. https://doi.org/10.1016/j.actbio.2015.02.018.

Montoro, Sérgio Roberto, Simone de Fátima Medeiros, and Gizelda Maria Alves. 2014. "Chapter 10 - Nanostructured Hydrogels." In *Nanostructured Polymer Blends Chandrasekharakurup*, edited by Sabu Thomas, Robert Shanks, and Sarathchandran BT, 325–55. Oxford: William Andrew Publishing. https://doi.org/10.1016/B978-1-4557-3159-6.00010-9.

Moretto, A, L Tesolin, F Marsilio, M Schiavon, M Berna, and FM Veronese. 2004. "Slow Release of Two Antibiotics of Veterinary Interest from PVA Hydrogels." *Farmaco (Societa Chimica Italiana : 1989)* 59 (1): 1–5. https://doi.org/10.1016/j.farmac.2003.11.003.

Morones, Jose Ruben, Jose Luis Elechiguerra, Alejandra Camacho, Katherine Holt, Juan B Kouri, Jose Tapia Ramírez, and Miguel Jose Yacaman. 2005. "The Bactericidal Effect of Silver Nanoparticles." *Nanotechnology* 16 (10): 2346. https://doi.org/10.1088/0957-4484/16/10/059.

Moskowitz, Ronald W, David S Howell, Roy D Altman, Joseph A Buckwalter, and Victor M Goldberg, eds. 2001. *Osteoarthritis: Diagnosis and Medical/Surgical Management*. Philadelphia: W.B. Saunders. https://books.google.rs/books?id=tCpsAAAAMAAJ.

Mosmann, Tim. 1983. "Rapid Colorimetric Assay for Cellular Growth and Survival: Application to Proliferation and Cytotoxicity Assays." *Journal of Immunological Methods* 65 (1): 55–63. https://doi.org/10.1016/0022-1759(83)90303-4.

Mozalewska, Wiktoria, Renata Czechowska-Biskup, Alicja K Olejnik, Radoslaw A Wach, Piotr Ulański, and Janusz M Rosiak. 2017. "Chitosan-Containing Hydrogel Wound Dressings Prepared by Radiation Technique." *Radiation Physics and Chemistry* 134: 1–7. https://doi.org/10.1016/j.radphyschem.2017.01.003.

Mulvaney, Paul. 1996. "Surface Plasmon Spectroscopy of Nanosized Metal Particles." *Langmuir* 12 (3): 788–800. https://doi.org/10.1021/la9502711.

Murali, Mohan, Y Kyungjae Lee, Thathan Premkumar, and Kurt E Geckeler. 2007. "Hydrogel Networks as Nanoreactors: A Novel Approach to Silver Nanoparticles for Antibacterial Applications." *Polymer* 48 (1): 158–64. https://doi.org/10.1016/j.polymer.2006.10.045.

Nacer Khodja, Assia, Mohamed Mahlous, Djamel Tahtat, Samah Benamer, Souad Larbi Youcef, Henni Chader, Latifa Mouhoub, et al. 2013. "Evaluation of Healing Activity of PVA/Chitosan Hydrogels on Deep Second Degree Burn: Pharmacological and Toxicological Tests." *Burns* 39 (1): 98–104. https://doi.org/10.1016/j.burns.2012.05.021.

Naseri-Nosar, Mahdi, and Zyta Maria Ziora. 2018. "Wound Dressings from Naturally-Occurring Polymers: A Review on Homopolysaccharide-Based Composites." *Carbohydrate Polymers* 189: 379–98. https://doi.org/10.1016/j.carbpol.2018.02.003.

Nedović, Viktor A, Bojana Obradović, Ida Leskošek-Čukalović, Olivera Trifunović, Radojica Pešić, and Branko Bugarski. 2001. "Electrostatic Generation of Alginate Microbeads Loaded with Brewing Yeast." *Process Biochemistry* 37 (1): 17–22. https://doi.org/10.1016/S0032-9592(01)00172-8.

Nedovic, Viktor A, Bojana Obradovic, Ida Leskosek-Cukalovic, and Gordana Vunjak-Novakovic. 2001. "Immobilized Yeast Bioreactor Systems for Brewing-Recent Achievements." In *Engineering and Manufacturing for Biotechnology*, edited by Marcel Hofman and Philippe Thonart, 277–92. Dordrecht: Springer Netherlands. https://doi.org/10.1007/0-306-46889-1_18.

Nešović, Katarina, Mohamed M Abudabbus, Kyong Yop Rhee, and Vesna Mišković-Stanković. 2017. "Graphene Based Composite Hydrogel for Biomedical Applications." *Croatica Chemica Acta* 90 (2): 207–13. https://doi.org/10.5562/cca3133.

Nešović, Katarina, Ana Janković, Vesna Kojić, Maja Vukašinović-Sekulić, Aleksandra Perić-Grujić, Kyong Yop Rhee, and Vesna Mišković-Stanković. 2018. "Silver/Poly(Vinyl Alcohol)/Chitosan/Graphene Hydrogels – Synthesis, Biological and Physicochemical Properties and Silver Release Kinetics." *Composites Part B: Engineering* 154: 175–85. https://doi.org/10.1016/j.compositesb.2018.08.005.

Nešović, Katarina, Ana Janković, Aleksandra Perić-Grujić, Maja Vukašinović-Sekulić, Tamara Radetić, Ljiljana Živković, Soo-Jin Park, Kyong Yop Rhee, and Vesna Mišković-Stanković. 2019. "Kinetic Models of Swelling and Thermal Stability of Silver/Poly(Vinyl Alcohol)/Chitosan/Graphene Hydrogels." *Journal of Industrial and Engineering Chemistry* 77: 83–96. https://doi.org/10.1016/j.jiec.2019.04.022.

Nešović, Katarina, Ana Janković, Tamara Radetić, Aleksandra Perić-Grujić, Maja Vukašinović-Sekulić, Vesna Kojić, Kyong Yop Rhee, and Vesna Mišković-Stanković. 2020. "Poly(Vinyl Alcohol)/Chitosan Hydrogels with Electrochemically Synthesized Silver Nanoparticles for Wound Dressing Applications." *Journal of Electrochemical Science and Engineering* 10 (2 SE-7th RSE SEE & 8th Kurt Schwabe symposium Special Issue): 185–98. https://doi.org/10.5599/jese.732.

Nešović, Katarina, Ana Janković, Tamara Radetić, Maja Vukašinović-Sekulić, Vesna Kojić, Ljiljana Živković, Aleksandra Perić-Grujić, Kyong Yop Rhee, and Vesna Mišković-Stanković. 2019. "Chitosan-Based Hydrogel Wound Dressings with Electrochemically Incorporated Silver Nanoparticles – In Vitro Study." *European Polymer Journal* 121: 109257. https://doi.org/10.1016/j.eurpolymj.2019.109257.

Nešović, Katarina, Vesna Kojić, Kyong Yop Rhee, and Vesna Mišković-Stanković. 2017. "Electrochemical Synthesis and Characterization of Silver Doped Poly(Vinyl Alcohol)/Chitosan Hydrogels." *Corrosion* 73 (12): 1437–47. https://doi.org/10.5006/2507.

Nešović, Katarina, and Vesna Mišković-Stanković. 2020. "A Comprehensive Review of the Polymer-Based Hydrogels with Electrochemically Synthesized Silver Nanoparticles for Wound Dressing Applications." *Polymer Engineering & Science* 60 (7): 1393–419. https://doi.org/10.1002/pen.25410.

———. 2022. "Silver/Poly(Vinyl Alcohol)/Graphene Hydrogels for Wound Dressing Applications: Understanding the Mechanism of Silver, Antibacterial Agent Release." *Journal of Vinyl and Additive Technology* 28 (1): 196–210. https://doi.org/10.1002/vnl.21882.

Neto, CGT, JA Giacometti, AE Job, FC Ferreira, JLC Fonseca, and MR Pereira. 2005. "Thermal Analysis of Chitosan Based Networks." *Carbohydrate Polymers* 62 (2): 97–103. https://doi.org/10.1016/j.carbpol.2005.02.022.

Nguyen, Nghi Thi-Phuong, Long Vuong-Hoang Nguyen, Nhi Tra Thanh, Vo Van Toi, Tran Ngoc Quyen, Phong A Tran, Hui-Min David Wang, and Thi-Hiep Nguyen. 2019. "Stabilization of Silver Nanoparticles in Chitosan and Gelatin Hydrogel and Its Applications." *Materials Letters* 248: 241–45. https://doi.org/10.1016/j.matlet.2019.03.103.

Nguyen, Ngoc-Thang, and Jui-Hsiang Liu. 2014. "A Green Method for in Situ Synthesis of Poly(Vinyl Alcohol)/Chitosan Hydrogel Thin Films with Entrapped Silver Nanoparticles." *Journal of the Taiwan Institute of Chemical Engineers* 45 (5): 2827–33. https://doi.org/10.1016/j.jtice.2014.06.017.

Nguyen, Thuy Thi Thu, Beomseok Tae, and Jun Seo Park. 2011. "Synthesis and Characterization of Nanofiber Webs of Chitosan/Poly(Vinyl Alcohol) Blends Incorporated with Silver Nanoparticles." *Journal of Materials Science* 46 (20): 6528–37. https://doi.org/10.1007/s10853-011-5599-0.

Nickerson, MT, AT Paulson, E Wagar, R Farnworth, SM Hodge, and D Rousseau. 2006. "Some Physical Properties of Crosslinked Gelatin–Maltodextrin Hydrogels." *Food Hydrocolloids* 20 (7): 1072–79. https://doi.org/10.1016/j.foodhyd.2005.12.003.

Nnamani, Petra Obioma, Franklin Chimaobi Kenechukwu, Chidinma L Anugwolu, Agubata Chukwuma Obumneme, and Anthony Amaechi Attama. 2013. "Characterization and Controlled Release of Gentamicin from Novel Hydrogels Based on Poloxamer 407 and Polyacrylic Acids." *African Journal of Pharmacy and Pharmacology* 7 (36): 2540–52. https://doi.org/10.5897/AJPP2013.3803.

Obradovic, B, and V Miskovic-Stankovic. 2013. "Silver Nanoparticles in Alginate Solutions and Hydrogels Aimed for Biomedical Applications." In *Silver Nanoparticles: Synthesis, Uses and Health Concerns*, edited by Ilaria Armentano and Jose Maria Kenny, 247–60. Hauppauge and New York: Nova Science Publishers.

Obradović, B, V Mišković-Stanković, Z Jovanovic, and J Stojkovska. 2015. "Obtaining Alginate Hydrogel Microparticles with Incorporated Silver Nanoparticles." Patent RS 53508 (B1)/2015, The Intellectual Property Office of the Republic of Serbia; RS20100499 (A2) —— 2012-06-30, EPO.

Obradovic, Bojana, Jasmina Stojkovska, Zeljka Jovanovic, and Vesna Miskovic-Stankovic. 2012. "Novel Alginate Based Nanocomposite Hydrogels with Incorporated Silver Nanoparticles." *Journal of Materials Science: Materials in Medicine* 23 (1): 99–107. https://doi.org/10.1007/s10856-011-4522-1.

Ohashi, Wakana, Kohshi Hattori, and Yuichi Hattori. 2015. "Control of Macrophage Dynamics as a Potential Therapeutic Approach for Clinical Disorders Involving Chronic Inflammation." *Journal of Pharmacology and Experimental Therapeutics* 354 (3): 240–250. https://doi.org/10.1124/jpet.115.225540.

Olewnik-Kruszkowska, E., Gierszewska, M., Jakubowska, E., Tarach, I., Sedlarik, V., Pummerova, M. 2019. Antibacterial films based on PVA and PVA-chitosan modified with poly(Hexamethylene Guanidine). *Polymers (Basel)* 11(12): 2093. doi: 10.3390/polym11122093. PMID: 31847274; PMCID: PMC6960635.

Oluwafemi, Oluwatobi S, John Leo Anyik, Nkosingiphile Excellent Zikalala, and El Hadji Mamour Sakho. 2019. "Biosynthesis of Silver Nanoparticles from Water Hyacinth Plant Leaves Extract for Colourimetric Sensing of Heavy Metals." *Nano-Structures & Nano-Objects* 20: 100387. https://doi.org/10.1016/j.nanoso.2019.100387.

Osmokrović, Andrea, Bojana Obradović, Diana Bugarski, Branko Bugarski, and Gordana Vunjak-Novakovic. 2006. "Development of a Packed Bed Bioreactor for Cartilage Tissue Engineering." *FME Transactions* 34: 65–70.

Păduraru, Oana Maria, Diana Ciolacu, Raluca Nicoleta Darie, and Cornelia Vasile. 2012. "Synthesis and Characterization of Polyvinyl Alcohol/Cellulose Cryogels and Their Testing as Carriers for a Bioactive Component." *Materials Science and Engineering: C* 32 (8): 2508–15. https://doi.org/10.1016/j.msec.2012.07.033.

Panáček, Aleš, Libor Kvítek, Robert Prucek, Milan Kolář, Renata Večeřová, Naděžda Pizúrová, Virender K Sharma, Tat'jana Nevěčná, and Radek Zbořil. 2006. "Silver Colloid Nanoparticles: Synthesis, Characterization, and Their Antibacterial Activity." *The Journal of Physical Chemistry B* 110 (33): 16248–53. https://doi.org/10.1021/jp063826h.

Pankongadisak, Porntipa, Suriyan Sangklin, Piyachat Chuysinuan, Orawan Suwantong, and Pitt Supaphol. 2019. "The Use of Electrospun Curcumin-Loaded Poly(L-Lactic Acid) Fiber Mats as Wound Dressing Materials." *Journal of Drug Delivery Science and Technology* 53: 101121. https://doi.org/10.1016/j.jddst.2019.06.018.

Park, Eun-Jung, Eunjoo Bae, Jongheop Yi, Younghun Kim, Kyunghee Choi, Sang Hee Lee, Junheon Yoon, Byung Chun Lee, and Kwangsik Park. 2010. "Repeated-Dose Toxicity and Inflammatory Responses in Mice by Oral Administration of Silver Nanoparticles." *Environmental Toxicology and Pharmacology* 30 (2): 162–68. https://doi.org/10.1016/j.etap.2010.05.004.

Park, Eun-Jung, Jongheop Yi, Younghun Kim, Kyunghee Choi, and Kwangsik Park. 2010. "Silver Nanoparticles Induce Cytotoxicity by a Trojan-Horse Type Mechanism." *Toxicology in Vitro* 24 (3): 872–78. https://doi.org/10.1016/j.tiv.2009.12.001.

Paul, Willi, Chandra P Sharma, and Chitra Tirunal. 2004. "Chitosan and Alginate Wound Dressings: A Short Review." *Trends in Biomaterials \& Artificial Organs* 18. https://api.semanticscholar.org/CorpusID:74098643.

Păunică-Panea, Georgeta, Mihaela Violeta Ghica, Ştefania Marin, Ana Maria Ene, Maria Minodora Marin, Elena Dănilă, Cornelia Niţipir, Mădălina Georgiana Albu, and Ioan Cristescu. 2015. "Collagen-Albumin-Gentamicin Hydrogels Usable for Infected Wound Healing." *Leather and Footwear Journal* 15 (4): 249–56. https://doi.org/10.24264/LFJ.15.4.4.

Pencheva, Daniela, Rayna Bryaskova, and Todor Kantardjiev. 2012. "Polyvinyl Alcohol/Silver Nanoparticles (PVA/AgNps) as a Model for Testing the Biological Activity of Hybrid Materials with Included Silver Nanoparticles." *Materials Science & Engineering. C, Materials for Biological Applications* 32 (7): 2048–51. https://doi.org/10.1016/j.msec.2012.05.016.

Peppas, Nikolaos A, and Shauna R Stauffer. 1991. "Reinforced Uncrosslinked Poly (Vinyl Alcohol) Gels Produced by Cyclic Freezing-Thawing Processes: A Short Review." *Journal of Controlled Release* 16 (3): 305–10. https://doi.org/10.1016/0168-3659(91)90007-Z.

Pereira, Anna Karla dos S, Davi T Reis, Keleen M Barbosa, Gessiel Newton Scheidt, Luelc Souza da Costa, and Lucas Samuel S Santos. 2020. "Antibacterial Effects and Ibuprofen Release Potential Using Chitosan Microspheres Loaded with Silver Nanoparticles." *Carbohydrate Research* 488: 107891. https://doi.org/10.1016/j.carres.2019.107891.

Pérez-Díaz, M, E Alvarado-Gomez, M Magaña-Aquino, R Sánchez-Sánchez, C Velasquillo, C Gonzalez, A Ganem-Rondero, G Martínez-Castañon, N Zavala-Alonso, and F Martinez-Gutierrez. 2016. "Anti-Biofilm Activity of Chitosan Gels Formulated with Silver Nanoparticles and Their Cytotoxic Effect on Human Fibroblasts." *Materials Science & Engineering. C, Materials for Biological Applications* 60 (March): 317–23. https://doi.org/10.1016/j.msec.2015.11.036.

Petráš, Ivo, and Richard L Magin. 2011. "Simulation of Drug Uptake in a Two Compartmental Fractional Model for a Biological System." *Communications in Nonlinear Science and Numerical Simulation* 16 (12): 4588–95. https://doi.org/10.1016/j.cnsns.2011.02.012.

Poncelet, D, VG Babak, RJ Neufeld, MFA Goosen, and B Burgarski. 1999. "Theory of Electrostatic Dispersion of Polymer Solutions in the Production of Microgel Beads Containing Biocatalyst." *Advances in Colloid and Interface Science* 79 (2): 213–28. https://doi.org/10.1016/S0001-8686(97)00037-7.

Powers, Jennifer Gloeckner, Laurel M Morton, and Tania J Phillips. 2013. "Dressings for Chronic Wounds." *Dermatologic Therapy* 26 (3): 197–206. https://doi.org/10.1111/dth.12055.

Puoci, Francesco, Cristiana Piangiolino, Francesco Givigliano, Ortensia Ilaria Parisi, Roberta Cassano, Sonia Trombino, Manuela Curcio, et al. 2012. "Ciprofloxacin-Collagen Conjugate in the Wound Healing Treatment." *Journal of Functional Biomaterials.* https://doi.org/10.3390/jfb3020361.

Qin, Yimin. 2005. "Silver-Containing Alginate Fibres and Dressings." *International Wound Journal* 2 (2): 172–76. https://doi.org/10.1111/j.1742-4801.2005.00101.x.

Queen, Douglas, Heather Orsted, Hiromi Sanada, and Geoff Sussman. 2004. "A Dressing History." *International Wound Journal* 1 (1): 59–77. https://doi.org/10.1111/j.1742-4801.2004.0009.x.

Rabea, Entsar I, Mohamed ET. Badawy, Christian V Stevens, Guy Smagghe, and Walter Steurbaut. 2003. "Chitosan as Antimicrobial Agent: Applications and Mode of Action." *Biomacromolecules* 4 (6): 1457–65. https://doi.org/10.1021/bm034130m.

Rai, Mahendra, Alka Yadav, and Aniket Gade. 2009. "Silver Nanoparticles as a New Generation of Antimicrobials." *Biotechnology Advances* 27 (1): 76–83. https://doi.org/10.1016/j.biotechadv.2008.09.002.

Rajan, Sabitha. 2012. "Skin and Soft-Tissue Infections: Classifying and Treating a Spectrum." *Cleveland Clinic Journal of Medicine* 79 (1): 57–66. https://doi.org/10.3949/ccjm.79a.11044.

Ran, Luoxiao, Yini Zou, Junwen Cheng, and Fei Lu. 2019. "Silver Nanoparticles in Situ Synthesized by Polysaccharides from Sanghuangporus Sanghuang and Composites with Chitosan to Prepare Scaffolds for the Regeneration of Infected Full-Thickness Skin Defects." *International Journal of Biological Macromolecules* 125: 392–403. https://doi.org/10.1016/j.ijbiomac.2018.12.052.

Ratner, Buddy D. 2016. "A Pore Way to Heal and Regenerate: 21st Century Thinking on Biocompatibility." *Regenerative Biomaterials* 3 (2): 107–10. https://doi.org/10.1093/rb/rbw006.

Rattanaruengsrikul, Vichayarat, Nuttaporn Pimpha, and Pitt Supaphol. 2009. "Development of Gelatin Hydrogel Pads as Antibacterial Wound Dressings." *Macromolecular Bioscience* 9 (10): 1004–15. https://doi.org/10.1002/mabi.200900131.

Regiel, Anna, Silvia Irusta, Agnieszka Kyzioł, Manuel Arruebo, and Jesus Santamaria. 2013. "Preparation and Characterization of Chitosan-Silver Nanocomposite Films and Their Antibacterial Activity against Staphylococcus Aureus." *Nanotechnology* 24 (1). https://doi.org/10.1088/0957-4484/24/1/015101.

Rehman, Syed Raza Ur, Robin Augustine, Alap Ali Zahid, Rashid Ahmed, Muhammad Tariq, and Anwarul Hasan. 2019. "Reduced Graphene Oxide Incorporated GelMA Hydrogel Promotes Angiogenesis For Wound Healing Applications." *International Journal of Nanomedicine* 14: 9603–17. https://doi.org/10.2147/IJN.S218120.

Reicha, Fikry M, Afaf Sarhan, Maysa I Abdel-Hamid, and Ibrahim M El-Sherbiny. 2012. "Preparation of Silver Nanoparticles in the Presence of Chitosan by Electrochemical Method." *Carbohydrate Polymers* 89 (1): 236–44. https://doi.org/10.1016/j.carbpol.2012.03.002.

Richards, Vernal N, Nigam P Rath, and William E Buhro. 2010. "Pathway from a Molecular Precursor to Silver Nanoparticles: The Prominent Role of Aggregative Growth." *Chemistry of Materials* 22 (11): 3556–67. https://doi.org/10.1021/cm100871g.

Ritger, Philip L, and Nikolaos A Peppas. 1987. "A Simple Equation for Description of Solute Release I. Fickian and Non-Fickian Release from Non-Swellable Devices in the Form of Slabs, Spheres, Cylinders or Discs." *Journal of Controlled Release* 5 (1): 23–36. https://doi.org/10.1016/0168-3659(87)90034-4.

Rodríguez-Sánchez, L, MC Blanco, and MA López-Quintela. 2000. "Electrochemical Synthesis of Silver Nanoparticles." *The Journal of Physical Chemistry B* 104 (41): 9683–88. https://doi.org/10.1021/jp001761r.

Roy, Daniel C, Seth Tomblyn, David M Burmeister, Nicole L Wrice, Sandra C Becerra, Luke R Burnett, Justin M Saul, and Robert J Christy. 2014. "Ciprofloxacin-Loaded Keratin Hydrogels Prevent Pseudomonas Aeruginosa Infection and Support Healing in a Porcine Full-Thickness Excisional Wound." *Advances in Wound Care* 4 (8): 457–68. https://doi.org/10.1089/wound.2014.0576.

Rubina, Margarita S, Ernest E Said-Galiev, Alexander V Naumkin, Alexandra V Shulenina, Olga A Belyakova, and Alexander Yu. Vasil'kov. 2019. "Preparation and Characterization of Biomedical Collagen–Chitosan Scaffolds with Entrapped Ibuprofen and Silver Nanoparticles." *Polymer Engineering & Science* 59 (12): 2479–87. https://doi.org/10.1002/pen.25122.

Rudko, Galyna Yu, Andrii O Kovalchuk, Volodymyr I Fediv, Weimin M Chen, and Irina A Buyanova. 2015. "Interfacial Bonding in a CdS/PVA Nanocomposite: A Raman Scattering Study." *Journal of Colloid and Interface Science* 452 (August): 33–37. https://doi.org/10.1016/j.jcis.2015.04.020.

Ryan, Catherine, Emma Alcock, Finbarr Buttimer, Michael Schmidt, David Clarke, Martyn Pemble, and Maria Bardosova. 2017. "Synthesis and Characterisation of Cross-Linked Chitosan Composites Functionalised with Silver and Gold Nanoparticles for Antimicrobial Applications." *Science and Technology of Advanced Materials* 18 (1): 528–40. https://doi.org/10.1080/14686996.2017.1344929.

Sabitha, M, and Sheeja Rajiv. 2015. "Preparation and Characterization of Ampicillin-Incorporated Electrospun Polyurethane Scaffolds for Wound Healing and Infection Control." *Polymer Engineering & Science* 55 (3): 541–48. https://doi.org/10.1002/pen.23917.

Salarizadeh, Parisa, Mehran Javanbakht, Mahdi Abdollahi, and Leila Naji. 2013. "Preparation, Characterization and Properties of Proton Exchange Nanocomposite Membranes Based on Poly(Vinyl Alcohol) and Poly(Sulfonic Acid)-Grafted Silica Nanoparticles." *International Journal of Hydrogen Energy* 38 (13): 5473–79. https://doi.org/10.1016/j.ijhydene.2012.07.079.

Salehi-Abari, Mahdis, Narjes Koupaei, and SA Hassanzadeh-Tabrizi. 2020. "Synthesis and Characterisation of Semi-Interpenetrating Network of Polycaprolactone/Polyethylene Glycol Diacrylate/Zeolite-CuO as Wound Dressing." *Materials Technology* 35 (5): 290–99. https://doi.org/10.1080/10667857.2019.1678088.

Sambhy, Varun, Megan M MacBride, Blake R Peterson, and Ayusman Sen. 2006. "Silver Bromide Nanoparticle/Polymer Composites: Dual Action Tunable Antimicrobial Materials." *Journal of the American Chemical Society* 128 (30): 9798–808. https://doi.org/10.1021/ja061442z.

Sangnim, Tanikan, Sontaya Limmatvapirat, Jurairat Nunthanid, Pornsak Sriamornsak, Wancheng Sittikijyothin, Sumalee Wannachaiyasit, and Kampanart Huanbutta. 2018. "Design and Characterization of Clindamycin-Loaded Nanofiber Patches Composed of Polyvinyl Alcohol and Tamarind Seed Gum and Fabricated by Electrohydrodynamic Atomization." *Asian Journal of Pharmaceutical Sciences* 13 (5): 450–58. https://doi.org/10.1016/j.ajps.2018.01.002.

Santos, Catherine M, Joey Mangadlao, Farid Ahmed, Alex Leon, Rigoberto C Advincula, and Debora F Rodrigues. 2012. "Graphene Nanocomposite for Biomedical Applications: Fabrication, Antimicrobial and Cytotoxic Investigations." *Nanotechnology* 23 (39): 395101. https://doi.org/10.1088/0957-4484/23/39/395101.

Santos, Tavares Pereira, Danielle dos Maria Helena Madruga Lima-Ribeiro, Ralph Santos-Oliveira, Carmelita de Lima Bezerra Cavalcanti, Nicodemos Teles de Pontes-Filho, Luana Cassandra Breitenbach Barroso Coelho, Ana Maria dos Anjos Carneiro-Leão, and Maria Tereza dos Santos Correia. 2012. "Topical Application Effect of the Isolectin Hydrogel (Cramoll 1,4) on Second-Degree Burns: Experimental Model." Edited by Monica Fedele. *Journal of Biomedicine and Biotechnology* 2012: 184538. https://doi.org/10.1155/2012/184538.

Schexnailder, Patrick, and Gudrun Schmidt. 2009. "Nanocomposite Polymer Hydrogels." *Colloid and Polymer Science* 287 (1): 1–11. https://doi.org/10.1007/s00396-008-1949-0.

Sciarretta, F V. 2013. "5 to 8 Years Follow-up of Knee Chondral Defects Treated by PVA-H Hydrogel Implants." *European Review for Medical and Pharmacological Sciences* 17 (22): 3031–38.

Seo, Song Yi, Ga Hyun Lee, Se Guen Lee, So Yeon Jung, Jeong Ok Lim, and Jin Hyun Choi. 2012. "Alginate-Based Composite Sponge Containing Silver Nanoparticles Synthesized in Situ." *Carbohydrate Polymers* 90 (1): 109–15. https://doi.org/10.1016/j.carbpol.2012.05.002.

Sharma, Jaishri, Monira Lizu, Mark Stewart, Kyle Zygula, Yang Lu, Rajat Chauhan, Xingru Yan, Zhanhu Guo, Evan K Wujcik, and Suying Wei. 2015. "Multifunctional Nanofibers towards Active Biomedical Therapeutics." *Polymers*. https://doi.org/10.3390/polym7020186.

Sharma, Parul, Garima Mathur, Sanjay R Dhakate, Subhash Chand, Navendu Goswami, Sanjeev K Sharma, and Ashwani Mathur. 2016. "Evaluation of Physicochemical and Biological Properties of Chitosan/Poly (Vinyl Alcohol) Polymer Blend Membranes and Their Correlation for Vero Cell Growth." *Carbohydrate Polymers* 137: 576–83. https://doi.org/10.1016/j.carbpol.2015.10.096.

Sharma, Shilpa, Pallab Sanpui, Arun Chattopadhyay, and Siddhartha Sankar Ghosh. 2012. "Fabrication of Antibacterial Silver Nanoparticle—Sodium Alginate–Chitosan Composite Films." *RSC Advances* 2 (13): 5837–43. https://doi.org/10.1039/C2RA00006G.

Sharma, Virender K, Ria A Yngard, and Yekaterina Lin. 2009. "Silver Nanoparticles: Green Synthesis and Their Antimicrobial Activities." *Advances in Colloid and Interface Science* 145 (1): 83–96. https://doi.org/10.1016/j.cis.2008.09.002.

Sheikh, Zeeshan, Patricia J Brooks, Oriyah Barzilay, Noah Fine, and Michael Glogauer. 2015. “Macrophages, Foreign Body Giant Cells and Their Response to Implantable Biomaterials.” *Materials*. https://doi.org/10.3390/ma8095269.

Shen, Mingchao, and Thomas A Horbett. 2001. “The Effects of Surface Chemistry and Adsorbed Proteins on Monocyte/Macrophage Adhesion to Chemically Modified Polystyrene Surfaces.” *Journal of Biomedical Materials Research* 57 (3): 336–45. https://doi.org/10.1002/1097-4636(20011205)57:3<336::AID-JBM1176>3.0.CO;2-E.

Shi, Guifang, Wenting Chen, Yu Zhang, Xiaomei Dai, Xinge Zhang, and Zhongming Wu. 2019. “An Antifouling Hydrogel Containing Silver Nanoparticles for Modulating the Therapeutic Immune Response in Chronic Wound Healing.” *Langmuir* 35 (5): 1837–45. https://doi.org/10.1021/acs.langmuir.8b01834.

Siepmann, J, and NA Peppas. 2001. “Modeling of Drug Release from Delivery Systems Based on Hydroxypropyl Methylcellulose (HPMC).” *Advanced Drug Delivery Reviews* 48 (2): 139–57. https://doi.org/10.1016/S0169-409X(01)00112-0.

———. 2011. “Higuchi Equation: Derivation, Applications, Use and Misuse.” *International Journal of Pharmaceutics* 418 (1): 6–12. https://doi.org/10.1016/j.ijpharm.2011.03.051.

Šileikaitė, Asta, Igoris Prosycevas, Judita Puišo, Algimantas Juraitis, and Asta Guobienė. 2006. “Analysis of Silver Nanoparticles Produced by Chemical Reduction of Silver Salt Solution.” *Materials Science (Medžiagotyra)* 12 (4): 287–91.

Simões, Déborah, Sónia P Miguel, Maximiano P Ribeiro, Paula Coutinho, António G Mendonça, and Ilídio J Correia. 2018. “Recent Advances on Antimicrobial Wound Dressing: A Review.” *European Journal of Pharmaceutics and Biopharmaceutics : Official Journal of Arbeitsgemeinschaft Fur Pharmazeutische Verfahrenstechnik e.V* 127 (June): 130–41. https://doi.org/10.1016/j.ejpb.2018.02.022.

Singh, Baljit, and Lok Pal. 2012. “Sterculia Crosslinked PVA and PVA-Poly(AAm) Hydrogel Wound Dressings for Slow Drug Delivery: Mechanical, Mucoadhesive, Biocompatible and Permeability Properties.” *Journal of the Mechanical Behavior of Biomedical Materials* 9: 9–21. https://doi.org/10.1016/j.jmbbm.2012.01.021.

Sirelkhatim, Amna, Shahrom Mahmud, Azman Seeni, Noor Haida Mohamad Kaus, Ling Chuo Ann, Siti Khadijah Mohd Bakhori, Habsah Hasan, and Dasmawati Mohamad. 2015. “Review on Zinc Oxide Nanoparticles: Antibacterial Activity and Toxicity Mechanism.” *Nano-Micro Letters* 7 (3): 219–42. https://doi.org/10.1007/s40820-015-0040-x.

Slistan-Grijalva, A, R Herrera-Urbina, JF Rivas-Silva, M Ávalos-Borja, FF Castillón-Barraza, and A Posada-Amarillas. 2005a. “Assessment of Growth of Silver Nanoparticles Synthesized from an Ethylene Glycol–Silver Nitrate–Polyvinylpyrrolidone Solution.” *Physica E: Low-Dimensional Systems and Nanostructures* 25 (4): 438–48. https://doi.org/10.1016/j.physe.2004.07.010.

———. 2005b. “Classical Theoretical Characterization of the Surface Plasmon Absorption Band for Silver Spherical Nanoparticles Suspended in Water and Ethylene Glycol.” *Physica E: Low-Dimensional Systems and Nanostructures* 27 (1): 104–12. https://doi.org/10.1016/j.physe.2004.10.014.

Song, Jae Yong, and Beom Soo Kim. 2009. “Rapid Biological Synthesis of Silver Nanoparticles Using Plant Leaf Extracts.” *Bioprocess and Biosystems Engineering* 32 (1): 79–84. https://doi.org/10.1007/s00449-008-0224-6.

Sood, Aditya, Mark S Granick, and Nancy L Tomaselli. 2013. “Wound Dressings and Comparative Effectiveness Data.” *Advances in Wound Care* 3 (8): 511–29. https://doi.org/10.1089/wound.2012.0401.

Spasojević, Jelena, Aleksandra Radosavljević, Jelena Krstić, Miodrag Mitrić, Maja Popović, Zlatko Rakočević, Melina Kalagasidis-Krušić, and Zorica Kačarević-Popović. 2017. "Structural Characteristics and Bonding Environment of Ag Nanoparticles Synthesized by Gamma Irradiation within Thermo-Responsive Poly(N-Isopropylacrylamide) Hydrogel." *Polymer Composites* 38 (5): 1014–26. https://doi.org/10.1002/pc.23665.

Sripriya, Ramasamy, Muthusamy Senthil Kumar, Mohamed Rafiuddin Ahmed, and Praveen Kumar Sehgal. 2007. "Collagen Bilayer Dressing with Ciprofloxacin, an Effective System for Infected Wound Healing." *Journal of Biomaterials Science, Polymer Edition* 18 (3): 335–51. https://doi.org/10.1163/156856207779996913.

Stashak, Ted S, Ellis Farstvedt, and Ashlee Othic. 2004. "Update on Wound Dressings: Indications and Best Use." *Clinical Techniques in Equine Practice* 3 (2): 148–63. https://doi.org/10.1053/j.ctep.2004.08.006.

Stevanović, Milena, Djošić, Marija, Janković, Ana, Nešović, Katarina, Kojić, Vesna, Stojanović, Jovica, Grujić, Svetlana, Matić Bujagić, Ivana, Yop Rhee, Kyong, Mišković-Stanković, Vesna. 2020. Assessing bioactivity of gentamicin preloaded hydroxyapatite/chitosan composite coating on titanium substrate. *ACS Omega* 5 (25): 15433–15445. https://dx.doi.org/10.1021/acsomega.0c01583

Stevanović, Milena, Djošić, Marija, Janković, Ana, Kojić, Vesna, Stojanović, Jovica, Grujić, Svetlana, Matić Bujagić, Ivana, Yop Rhee, Kyong, Mišković-Stanković, Vesna. 2021. The chitosan-based bioactive composite coating on titanium. *Journal of Materials Research and Technology* 15: 4461–4474. https://doi.org/10.1016/j.jmrt.2021.10.072

Stojkovska, Jasmina, Branko Bugarski, and Bojana Obradovic. 2010. "Evaluation of Alginate Hydrogels under in Vivo–like Bioreactor Conditions for Cartilage Tissue Engineering." *Journal of Materials Science: Materials in Medicine* 21 (10): 2869–79. https://doi.org/10.1007/s10856-010-4135-0.

Stojkovska, Jasmina, Zeljka Djurdjevic, Ivan Jancic, Biljana Bufan, Marina Milenkovic, Radmila Jankovic, Vesna Miskovic-Stankovic, and Bojana Obradovic. 2018. "Comparative in Vivo Evaluation of Novel Formulations Based on Alginate and Silver Nanoparticles for Wound Treatments." *Journal of Biomaterials Applications* 32 (9): 1197–211. https://doi.org/10.1177/0885328218759564.

Stojkovska, Jasmina, Z Jovanovic, I Jancic, B Bufan, M Milenkovic, V Miškovic-Stankovic, and B Obradovic. 2013. "Novel Ag/Alginate Nanocomposites for Wound Treatments: Animal Studies." *Rane* 4: 17–22.

Stojkovska, Jasmina, Danijela Kostić, Željka Jovanović, Maja Vukašinović-Sekulić, Vesna Mišković-Stanković, and Bojana Obradović. 2014. "A Comprehensive Approach to in Vitro Functional Evaluation of Ag/Alginate Nanocomposite Hydrogels." *Carbohydrate Polymers* 111: 305–14. https://doi.org/10.1016/j.carbpol.2014.04.063.

Stojkovska, Jasmina, Jovana Zvicer, Željka Jovanović, Vesna Mišković-Stanković, and Bojana Obradović. 2012. "Controlled Production of Alginate Nanocomposites with Incorporated Silver Nanoparticles Aimed for Biomedical Applications." *Journal of the Serbian Chemical Society* 77 (12): 1709–22. https://doi.org/10.2298/JSC121108148S.

Sun, Jinchen, and Huaping Tan. 2013. "Alginate-Based Biomaterials for Regenerative Medicine Applications." *Materials*. https://doi.org/10.3390/ma6041285.

Sur, Srija, Aishwarya Rathore, Vivek Dave, Kakarla Raghava Reddy, Raghuraj Singh Chouhan, and Veera Sadhu. 2019. "Recent Developments in Functionalized Polymer Nanoparticles for Efficient Drug Delivery System." *Nano-Structures & Nano-Objects* 20: 100397. https://doi.org/10.1016/j.nanoso.2019.100397.

Surudžić, Rade, Željka Jovanović, Nataša Bibić, Branislav Nikolić, and Vesna Miskovic-Stankovic. 2013. "Electrochemical Synthesis of Silver Nanoparticles in Poly(Vinyl Alcohol) Solution." *Journal of the Serbian Chemical Society* 78 (12): 2087–98. https://doi.org/10.2298/JSC131017124S.

Surudžić, Rade, Ana Janković, Nataša Bibić, Maja Vukašinović-Sekulić, Aleksandra Perić-Grujić, Vesna Mišković-Stanković, Soo Jin Park, and Kyong Yop Rhee. 2016. "Physico–Chemical and Mechanical Properties and Antibacterial Activity of Silver/Poly(Vinyl Alcohol)/Graphene Nanocomposites Obtained by Electrochemical Method." *Composites Part B: Engineering* 85: 102–12. https://doi.org/10.1016/j.compositesb.2015.09.029.

Surudžić, Rade, Ana Janković, Miodrag Mitrić, Ivana Matić, Zorica D Juranić, Ljiljana Živković, Vesna Mišković-Stanković, Kyong Yop Rhee, Soo Jin Park, and David Hui. 2016. "The Effect of Graphene Loading on Mechanical, Thermal and Biological Properties of Poly(Vinyl Alcohol)/Graphene Nanocomposites." *Journal of Industrial and Engineering Chemistry* 34: 250–57. https://doi.org/10.1016/j.jiec.2015.11.016.

Taleb, C, S Berner, and G Mantovani Ruggiero. 2014. "First Metacarpal Resurfacing with Polyvinyl Alcohol Implant in Osteoarthritis: Preliminary Study." *Chirurgie de La Main* 33 (3): 189–95. https://doi.org/10.1016/j.main.2014.03.001.

Tanpichai, Supachok, and Kristiina Oksman. 2016. "Cross-Linked Nanocomposite Hydrogels Based on Cellulose Nanocrystals and PVA: Mechanical Properties and Creep Recovery." *Composites Part A: Applied Science and Manufacturing* 88: 226–33. https://doi.org/10.1016/j.compositesa.2016.06.002.

Thompson, Brianna C, Eoin Murray, and Gordon G Wallace. 2015. "Graphite Oxide to Graphene. Biomaterials to Bionics." *Advanced Materials* 27 (46): 7563–82. https://doi.org/10.1002/adma.201500411.

Torres-Giner, Sergio, Rocío Pérez-Masiá, and Jose M Lagaron. 2016. "A Review on Electrospun Polymer Nanostructures as Advanced Bioactive Platforms." *Polymer Engineering & Science* 56 (5): 500–27. https://doi.org/10.1002/pen.24274.

Tran, Hoang Vinh, Lam Dai Tran, Cham Thi Ba, Hoang Dinh Vu, Thinh Ngoc Nguyen, Dien Gia Pham, and Phuc Xuan Nguyen. 2010. "Synthesis, Characterization, Antibacterial and Antiproliferative Activities of Monodisperse Chitosan- Based Silver Nanoparticles." *Colloids and Surfaces A: Physicochemical and Engineering Aspects* 360 (1): 32–40. https://doi.org/10.1016/j.colsurfa.2010.02.007.

Trindade, Ricardo, Tomas Albrektsson, Pentti Tengvall, and Ann Wennerberg. 2016. "Foreign Body Reaction to Biomaterials: On Mechanisms for Buildup and Breakdown of Osseointegration." *Clinical Implant Dentistry and Related Research* 18 (1): 192–203. https://doi.org/10.1111/cid.12274.

Twu, Yawo-Kuo, Yu-Wan Chen, and Chao-Ming Shih. 2008. "Preparation of Silver Nanoparticles Using Chitosan Suspensions." *Powder Technology* 185 (3): 251–57. https://doi.org/10.1016/j.powtec.2007.10.025.

Tyliszczak, Bożena, Anna Drabczyk, Sonia Kudłacik-Kramarczyk, Katarzyna Bialik-Wąs, Regina Kijkowska, and Agnieszka Sobczak-Kupiec. 2017. "Preparation and Cytotoxicity of Chitosan-Based Hydrogels Modified with Silver Nanoparticles." *Colloids and Surfaces. B, Biointerfaces* 160 (December): 325–30. https://doi.org/10.1016/j.colsurfb.2017.09.044.

Ueno, Hiroshi, Takashi Mori, and Toru Fujinaga. 2001. "Topical Formulations and Wound Healing Applications of Chitosan." *Advanced Drug Delivery Reviews* 52 (2): 105–15. https://doi.org/10.1016/S0169-409X(01)00189-2.

Uttayarat, Pimpon, Jarurattana Eamsiri, Theeranan Tangthong, and Phiriyatorn Suwanmala. 2015. "Radiolytic Synthesis of Colloidal Silver Nanoparticles for Antibacterial Wound Dressings." Edited by Erwan Rauwel. *Advances in Materials Science and Engineering* 2015: 376082. https://doi.org/10.1155/2015/376082.

Venkatesan, Jayachandran, Jin-Young Lee, Dong Seop Kang, Sukumaran Anil, Se-Kwon Kim, Min Suk Shim, and Dong Gyu Kim. 2017. "Antimicrobial and Anticancer Activities of Porous Chitosan-Alginate Biosynthesized Silver Nanoparticles." *International Journal of Biological Macromolecules* 98: 515–25. https://doi.org/10.1016/j.ijbiomac.2017.01.120.

Verma, Jyoti, Jovita Kanoujia, Poonam Parashar, Chandra Bhusan Tripathi, and Shubhini A Saraf. 2017. "Wound Healing Applications of Sericin/Chitosan-Capped Silver Nanoparticles Incorporated Hydrogel." *Drug Delivery and Translational Research* 7 (1): 77–88. https://doi.org/10.1007/s13346-016-0322-y.

Vo, Thanh Truc, Thi Thanh Ngan Nguyen, Thi Thanh Tam Huynh, Thi Thuy Trang Vo, Thi Thuy Nhung Nguyen, Dinh Truong Nguyen, Van Su Dang, Chi Hien Dang, and Thanh Danh Nguyen. 2019. "Biosynthesis of Silver and Gold Nanoparticles Using Aqueous Extract from Crinum Latifolium Leaf and Their Applications Forward Antibacterial Effect and Wastewater Treatment." *Journal of Nanomaterials* 2019. https://doi.org/10.1155/2019/8385935.

Wahid, Fazli, Hai-Song Wang, Cheng Zhong, and Li-Qiang Chu. 2017. "Facile Fabrication of Moldable Antibacterial Carboxymethyl Chitosan Supramolecular Hydrogels Cross-Linked by Metal Ions Complexation." *Carbohydrate Polymers* 165: 455–61. https://doi.org/10.1016/j.carbpol.2017.02.085.

Wang, Tao, and Sundaram Gunasekaran. 2006. "State of Water in Chitosan–PVA Hydrogel." *Journal of Applied Polymer Science* 101 (5): 3227–32. https://doi.org/10.1002/app.23526.

Wang, Tom C, Michael F Rubner, and Robert E Cohen. 2002. "Polyelectrolyte Multilayer Nanoreactors for Preparing Silver Nanoparticle Composites: Controlling Metal Concentration and Nanoparticle Size." *Langmuir* 18 (8): 3370–75. https://doi.org/10.1021/la015725a.

Wang, ZL. 2000. "Transmission Electron Microscopy of Shape-Controlled Nanocrystals and Their Assemblies." *The Journal of Physical Chemistry B* 104 (6): 1153–75. https://doi.org/10.1021/jp993593c.

Ward, W Kenneth, Emily P Slobodzian, Kenneth L Tiekotter, and Michael D Wood. 2002. "The Effect of Microgeometry, Implant Thickness and Polyurethane Chemistry on the Foreign Body Response to Subcutaneous Implants." *Biomaterials* 23 (21): 4185–92. https://doi.org/10.1016/S0142-9612(02)00160-6.

Wei, Dongwei, Wuyong Sun, Weiping Qian, Yongzhong Ye, and Xiaoyuan Ma. 2009. "The Synthesis of Chitosan-Based Silver Nanoparticles and Their Antibacterial Activity." *Carbohydrate Research* 344 (17): 2375–82. https://doi.org/10.1016/j.carres.2009.09.001.

Wujcik, Evan K, and Chelsea N Monty. 2013. "Nanotechnology for Implantable Sensors: Carbon Nanotubes and Graphene in Medicine." *WIREs Nanomedicine and Nanobiotechnology* 5 (3): 233–49. https://doi.org/10.1002/wnan.1213.

Xie, Yajuan, Xiaozhu Liao, Jingxiang Zhang, Feiwen Yang, and Zengjie Fan. 2018. "Novel Chitosan Hydrogels Reinforced by Silver Nanoparticles with Ultrahigh Mechanical and High Antibacterial Properties for Accelerating Wound Healing." *International Journal of Biological Macromolecules* 119: 402–12. https://doi.org/10.1016/j.ijbiomac.2018.07.060.

Xu, Hengyi, Feng Qu, Hong Xu, Weihua Lai, Y Andrew Wang, Zoraida P Aguilar, and Hua Wei. 2012. "Role of Reactive Oxygen Species in the Antibacterial Mechanism of Silver Nanoparticles on Escherichia Coli O157:H7." *BioMetals* 25 (1): 45–53. https://doi.org/10.1007/s10534-011-9482-x.

Xu, Xiaoyi, Qingbiao Yang, Yongzhi Wang, Haijun Yu, Xuesi Chen, and Xiabin Jing. 2006. "Biodegradable Electrospun Poly(l-Lactide) Fibers Containing Antibacterial Silver Nanoparticles." *European Polymer Journal* 42 (9): 2081–87. https://doi.org/10.1016/j.eurpolymj.2006.03.032.

Yang, Chih-Hui, Lung-Shuo Wang, Szu-Yu Chen, Mao-Chen Huang, Ya-Hua Li, Yun-Chul Lin, Pei-Fan Chen, Jei-Fu Shaw, and Keng-Shiang Huang. 2016. "Microfluidic Assisted Synthesis of Silver Nanoparticle–Chitosan Composite Microparticles for Antibacterial Applications." *International Journal of Pharmaceutics* 510 (2): 493–500. https://doi.org/10.1016/j.ijpharm.2016.01.010.

Yang, Xiao, Wen Liu, Guanghui Xi, Mingshan Wang, Bin Liang, Yifen Shi, Yakai Feng, Xiangkui Ren, and Changcan Shi. 2019. "Fabricating Antimicrobial Peptide-Immobilized Starch Sponges for Hemorrhage Control and Antibacterial Treatment." *Carbohydrate Polymers* 222: 115012. https://doi.org/10.1016/j.carbpol.2019.115012.

Yang, Xiaomin, Qi Liu, Xiliang Chen, Feng Yu, and Zhiyong Zhu. 2008. "Investigation of PVA/Ws-Chitosan Hydrogels Prepared by Combined γ-Irradiation and Freeze-Thawing." *Carbohydrate Polymers* 73 (3): 401–8. https://doi.org/10.1016/j.carbpol.2007.12.008.

Yao, Kang De, Tao Peng, Han Bao Feng, and Yu Ying He. 1994. "Swelling Kinetics and Release Characteristic of Crosslinked Chitosan: Polyether Polymer Network (Semi-IPN) Hydrogels." *Journal of Polymer Science Part A: Polymer Chemistry* 32 (7): 1213–23. https://doi.org/10.1002/pola.1994.080320702.

Ye, Qingsong, Martin C Harmsen, Marja JA van Luyn, and Ruud A Bank. 2010. "The Relationship between Collagen Scaffold Cross-Linking Agents and Neutrophils in the Foreign Body Reaction." *Biomaterials* 31 (35): 9192–201. https://doi.org/10.1016/j.biomaterials.2010.08.049.

Yenier, Zafer, Yoldas Seki, İbrahim Şen, Kutlay Sever, Ömer Mermer, and Mehmet Sarikanat. 2016. "Manufacturing and Mechanical, Thermal and Electrical Characterization of Graphene Loaded Chitosan Composites." *Composites Part B: Engineering* 98: 281–87. https://doi.org/10.1016/j.compositesb.2016.04.072.

Yin, Bingsheng, Houyi Ma, Shuyun Wang, and Shenhao Chen. 2003. "Electrochemical Synthesis of Silver Nanoparticles under Protection of Poly(N-Vinylpyrrolidone)." *The Journal of Physical Chemistry B* 107 (34): 8898–904. https://doi.org/10.1021/jp0349031.

Ying, Huiyan, Juan Zhou, Mingyu Wang, Dandan Su, Qiaoqiao Ma, Guozhong Lv, and Jinghua Chen. 2019. "In Situ Formed Collagen-Hyaluronic Acid Hydrogel as Biomimetic Dressing for Promoting Spontaneous Wound Healing." *Materials Science and Engineering: C* 101: 487–98. https://doi.org/10.1016/j.msec.2019.03.093.

Yokoyama, F, I Masada, K Shimamura, T Ikawa, and K Monobe. 1986. "Morphology and Structure of Highly Elastic Poly(Vinyl Alcohol) Hydrogel Prepared by Repeated Freezing-and-Melting." *Colloid and Polymer Science* 264 (7): 595–601. https://doi.org/10.1007/BF01412597.

Yuan, Xiaoya. 2011. "Enhanced Interfacial Interaction for Effective Reinforcement of Poly(Vinyl Alcohol) Nanocomposites at Low Loading of Graphene." *Polymer Bulletin* 67 (9): 1785–97. https://doi.org/10.1007/s00289-011-0506-z.

Zawadzki, Jerzy, and Halina Kaczmarek. 2010. "Thermal Treatment of Chitosan in Various Conditions." *Carbohydrate Polymers* 80 (2): 394–400. https://doi.org/10.1016/j.carbpol.2009.11.037.

Zhang, Shaohan, Jingyi Hou, Qijuan Yuan, Peikun Xin, Huitong Cheng, Zhipeng Gu, and Jun Wu. 2020. "Arginine Derivatives Assist Dopamine-Hyaluronic Acid Hybrid Hydrogels to Have Enhanced Antioxidant Activity for Wound Healing." *Chemical Engineering Journal* 392: 123775. https://doi.org/10.1016/j.cej.2019.123775.

Zhang Di, Wei Zhou, Bing Wei, Xin Wang, Rupei Tang, Jiemin Nie, and Jun Wang. 2015. "Carboxyl-Modified Poly(Vinyl Alcohol)-Crosslinked Chitosan Hydrogel Films for Potential Wound Dressing." *Carbohydrate Polymers* 125: 189–99. https://doi.org/10.1016/j.carbpol.2015.02.034.

Zheng, Lian-Ying, and Jiang-Feng Zhu. 2003. "Study on Antimicrobial Activity of Chitosan with Different Molecular Weights." *Carbohydrate Polymers* 54 (4): 527–30. https://doi.org/10.1016/j.carbpol.2003.07.009.

Zhou, Yingshan, Qi Dong, Hongjun Yang, Xin Liu, Xianze Yin, Yongzhen Tao, Zikui Bai, and Weilin Xu. 2017. "Photocrosslinked Maleilated Chitosan/Methacrylated Poly (Vinyl Alcohol) Bicomponent Nanofibrous Scaffolds for Use as Potential Wound Dressings." *Carbohydrate Polymers* 168: 220–26. https://doi.org/10.1016/j.carbpol.2017.03.044.

Zhu, Jie, Faxue Li, Xueli Wang, Jianyong Yu, and Dequn Wu. 2018. "Hyaluronic Acid and Polyethylene Glycol Hybrid Hydrogel Encapsulating Nanogel with Hemostasis and Sustainable Antibacterial Property for Wound Healing." *ACS Applied Materials & Interfaces* 10 (16): 13304–16. https://doi.org/10.1021/acsami.7b18927.

3 Hydroxyapatite-Based Coatings Aimed for Hard Tissue Implants

Traditional metallic implants are irreplaceable in repairing damaged bone tissue, but the greatest concern is their gradual electrochemical degradation (Manivasagam, Dhinasekaran, and Rajamanickam 2010). Bone fractures are one of the most common forms of injury along with bone diseases and that is why metallic implants with bioactive and biocompatible-coated materials are often used in order to enhance the bone healing process (Eftekhari et al. 2014). Synthetic hydroxyapatite (HAP, $Ca_{10}(PO_4)_6(OH)_2$) has long been known as one of the best coating materials for metallic implants due to its biocompatible, osteoconductive, and osteoinductive properties (Fidancevska et al. 2007). Besides controlling the stoichiometry of synthetic HAP, the control of crystallinity, porosity, particle shape, surface area, and agglomeration characteristics are of great interest (M S Djošić et al. 2008; V. B. Mišković-Stanković 2014). Materials implanted in the human body face an environment that is extremely delicate but at the same time hostile. The implants confront a severe corrosive environment that includes blood and body fluid composed of several constituents (water, sodium, chlorine, proteins, plasma, and amino acids) along with mucin in the case of saliva. The noncompatible metal ions released by the implants into the body are found to cause allergic and toxic reactions. To minimize direct contact between metal and body fluids, and to limit the release of undesired metallic ions in the body, biocompatible and bioactive coatings on the metallic substrate, such as HAP, are suggested by many researchers (Rath et al. 2012; M. Geetha et al. 2009; Swetha et al. 2010).

Titanium and its alloys have become the material of choice for long-term implant application for their favorable corrosion resistance as well as their low toxicity, biocompatibility, and good mechanical properties, such as high strength, durability, and light weight (C. X. Wang, Wang, and Zhou 2002; García, Ceré, and Durán 2006; Kung, Lee, and Lui 2010; Moseke et al. 2011). Hence, a good combination of the biocompatibility of hydroxyapatite and the excellent mechanical properties of titanium is considered a promising approach to fabricate more suitable bone implants. The concept of coating titanium implant surfaces with HAP combines the mechanical benefits of metal alloys with the biocompatibility of HAP (Stoch et al. 2001).

Postoperative infections are the result of bacterial adhesion to the implant surface and subsequent biofilm formation at the implantation site (Mouriño, Cattalini, and Boccaccini 2012). To stop bacterial infection, it is crucial to inhibit bacterial adhesion since biofilm can be very resistant to immune response and antibiotics (Rameshbabu

DOI: 10.1201/9781032668895-3

et al. 2007). The antimicrobial activity of silver and silver ions has been known for a very long time; additionally, silver cation does not develop bacterial resistance, and, at the same time, it shows low toxicity to human cells (Lee et al. 2006; Pang and Zhitomirsky 2008). Therefore, the possibility to prevent bone implant infections by using antimicrobial properties of Ag has generated great interest in the development of silver-doped HAP coatings (Simchi et al. 2011).

There are various methods to deposit ceramic coatings on metal surfaces, including plasma spraying, sputtering, pulsed laser deposition, sol-gel, electrophoresis, and electrodeposition (Song, Shan, and Han 2008). Among these, electrophoretic deposition (EPD) emerges as a method of choice due to its simple setup and formation of uniform coatings, even on substrates of complex shape (V. B. Mišković-Stanković 2014; Boccaccini, Keim et al. 2010; Corni, Ryan, and Boccaccini 2008; Boccaccini, Cho et al. 2010; Kaya, Singh, and Boccaccini 2008). Other advantages are that EPD represents an inexpensive electrochemical technique that can be carried out at room temperature with the possibility of coating thickness and morphology controlled by adjusting deposition parameters. The necessary condition that enables successful EPD is a stable suspension/sol, where the particles have a high zeta potential while the ionic conductivity of the suspension is kept at a low value (V. B. Mišković-Stanković 2014; Van der Biest and Vandeperre 1999; Božić et al. 2023).

In recent years, research has been focused on improving the biocomposite HAP/polymer coatings and other functional properties of the implant, such as good adhesion properties, chemical stability, bioactivity, biocompatibility, and antimicrobial properties. Biodegradable natural or synthetic polymers are used to develop new biocomposite coatings. Use of the polymer dictates that thermal treatment of the composite material be performed at lower sintering temperatures (Shuai et al. 2012). Development of HAP/biopolymer coatings is especially important for applications in medicine, specifically transplantation surgery, because their mechanical properties are most similar to natural bone tissue (Alves Cardoso, Jansen, and G. Leeuwenburgh 2012). Other characteristics of biocomposite coating that make it biocompatible are non-toxicity, corrosion stability, and controlled biodegradibility as well as elastic modulus, therefore it is suitable for specific biomedical applications. The use of natural biopolymers, such as polysaccharides – alginate, chitosan/chitin and hyaluronic acid, proteins – collagen and silk, as well as different biofibers – lignin and cellulose – offers the advantage of improving the adhesion of bioceramic coating by decreasing its brittleness (Alves Cardoso, Jansen, and G. Leeuwenburgh 2012). Significant interest was shown and investigations were focused on the fabrication of composite coatings: HAP/chitosan (Simchi et al. 2011; Boccaccini, Keim et al. 2010; J. Wang, de Boer, and de Groot 2004; Martin et al. 2008; Xianmiao et al. 2009; Gebhardt et al. 2012; Mahmoodi et al. 2013), HAP/chitosan/carbon nanotubes (Batmanghelich and Ghorbani 2013), aluminosilicate nanotubes/HAP/hyaluronic acid (Deen and Zhitomirsky 2014), HAP/alginate (Cheong and Zhitomirsky 2008), Bioglass®/HAP/chitosan and Bioglass®/HAP/alginate coatings (D. Zhitomirsky et al. 2009), HAP/glucose (P. Li et al. 2009), Y_2O_3/HAP (Parente et al. 2013), HAP/lignin (Raschip et al. 2007; Y. Park, Doherty, and Halley 2008; Mansur, Mansur, and Bicallho 2005; Martinez, Pacheco, and Vargas 2009; Erakovic et al. 2009; Eraković et al. 2012; Eraković, Janković, Veljović et al. 2013; Eraković, Janković, Matić et al. 2013; Erakovic et al. 2014), HAP/graphene (Janković, Eraković, Mitrić et al. 2015; Janković, Eraković, Vukašinović-Sekulić et al. 2015), HAP/TiO_2 (Pantović Pavlović et al. 2019), HAP/chitosan oligosaccharide lactate (Pantović Pavlović et al. 2020, 2021, 2023).

3.1 HYDROXYAPATITE-BASED COATINGS WITH SILVER NANOPARTICLES AIMED FOR HARD TISSUE IMPLANTS

3.1.1 Hydroxyapatite/Lignin Coatings

3.1.1.1 Synthesis and Characterization

Organosolv lignin emerged as a suitable candidate for composite hydroxyapatite/natural polymer coatings. Lignin (Lig) is a complex natural polyphenolic polymer connected with a variety of chemical bonds. Lignin possesses antioxidant and antimicrobial properties; therefore, its incorporation in different materials is attractive in medical applications due to its biocompatibility, hydrophilicity, and thermal stability. Among the functional groups present in lignin, the most reactive chemical sites are phenolic hydroxyl groups. Other major chemical functional groups in lignins include methoxyl, carbonyl, and carboxyl groups, varying on the plant origin and the applied pulping processes. Organosolv lignins are being examined because they show significantly improved solubility and thermal properties compared to sulfite or kraft lignins. Biocomposite hydroxyapatite/lignin as a 3D scaffold was first studied by Mansur et al. (Mansur, Mansur, and Bicallho 2005) where organosolv lignin polymer was used. Pan et al. (Pan et al. 2006) examined the solubility and physicochemical properties of extracted organosolv lignin. Excellent solubility of lignin, more than 90%, is obtained from the solution that contained more than 65% of ethanol. For the same reason, the HAP/Lig coatings on titanium were precipitated from ethanol suspensions.

Hydroxyapatite/lignin (HAP/Lig) and silver/hydroxyapatite/lignin (Ag/HAP/Lig) biocomposite coatings on titanium were deposited by EPD, mimicking the structure and properties of natural bone (Erakovic et al. 2009; Eraković et al. 2012; Eraković, Janković, Veljović et al. 2013; Eraković, Janković, Matić et al. 2013; Erakovic et al. 2014) with the aim to improve porosity structure to prompt osteogenesis. Organosolv Alcell lignin was extracted from a mixture of North American hardwoods (maple, birch, and poplar) by an organosolv process using a mixture of ethanol and water. A nanosized HAP powder was obtained using a modified chemical precipitation method by the reaction of calcium oxide with phosphoric acid described elsewhere (Palcevskis et al. 2005; Veljović et al. 2009). A modified chemical precipitation method was also employed for preparing the Ag/HAP powder ($Ca_{9.95}Ag_{0.05}(PO_4)_6(OH)_2$) using calcium oxide and $AgNO_3$ solution, yielding a final concentration of silver ion of 0.4 ± 0.1 wt. % (Erakovic et al. 2009; Eraković, Janković, Veljović et al. 2013).

The particle size distribution (PSD) measurement of HAP/Lig and Ag/HAP/Lig with 1 wt. % Lig suspensions was made by using a dynamic light-scattering technique. The obtained average particle size is around 363.0 nm, for HAP/Lig suspension, and 207.3 nm, for Ag/HAP/Lig suspension (Erakovic et al. 2009; Eraković, Janković, Veljović et al. 2013). It was assumed for both suspensions that bigger particles are agglomerates of smaller ones, since transmission electron microscopy images of the HAP powder demonstrated that HAP particles are nanosized in the range of 50–100 nm (Palcevskis et al. 2005). Also, it was noticed that pure HAP suspension had much higher average particle size value (1500 nm) compared to HAP/Lig suspension (Erakovic et al. 2009). Therefore, it can be concluded that lignin decreases agglomeration of HAP nanoparticles.

The ζ-potential is a measure of the strength of interactions between colloid particles, and, hence, it relates to colloid solution stability. A biomaterial's ζ -potential indicates its electric surface properties; bioceramic particles must be electrically charged for electrophoretic deposition on metal substrates. High positive values ζ-potential of HAP/Lig and Ag/HAP/Lig suspensions of 28 and 29 mV, respectively, indicate positively charged particle surfaces of HAP/Lig and Ag/HAP/Lig particles, thus enabling the attraction of particles by negatively charged cathode and successful electrophoretic deposition of coatings on titanium substrate (Eraković et al. 2012; Eraković, Janković, Veljović et al. 2013).

Electrophoretic deposition of HAP/Lig and Ag/HAP/Lig coatings on titanium was performed from ethanol suspensions (Erakovic et al. 2009; Eraković et al. 2012; Eraković, Janković, Veljović et al. 2013; Eraković, Janković, Matić et al. 2013). The deposition parameters, applied voltage, and deposition time significantly influence the coating morphology and thickness. The process was optimized by varying EPD voltage from 50 to 100 V at different deposition times of 30 s to 5 min (Erakovic et al. 2009). Increase in deposition time up to 5 min at constant voltage of 60 V enhances the mass of HAP/Lig and Ag/HAP/Lig coatings since more particles are reaching the cathode. On the other hand, the obtained coatings are more porous since greater amounts of hydrogen evolved from the cathode, leaving more vacancies in the deposited coatings. Therefore, the optimal ratio of coating mass and porosity in both composite coatings was achieved at constant voltage of 60 V for 45 s (Erakovic et al. 2009).

The influence of the lignin concentration in the range of 0.5–10 wt.% Lig on the microstructure, morphology (Figure 3.1), phase composition, thermal behavior, antimicrobial activity, and cytotoxicity of composite HAP/Lig coatings electrodeposited on titanium was investigated in order to find the optimal lignin concentration for producing HAP/Lig composite coatings (Erakovic et al. 2009; Eraković et al. 2012; Erakovic et al. 2014). FE-SEM micrograph of sintered HAP/Lig coating with 1 wt. % Lig (Figure 3.1b) shows homogeneous fracture-free surface. Comparing the micrographs of the sintered HAP coatings with different amount of incorporated lignin, HAP/Lig coating with 1 wt.% Lig indicated that lignin strengthens the bonding between HAP particles and the substrate surface. Based on these results, the optimal lignin concentration to obtain coatings with a smooth surfaces without fractures was 1 wt. %. Four types of hydrogen bonding were proposed as possible interactions

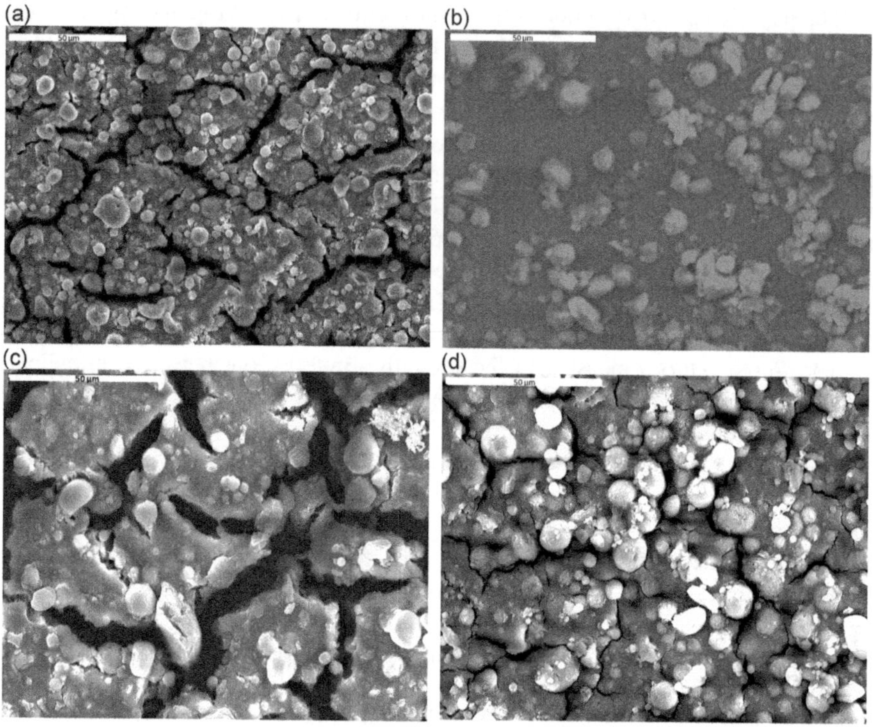

FIGURE 3.1 FE-SEM micrographs of sintered HAP/Lig coatings with (a) 0.5, (b) 1, (c) 3, and (d) 10 wt.% Lig (reprinted from (Erakovic et al. 2014) with permission from MDPI)

between HAP and lignin (Erakovic et al. 2009): between phenolic hydroxyl –OH from lignin and –OH from HAP, between α-carbonyl from lignin side chain –C=O and –OH from HAP, between –OH from lignin and PO_4^{3-} from HAP, and between ether bond oxygen from lignin C–O–C and –OH from HAP.

The phase composition and structure of HAP and HAP/Lig coatings were investigated by XRD analysis (Erakovic et al. 2009; Eraković et al. 2012). All the peaks in XRD patterns of the non-sintered HAP/Lig coatings (0.5–10 wt.% Lig) corresponded to the hydroxyapatite. After sintering, the diffraction peaks of all HAP/Lig coatings become sharper and of higher intensity with a decrease in peak width, indicating that sintered coatings had a better crystallinity (Eraković et al. 2012). A higher degree of crystallinity would make coatings less prone to dissolution in body fluids (Kwok et al. 2009). The sintering depends on the characteristics of the initial HAP powder, and the smaller particles have a tendency to aggregate in order to minimize their high free surface energy, resulting in densification and an increase in the grain size (Landi et al. 2000; Mostafa 2005). Therefore, the initial nanosized HAP powder was successfully sintered at a temperature of 900 °C and the same temperature was applied as thermal treatment of all composite HAP/Lig coatings, although the usually applied sintering temperature is in a range between 1000 °C and 1300 °C.

Comparing the XRD patterns of sintered HAP and HAP/Lig coatings, the partial HAP decomposition during thermal treatment at 900 °C was observed only for pure HAP coating and HAP/Lig coating with 0.5 wt.% Lig, while HAP/Lig coatings containing 1, 3, and 10 wt.% Lig did not show any new crystalline phase (Erakovic et al. 2009, 2012). As an example, in the case of pure HAP coating, beside the main peaks corresponding to HAP, the observed new diffraction peaks for CaO, $Ca(OH)_2$, and $CaCO_3$ crystalline phases indicated the HAP coating decomposition that were not observed for HAP/Lig coating with 1 wt.% Lig. It can be explained by reaction of CaO, generated during HAP decomposition at sintering temperature, with traces of atmospheric water and CO_2, yielding $Ca(OH)_2$ and $CaCO_3$, respectively (Ye, Liu, and Hong 2009a). In the case of sintered HAP/Lig coating with 0.5 wt.% Lig, beside these peaks a new phase TiP appeared (Eraković et al. 2012), which could be explained by the diffusion of phosphorous ions into the Ti surface as a result of HAP decomposition. It was reported that during the thermal treatments, the diffusion of calcium (limited diffusion) and phosphorus (profuse diffusion) ions into the Ti substrate occur, resulting in the HAP decomposition (Eraković et al. 2012; Filiaggi, Pilliar, and Coombs 1993). By comparing the diffraction patterns of all sintered HAP/Lig coatings, it can be concluded that degradation of hydroxyapatite did not occur for lignin concentrations of 1 wt.% and higher, meaning that higher lignin concentrations protect the HAP lattice from decomposition during sintering.

The mean crystallite domain size, D_p, of the HAP/Lig coatings was calculated using the Scherrer equation (3.1.) and half height width, $\beta_{1/2}$, of XRD reflection of (002) plane at $2\theta \approx 26°$:

$$D_P = \frac{K\lambda}{\beta_{1/2} \cos ,} \tag{3.1}$$

where λ is the wavelength of the X-ray radiation, K is the shape coefficient equal to 0.9, and θ is the diffraction angle. No microstrain corrections were taken into account. The values of mean crystallite domain size were calculated to be between 35 and 39 nm for HAP/Lig coatings with 0.5, 1, 3, and 10 wt.% Lig, indicating that mean crystallite domain size does not depend on the lignin concentration.

The qualitative analysis of the XPS spectra of pure HAP and HAP/Lig coatings revealed certain differences between non-sintered and sintered coatings (Erakovic et al. 2009; Eraković et al. 2012). The quantitative analysis data of the XPS spectra obtained from high-resolution measurements are presented in Table 3.1.

The carbon content of non-sintered HAP/Lig coating with 1 wt.% Lig is higher than that of non-sintered HAP coating, which confirms the presence of lignin. On the other hand, the carbon content of the non-sintered HAP/Lig coatings increased with increasing lignin concentration, proving that lignin was bonded to the HAP lattice. However, the highest increase in the carbon content after sintering was evidenced for pure HAP and HAP/Lig coating with 0.5 wt.% Lig, which could be explained by $CaCO_3$ formation by reaction between CaO with atmospheric CO_2. XRD analysis also confirmed the decomposition of HAP and HAP/Lig coating with 0.5 wt.% Lig. A small increase in the carbon content for sintered HAP/Lig coatings with 1 and

TABLE 3.1
Quantitative XPS Analysis Data for HAP and HAP/Lig Coatings (Reprinted from Erakovic et al. 2014 with Permission from MDPI)

HAP/Lig (wt. % Lig)		Ca	P	C	Ca/P
0 (Pure HAP)	Non-sintered	19.4	11.3	7.2	1.72
	Sintered	16.5	5.5	21.7	3.00
0.5	Non-sintered	19.1	11.3	8.2	1.69
	Sintered	18.4	7.9	15.9	2.33
1	Non-sintered	19.3	10.8	10.5	1.79
	Sintered	18.7	8.9	11.3	2.10
3	Non-sintered	18.4	12.0	11.7	1.53
	Sintered	18.8	10.8	12.9	1.74
10	Non-sintered	15.8	10.3	21.3	1.53
	Sintered	17.1	9.6	18.9	1.78

3 wt.% Lig, and decrease in carbon content for sintered HAP/Lig coatings with 10 wt.% Lig compared to non-sintered coatings, indicated the absence of HAP decomposition during sintering. This means that lignin limited the formation of $CaCO_3$. XPS results are in accordance with the XRD results obtained for HAP/Lig coatings with lignin concentration higher than 0.5 wt.%, pointing to the absence of HAP lattice decomposition during sintering. The calculated Ca/P ratio varied in the range of 1.53–1.69 for the non-sintered HAP and HAP/Lig coatings, which is similar to the Ca/P ratio for stoichiometric HAP (1.67). According to the literature (Caroline Victoria and Gnanam 2002), stable HAP phases correspond to Ca/P ratio within a range of 1.3–1.8. It could be observed that the Ca/P ratios of the sintered HAP/Lig coatings were higher than those of the non-sintered (Table 3.1.). The highest increase in Ca/P ratio to 3.00 for sintered HAP coating and 2.33 for sintered HAP/Lig coating with 0.5 wt.% Lig can be explained by diffusion of phosphorus ions, resulting in the partial HAP decomposition and also the presence of a new TiP peak in XRD pattern (Eraković et al. 2012). It could be concluded that lignin limited the decomposition of the HAP lattice of sintered HAP/Lig coatings with 1–10 wt.% Lig as indicated by the smaller increase in carbon content and smaller Ca/P ratio, compared to pure HAP coating and HAP/Lig coating with 0.5 wt.% Lig. This is in accordance with XRD results.

ATR-FTIR measurements were used to identify and verify the presence of specific functional groups on the surfaces of non-sintered and sintered HAP and HAP/Lig coatings (Erakovic et al. 2009, 2012). The spectra of non-sintered HAP and HAP/Lig coatings with different lignin concentration exhibit characteristic $\upsilon_1 PO_4^{3-}$, $\upsilon_3 PO_4^{3-}$, and $\upsilon_4 PO_4^{3-}$ bands typical for the PO_4^{3-} group. In addition, the characteristic band at 630 cm^{-1} corresponds to the vibration of structural OH^- groups (Kaya, Singh, and Boccaccini 2008). The ATR-FTIR spectra of HAP/Lig coatings before sintering are very similar to the ATR-FTIR spectrum of pure HAP coating with respect to the functional groups, which indicates that the lignin in HAP/Lig coatings does not significantly alter the structure of the hydroxyapatite lattice (Erakovic et al. 2009, 2012). However, in the ATR-FTIR spectrum of HAP/Lig coatings, the appearance of C–H deformation vibration corresponds to C–H bonds in the aromatic rings, as well as to bands for the methoxy group of lignin. This implies that lignin in the HAP/Lig coating did not change the formation and structure of the HAP lattice. Most of the lignin hydroxyl groups are phenolic hydroxyl groups, which have a strong ability to form hydrogen bonds with the carbonyl groups and would induce an obvious shift of the band position to lower wavenumbers. The appearance of ν(O–H) vibrations in OH^- groups from HAP occurred at a lower wavelength than expected, confirming the intermolecular hydrogen bonds (P–O···OH) between OH^- groups from lignin and PO_4^{3-} groups from hydroxyapatite. By comparing the ATR-FTIR spectra for sintered HAP/Lig coatings, it was observed that HAP decomposition during sintering does not occur for coatings with lignin concentration 1, 3, and 10 wt.% Lig. In other words, lignin concentrations of 1 wt.% and higher prevent HAP decomposition and/or diffusion of phosphorus ions into the Ti surface due to the established hydrogen bonds.

3.1.1.2 Biomechanical Properties

Nanoindentation technique has become a method of choice for studies of mechanical characteristics of bicomposite coatings due to its many advantages: the test depth can be less than coating thickness, the nanomechanical response of the coated system can be measured on the substrate *in situ*, and the test can be performed at variable displacements. The technique thus represents a unique way of ascertaining elastic, plastic, and fracture responses of surfaces (Roop Kumar and Wang 2002).

The elastic modulus and hardness of sintered HAP coating and HAP/Lig coating with 1 wt.% lignin were analyzed by nanoindentation test (Erakovic et al. 2014). The mean hardness, H, was measured to be 7.40 GPa for the HAP coating, while the mean reduced elastic modulus, E_r, was found to be 132 GPa. These values are in agreement with published data (Roop Kumar and Wang 2002) for bulk hydroxyapatite ($H = 6.19$ GPa–6.76 GPa and $E_r = 122$ GPa–125 GPa) as well as for thin film coatings. The HAP/Lig (1 wt.% Lig) coating showed mean hardness of 6.90 GPa and mean reduced elastic modulus of 134 GPa, which were comparable to those of the pure HAP coating. In general, for biomedical metallic implants aimed for total hip and knee replacements, the bonding strength (or inter-laminar shear strength) between implant and coating layer is the most important issue for lifespan of replaced implant. Therefore, the obtained E_r and H results for HAP/Lig coating leads to the conclusion that lignin does not significantly affect the mechanical properties of the composite, probably due to small concentrations of incorporated lignin.

3.1.1.3 Cytotoxicity and Antibacterial Activity

Cell survival was determined using the 3-(4,5-dimethylthiazol-2-yl)-2,5-dipheny ltetrazolium bromide (MTT) test (Erakovic et al. 2014) according to the method of Mosmann (Mosmann 1983), which was modified by Ohno and Abe (Ohno and Abe

1991). The MTT test is based on 3-(4,5-dimethylthiazol-2-yl)-2,5-diphenyltetrazolium bromide to assess the activity of living cells by their mitochondrial dehydrogenase activity. The nutrient medium was RPM1 1640 medium supplemented with 10% heat-inactivated bovine serum, penicillin (100 IU mL^{-1}), streptomycin (100 μg mL^{-1}), L-glutamine (3 mM), and 25 mM Hepes. To analyze the biological effects of HAP and HAP/Lig coatings on human cells, cytotoxicity experiments were conducted on human peripheral blood mononuclear cells (PBMC) after stimulation to proliferation with mitogen phytohemagglutinin (PHA). The survival of PHA-stimulated PBMC in the control sample and in the presence of pure HAP and HAP/Lig coatings (1 and 10 wt.% Lig) were investigated 72 h after seeding.

Cell survival, *S* (%), is defined as the ratio of the number of cells grown in nutrient medium with coating and the number of cells grown in control wells containing nutrient medium without coating, multiplied by 100. As the number of live cells is directly proportional to the absorbance of live metabolically active MTT-treated cells, for the calculation of cell survival, absorbance of the newly formed formazan was used instead of the number of live cells. Therefore, cell survival can be calculated as the ratio of absorbance of the cells grown in the presence of coating and absorbance of the cells of the control sample. The absorbance of the blank was always subtracted from the absorbance of the corresponding cell sample. The results are reported as the average value ± standard deviation (SD) from three independent experiments. The survival of PBMC stimulated to proliferate with mitogen phytohemagglutinin (PHA) in control sample and in the presence of sintered HAP and HAP/Lig coatings with 1 and 10 wt. % Lig (Table 3.2) show that the survival of the PHA-stimulated PBMC did not decrease significantly with increasing lignin concentration (Eraković et al. 2012). MTT results indicate that HAP and both HAP/

TABLE 3.2
Cell Survival of PBMC and PHA-Stimulated PBMC Cells in the Presence of Sintered HAP, HAP/Lig, and Ag/HAP/Lig Coatings (Reprinted from Eraković et al. 2012 with Permission from Elsevier and Erakovic et al. 2014 with Permission from MDPI)

Cell Type	PHA-Stimulated Peripheral Blood Mononuclear Cells (PBMC)			PHA-Stimulated Peripheral Blood Mononuclear Cells (PBMC)	Peripheral Blood Mononuclear Cells (PBMC)
Coating	HAP	HAP/Lig (1 wt. % Lig)	HAP/Lig (10 wt. % Lig)	Ag/HAP/Lig (1 wt. % Lig)	Ag/HAP/Lig (1 wt. % Lig)
Cell survival (*S*), %	93.4 ± 4.0	90.4 ± 8.2	83.7± 5.8	83.8 ± 6.3	89.4 ± 3.5
Classification	Non-cytotoxic	Non-cytotoxic	Slightly cytotoxic	Non-cytotoxic	Non-cytotoxic

Lig coatings could induce a mild decrease in survival of healthy immunocompetent PHA-stimulated PBMC but that all the results were similar to that of the control sample ($S = 100$ %). According to the literature (Sjögren, Sletten, and Dahl 2000), HAP coating and HAP/Lig coating with 1 wt.% Lig can be classified as non-toxic, while HAP/Lig coating with 10 wt.% Lig as slightly cytotoxic. The reason for the slight lignin cytotoxicity could be due to its known absorption capability, i.e. it could slightly non-specifically absorb some of the micronutrient constituents needed for sustaining tested PBMC proliferation, but also due to lignin antioxidant activity, as shown in tests on human keratinocytes and mouse fibroblasts (Ugartondo, Mitjans, and Vinardell 2008).

Post-surgical infections of the implantation site are the major problem and inevitably lead to revision surgeries. Antibacterial activities of the samples were tested for microorganisms that are responsible for most of the inter-hospital infections. Gram-positive bacterium *Staphylococcus aureus* (*S. aureus*) and Gram-negative bacterium *Escherichia coli* (*E. coli*) can cause serious infections. The antibacterial activity of sintered HAP and HAP/Lig (1 wt.% Lig) coatings on titanium was tested on two bacteria types, bacterial strains *E. coli* (ATCC-25922) and *S. aureus* TL by using the agar diffusion method (Erakovic et al. 2014). The results of antimicrobial activity were estimated by measuring the inhibition zone of bacterial growth formed around the samples (mm). There was no light zone around the HAP coating and HAP/Lig coating (1 wt.% Lig) after 24 hours of incubation in the case of both bacterial strains, meaning that both pure HAP and HAP/Lig coating with 1 wt.% Lig did not exhibit antimicrobial activity. Therefore, the subsequent course of research aimed to obtain biocomposite coating doped with silver ions, a major antimicrobial agent.

3.1.2 Sintered Silver/Hydroxyapatite/Lignin Coatings

3.1.2.1 *In Vitro* Bioactivity

In vitro bioactivity of silver-doped hydroxyapatite/lignin (Ag/HAP/Lig) coating electrodeposited on Ti was tested by immersion in simulated body fluid (SBF) solution. The influence of silver on the microstructure, morphology, phase composition, thermal behavior, antimicrobial activity, and cytotoxicity as well as on bioactivity of Ag/HAP/Lig coating with 0.5 wt.% Ag and 1 wt.% Lig was investigated (Eraković, Janković, Veljović et al. 2013). After seven days in SBF the samples were characterized by FE-SEM, XRD, and ATR-FTIR.

The FE-SEM micrographs revealed newly formed plate-shaped apatite crystals after immersion in SBF solution. A relatively high porosity of implant surface along with improved mechanical stability provides better cell adhesion that facilitates osteointegration. The key point is that high interconnected porosity structures enable the penetration of osteoblasts, leading to better connection between the implant and the bone (García, Ceré, and Durán 2006). The composition of new plate-shaped crystals was revealed by ATR-FTIR and XRD analysis (Eraković, Janković, Veljović et al. 2013), while the formation of apatite has been previously explained by Sun et al. (Sun et al. 2006). Briefly, the negatively charged hydroxyapatite surface interacts with Ca^{2+} ions from SBF, forming an amorphous positive Ca-rich surface. Subsequently, thus formed surfaces interact with the negative PO_4^{3-} ions in the SBF to form Ca-poor apatite, which gradually crystallizes into bone-like apatite. Once formed in SBF, the apatite grows spontaneously, consuming the calcium and phosphate ions, incorporating ions such as sodium, magnesium, and carbonate, and thereby developing a bone mineral-like compositional and structural feature (Kim et al. 2005).

XRD analysis was performed to determine the phase composition and structure of Ag/HAP/Lig coatings before and after immersion in SBF. XRD diffractograms of Ag/HAP/Lig coating before immersion in SBF showed only characteristic hydroxyapatite peaks without any additional crystalline phases even after sintering, meaning that lignin protected Ag/HAP lattice during sintering. Labeled XRD peaks match very well hydroxyapatite, but incorporation of Ag in the hydroxyapatite crystal lattice caused a shift of specific HAP peaks toward smaller 2θ values, confirming the silver substitution for calcium (Eraković, Janković, Veljović et al. 2013). The Ag presence was verified through the shift of characteristic HAP peaks (crystal planes (002), (211), (112), and (300)) toward smaller angles for the Ag/HAP coating before immersion in SBF compared to the pure HAP coating. The additional peaks that originate from the Ti substrate indicate the suboxide of titanium, Ti_3O, which is classified as a nonstoichiometric oxide deficient in oxygen. The complex valence status of Ti appears to be due to the oxygen diffusion from the exterior surface to the inside during sintering. According to Ye et al. (Ye, Liu, and Hong 2009b), Ti metal and Ti suboxides on the composite surfaces are believed to be more active than TiO_2 in the physiological environment and can activate chemical bonding between the implant surface and adjacent biomolecules. After seven days of immersion in SBF solution, a new phase was detected by observing the shift in characteristic HAP peaks toward higher angles. These findings were attributed to carbonate ions in the lattice and confirmed, therefore, the growth of carbonated HAP onto the surface of Ag/HAP/Lig coating. The mean crystallite domain size, D_p, was calculated at $2\theta \approx 26°$ by Eq. 3.1. The crystallite domain size of Ag/HAP/Lig coating before and after soaking in SBF was calculated to be almost the same, 20.8 and 22.0 nm, respectively, indicating the homogeneous surface. Small difference between the crystallite size before and after immersion is probably due to the incorporation of CO_3^{2-} ions into the apatite lattice by occupying the OH^- sites or the PO_4^{3-} positions.

The presence of CO_3^{2-} bands in ATR-FTIR spectrum is clear evidence of its incorporation in the HAP layer, since it is well known that the biological hydroxyapatite contains carbonate groups (Pecheva et al. 2004). Ag/HAP/Lig coating was investigated by the ATR-FTIR method before and after immersion in SBF solution (Eraković, Janković, Veljović et al. 2013). Before immersion in SBF, the ATR-FTIR spectrum exhibited characteristic hydroxyapatite bands. The presence of phosphate groups was confirmed by vibrational bands at 960, 1016, and 1089 cm^{-1}. Also, the weak characteristic bands at around 3573 and 627 cm^{-1} corresponding to the vibration of structural OH– groups have been found in the hydroxyapatite lattice. The absence of a low-intensity wide band at wavenumbers between 1400 and 1585 cm^{-1} before immersion in SBF confirmed that there was no decomposition of hydroxyapatite, as also has been detected by XRD. After seven days of immersion in SBF at

37 °C carbonated apatite was formed, which could be seen from three peaks at 1640, 1476, and 1420 cm^{-1}, attributed to the vibrational bands of CO_3^{2-} groups. According to the literature, B-type carbonated apatite appears on the surface after soaking in SBF solution (Ye, Liu, and Hong 2009b; Dong, Li, and Zou 2009). The spectrum of bone-like apatite showed a high concentration of OH^- and PO_4^{3-} groups compared to the peaks appearing in the spectrum of Ag/HAP/Lig coating before immersion in SBF, which allows the coating surface to exhibit the negative surface potentials required for apatite nucleation. Therefore, the formation of carbonated HAP is very beneficial due to its weak crystalline form that resembles human bone, a property that facilities osteointegration.

The chemical composition of the outermost coating surface level is important because it would be in direct contact with the bone tissue and dissolve first at the initial stage of implantation. It has been shown that the optimum Ca/P ratio is 1.67–1.76 (Bai et al. 2009). From a semi-quantitative XPS analysis of Ag/HAP/Lig coating, Ca/P ratio was calculated to be 1.62 (Eraković, Janković, Veljović et al. 2013).

Electrochemical impedance spectroscopy (EIS) was employed to investigate the bioactivity of Ag/HAP/Lig coating in the physiological environment. The Nyquist plots in complex plane for the impedance of Ag/HAP/Lig coating deposited on titanium after a prolonged exposure time in SBF solution at 37 °C were obtained, where the high-frequency range is attributed to the coating, while the low-frequency range describes the characteristics of the passive oxide layer on titanium (Eraković, Janković, Veljović et al. 2013). Fitting of the experimental data obtained from Nyquist plots in complex plane for 14 days in SBF was accomplished by using the equivalent electrical circuit (EEC) shown in Figure 3.2a, consisting of the electrolyte resistance, R_s, the coating pore resistance, R_p, and constant phase elements, CPE_c and CPE_{ox}, which represent all the frequency-dependent electrochemical phenomena, i.e. the coating capacitance, C_c, and the passive oxide film capacitance, C_{ox}, respectively. CPE is used in these models to compensate for non-homogeneity in the system and is defined by two parameters, Y_0 and n. The impedance of CPE is represented by the following equation (Orazem and Tribollet 2008):

$$Z_{CPE} = Y_0^{-1} \times (j\omega)^{-n} \tag{3.2}$$

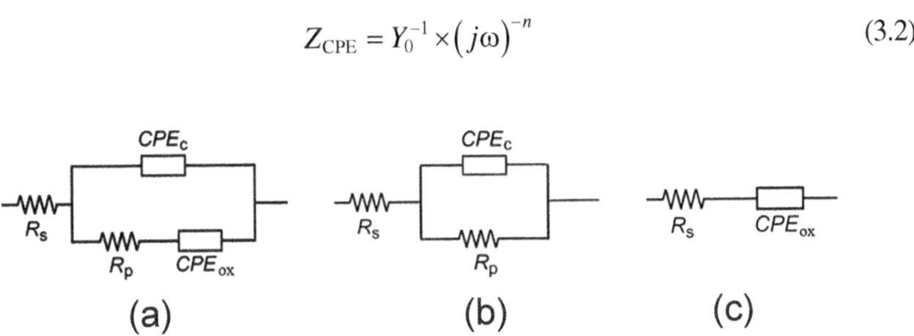

FIGURE 3.2 Equivalent electrical circuits for fitting of experimental Nyquist impedance plots in complex plane (adapted from Eraković, Janković, Matić et al. 2013 with permission from Elsevier)

where $j = (-1)^{1/2}$, $\omega = 2\pi f$ is frequency in rad s^{-1} and f is the frequency in Hz. If n values range from 0.8 to 1, the impedance of CPE can be considered to be the one of the pure capacitor:

$$Z_{CPE} = \left(j\omega C\right)^{-n} \tag{3.3}$$

In this case Y_0 gives a pure capacitance (C). The impedance data in the complex plane were well fitted by the proposed EEC and three basic criteria were used to evaluate the general accuracy of the fit: visual fit to Nyquist plots, low goodness of fit and low relative standard errors for every circuit element (Orazem and Tribollet 2008). The obtained fitting results are listed in Table 3.3.

As seen in Table 3.3, n_c and n_{ox} values for sintered Ag/HAP/Lig coating are close to 0.8; therefore, CPE_c can be considered as coating capacitance, C_c, while CPE_{ox} can

TABLE 3.3
The Fitting Values of Equivalent Electrical Circuits Parameters for Sintered Ag/HAP/Lig (1 wt.% Lig) Coating (Reprinted from Erakovic et al. 2014 with Permission from MDPI) and Non-Sintered Ag/HAP/Lig (1 wt.% Lig) (Reprinted from Eraković, Janković, Matić et al. 2013 with Permission from Elsevier).

Coating	t/h	R_s/Ω cm²	CPE_{ox}/μF cm⁻²	n_{ox}	CPE_c /μF cm⁻²	n_c	R_p/kΩ cm²
Sintered Ag/HAP/Lig (1 wt.% Lig)	1	43.3	1030.0	0.76	745.2	0.88	4.3
	3	44.5	1046.0	0.80	697.6	0.88	5.2
	6	44.5	1010.0	0.81	667.9	0.88	5.9
	8	44.1	880.1	0.77	655.8	0.88	6.1
	24	29.2	620.8	0.70	627.2	0.88	5.6
	72	23.1	821.3	0.76	588.2	0.88	6.4
	120	31.5	610.4	0.74	560.6	0.89	5.9
	168	18.8	782.4	0.77	559.3	0.88	5.8
	240	21.8	522.0	0.74	543.5	0.88	6.3
	288	21.3	475.8	0.70	529.0	0.88	6.9
	336	17.7	403.2	0.71	547.1	0.87	6.3
Non-sintered Ag/HAP/Lig (1 wt.% Lig)	1	29.4	118.0	0.91	33.3	0.88	10.4
	72	50.6	101.9	0.91	34.4	0.88	13.0
	120	87.8	75.8	1.00	36.4	0.87	110.3
	168	82.0	-	-	35.4	0.86	634.7
Bare titanium	1	21.1	33.2	0.88	-	-	-
	72	72.9	26.8	0.89	-	-	-
	120	13.9	25.7	0.90	-	-	-
	168	29.7	24.1	0.90	-	-	-

be considered as capacitance of oxide film on the titanium surface beneath Ag/HAP/Lig coating, C_{ox}. The time dependence of coating pore resistance, R_p, and the coating capacitance, C_c, of the Ag/HAP/Lig coating during 14 days in SBF are presented in Table 3.3. It can be noticed that the coating pore resistance, R_p, increased and the coating capacitance, C_c, decreased during the exposure to SBF, which is related to the growth of the newly formed apatite layer on the coating surface. The continuous increase in R_p up to 6.3 kΩ cm^2 and decrease in C_c up to 547.1 μF cm^{-2} reflect the process of the apatite nucleation after prolonged time in SBF, in accordance with FE-SEM, XRD, and ATR-FTIR analysis. This suggests that Ag/HAP/Lig coating surface represented the site of nucleation and the growth of a new carbonated apatite layer able to induce stable bonding to bone.

3.1.2.2 Biomechanical Properties

Ag/HAP coating had reduced elastic modulus, E_r, and mean hardness, H, of 172 GPa and 14.5 GPa, respectively, while Ag/HAP/Lig coating with 1 wt.% lignin had slightly higher H and lower E_r values of 173 GPa and 13.3 GPa, respectively (Erakovic et al. 2014). Comparing HAP and HAP/Lig coating and their counterparts with silver, it was observed that the addition of Ag contributed to the increase of both E_r (172 GPa *vs.* 132 GPa) and H (14.5 GPa *vs.* 7.40 GPa).

An evaluation of E/H value is a prerequisite for the evaluation of fracture toughness. In the case of pure HAP and Ag/HAP coatings, E_r/H ratios were 17.86 and 11.87, respectively, while in the case of HAP/Lig and Ag/HAP/Lig coatings E_r/H ratios were 19.34 and 13.00, respectively, indicating that Ag reinforcement caused decrements in the value of E_r/H, implying that toughness values may be affected with Ag addition. On the other hand, calculated E_r/H ratio for HAP and HAP/Lig coatings was 17.86 and 19.34, respectively, and for Ag/HAP and Ag/HAP/Lig was 11.87 and 13.00, respectively. It can be concluded that the E_r/H ratio was similar for coatings with and without lignin, meaning the small concentration of 1 wt.% lignin does not affect mechanical properties of composite coatings.

3.1.2.3 Cytotoxicity and Antibacterial Activity

Cytotoxicity of Ag/HAP/Lig (1 wt.% Lig) coating was determined by MTT test against PBMC and PHA-stimulated PBMC cells (Eraković, Janković, Veljović et al. 2013; Erakovic et al. 2014) since it is important to produce the biomaterials that will not exert toxic effects against cells of the surrounding tissue as well as against healthy immunocompetent PBMC, components of the immune response. Examination of cytotoxic effects of the investigated Ag/HAP/Lig coating with 1 wt.% Lig (Table 3.2) showed a mild decrease in survival of healthy immunocompetent PBMC, unstimulated (89.4%) and PHA-stimulated (83.8%) compared to the control cell sample (S = 100%), while cell survival of PHA-stimulated PBMC in the presence of HAP/Lig coating was 90.4%. According to cytotoxicity classification (Sjögren, Sletten, and Dahl 2000), both Ag/HAP and Ag/HAP/Lig coating with 1 wt.% Lig was displayed as non-cytotoxic against target PBMC cells.

Recently, research in orthopedic surgery has focused on the development of surface modified devices that are capable of releasing drugs adapted to the clinical situation (antibiotics, antimicrobial agents, etc.) in a controlled and predictable manner, according to established kinetic laws. Silver, as Ag ions and Ag nanoparticles, are well known as primary inorganic antimicrobial agents that have been widely used in different fields of medicine. Although not completely revealed, it is assumed that Ag ion disrupts the bacterial cell integrity by binding to the enzymes and proteins within the bacteria, thus accelerating their death. The antibacterial activity of sintered Ag/HAP/Lig (1 wt. % Lig) coatings was tested against pathogenic Gram-positive bacteria strain *S. aureus* TL (Erakovic et al. 2014) and was noticed immediately after inoculation of samples and further reduction of cell viability for two logarithmic units is achieved after just one hour of incubation when compared to the initial number of cells in suspensions (from 1.0×10^5 CFU mL^{-1} to 2.0×10^3 CFU mL^{-1}). Based on silver ion release results, the concentration of silver ions after one hour was 0.4493 ppm (Eraković, Janković, Matić et al. 2013), which is a sufficiently small concentration to achieve antibacterial effect without causing cytotoxicity. The total reduction in the bacterial numbers after 24 hours indicated antimicrobial activity of 0.5 wt.% Ag in Ag/HAP/Lig coating, providing good protection against infection. Moreover, an immediate silver ion release provided for the imminent drop in CFU numbers even after one hour of exposure, which is the bactericidal effect needed for prevention of biofilm formation (Jamuna-Thevi et al. 2011).

3.1.3 Non-Sintered Silver/Hydroxyapatite/Lignin Coatings

3.1.3.1 *In Vitro* Bioactivity

FE-SEM microphotographs revealed the surface homogeneity of non-sintered Ag/HAP/Lig (1 wt.% Lig) coating before immersion in SBF, while newly formed plate-shaped apatite crystals are evident after soaking in SBF solution. The composition of new apatite crystals was revealed by ATR-FTIR and XRD analysis (Eraković, Janković, Matić et al. 2013). Before immersion in SBF, the ATR-FTIR spectrum exhibited characteristic hydroxyapatite bands, while PO_4^{3-} groups were confirmed by vibrational bands at 963, 1021, and 1086 cm^{-1} in ATR-FTIR spectrum. The appearance of a small peak around 3600 cm^{-1} along with broad band at 1600 cm^{-1} corresponds to the OH^- stretching in the hydroxyapatite lattice. Two peaks at 1420 and 1448 cm^{-1} characteristic for methoxy groups revealed the presence of biopolymer lignin in Ag/HAP/Lig coating. Lignin can be traced through the appearance of the slight shoulder at 875 cm^{-1} from the C–H vibration in the aromatic rings. The band at 635 cm^{-1} for OH^- vibrations from HAP lattice indicates the intermolecular hydrogen bonds between HAP and Lig (El-Hendawy 2006). The appearance of absorption peak at 1101 cm^{-1} due to (P–O) stretching of the phosphorous group also proposed that intermolecular hydrogen bonds between OH^- groups from lignin and PO_4^{3-} groups from HAP were established. The ATR-FTIR spectrum of the non-sintered Ag/HAP/Lig coating after seven days immersion in SBF solution exhibited the broad absorbance band at 3380 cm^{-1} attributed to the OH^- stretching with higher intensity than the intensity before immersion, revealing the formation of a new bone-like apatite layer on the coating surface (Sun et al. 2006). Three peaks at 1642, 1460, and 1424 cm^{-1} attributed to the vibrational bands of CO_3^{2-} groups (B-type carbonated apatite) confirmed formation of biological apatite (Eraković, Janković, Veljović et al. 2013).

The XRD patterns of non-sintered Ag/HAP/Lig coating before immersion in SBF exhibited characteristic hydroxyapatite peaks at (002), (211), and (300) crystal planes at 2θ = 25.740°, 31.56°, and 32.47°, respectively (Eraković, Janković, Matić et al. 2013). After seven days of immersion in SBF, the new carbonated HAP phase was detected by the shift in characteristic HAP peaks at (002), (211), and (300) crystal planes toward higher angles, which is beneficial due to its weak crystalline form that resembles human bone and facilities osetointegration (Stoch et al. 1999).

Surface analysis was performed by XPS measurements on non-sintered Ag/HAP/Lig coating (Eraković, Janković, Matić et al. 2013) before soaking in SBF and obtained deconvoluted spectra corresponded to characteristic elements for hydroxyapatite (Ca and P). The measured binding energy (BE) values were calibrated by the C1s (hydrocarbon C–C, C–H) of 285 eV. The Ca 2p spectrum of the Ag/HAP/Lig coating has doublet Ca 2p 3/2 (BE of 347.1 eV) and Ca 2p 1/2 (BE of 350.6 eV) peaks and the P 2p spectrum has single P 2p 3/2 peak at BE position of 133.6 eV, indicating the presence of hydroxyapatite (Yao et al. 2010). The deconvoluted elements of the C 1s had four components with peak positions at 285 eV, 286.7 eV, 288.2 eV, and 289.3 eV, which correspond to aromatic hydrocarbons, alcoxy, and $RCOO^-$ groups, respectively (Battistoni et al. 2000). Concerning the C 1s line, the new peak occurred at 289.3 eV (C=O bonds), suggesting the presence of lignin (Dupraz et al. 1999). In addition, the interaction mechanism of hydrogen bonding can be detected by XPS. The hydrogen bonding between C=O and –OH groups represented by an increase in O 1s BE of the C=O groups and decrease in O 1s BE of the –OH groups. The O 1s signal at 533.1 eV may be attributed to PO_4^{3-} groups, while at 532.4 eV corresponds to –OH groups from HAP (Dupraz et al. 1999; Viornery et al. 2002). Therefore, the O 1s lines is at higher BE than it is for O 1s for PO_4^{3-} groups, indicating hydrogen bonding between lignin and HAP lattice. From semi-quantitative XPS analysis the atomic percentages of elements were calculated to be 5.5% C1s, 63.9% O1s, 18.3% Ca $2p_{3/2}$, and 11.3% P 2p, while Ca/P ratio was calculated to be 1.62, similar to the value of Ca/P ratio in stoichiometric hydroxyapatite (1.67). The stable hydroxyapatite has to be within a range of 1.3 – 1.8 for Ca/P ratio (Bai et al. 2009).

EIS measurements were performed in order to study the bioactivity of non-sintered Ag/HAP/Lig coating during exposure to SBF solution at 37 °C. The Nyquist impedance plots of Ag/HAP/Lig coating on titanium and bare titanium used as reference, after three, five, and seven days in SBF are presented in Figures 3.3a and b, respectively. The inset in Figure 3.3a provides Nyquist plots of Ag/HAP/Lig coating in the high-frequency range. High-frequency range is attributed to the Ag/HAP/Lig coating, while the low-frequency range represents the characteristics of the passive titanium oxide film beneath the coating.

The Nyquist impedance plots were fitted with the equivalent electrical circuits shown in Figure 3.2. The equivalent circuit used for the fitting of impedance data for Ag/HAP/Lig coating during initial time of exposure (Figure 3.2a) consists of the electrolyte resistance, R_s, the coating pore resistance, R_p, the constant phase elements CPE_c and CPE_{ox}, which include all the frequency-dependent electrochemical

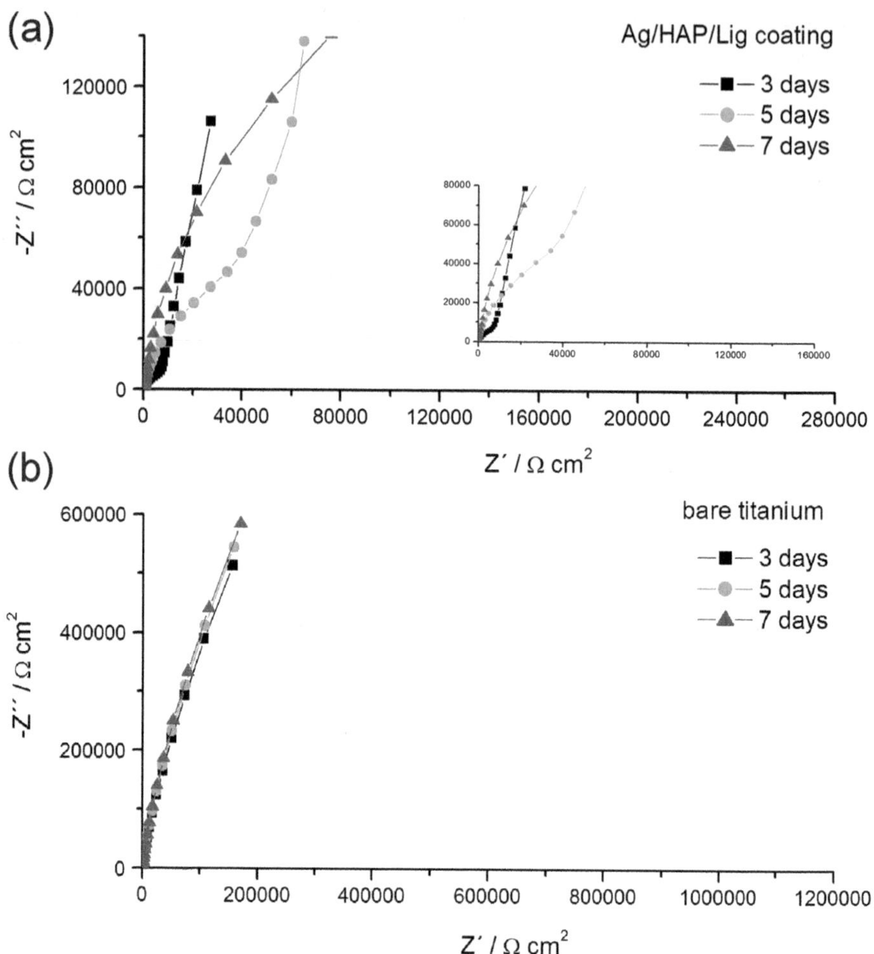

FIGURE 3.3 The Nyquist plots of (a) non-sintered Ag/HAP/Lig (1 wt.% Lig) coating on titanium and (b) bare titanium, after different times of exposure to SBF at 37 °C (reprinted from Eraković, Janković, Matić et al. 2013 with permission from Elsevier)

phenomena, namely coating capacitance, C_c, and capacitance of passive oxide film beneath Ag/HAP/Lig coating, C_{ox}, respectively, and diffusion processes. The equivalent circuit used for the fitting of impedance data for Ag/HAP/Lig coating during prolonged time of exposure (Figure 3.2b) consists of the electrolyte resistance, R_s, the coating pore resistance, R_p, and the constant phase element CPE_c. For impedance analysis of bare titanium, the equivalent circuit represented in Figure 3.2c was used, where R_s is the electrolyte resistance and CPE_{ox} is the constant phase element for passive oxide film on titanium surface. The fitting results are listed in Table 3.3.

It can be seen from Table 3.3 that n_c and n_{ox} values for non-sintered Ag/HAP/Lig coating and bare titanium are higher than 0.8; therefore, CPE_c can be considered as coating capacitance, C_c, while CPE_{ox} can be considered as capacitance of oxide film on the titanium surface beneath Ag/HAP/Lig coating, C_{ox}. An equivalent electrical circuit shown in Figure 3.2a was used for fitting of Nyquist plots of Ag/HAP/Lig coating during five days of exposure to SBF solution. According to these results, R_p and C_c remain almost constant during the first three days of exposure to SBF solution, while after the fifth day the R_p value was ten times higher, indicating the beginning of the formation of a new apatite layer. After the seventh day the impedance Nyquist plot could not be fitted more with equivalent circuit shown in Figure 3.2a and instead the equivalent circuit in Figure 3.2b was used. After seven days in SBF solution the calculated value of R_p was 634.7 kΩ cm^2, indicating the new carbonated HAP on the coating surface. This was already confirmed by FE-SEM, ATR-FTIR, and XRD results.

EIS spectra of bare titanium (Figure 3.3b) exposed to SBF solution were fitted with equivalent electrical circuit shown in Figure 3.2c and exhibit behavior typical of a thin passive oxide film on titanium surface. Furthermore, the slight decrease in C_{ox} during immersion time (Table 3.3) corresponded to a slow growth of the titanium oxide film, indicating a long-term stability of the thin oxide film in SBF solution.

3.1.3.2 Cytotoxicity

The coatings doped with silver ions provided high initial concentration of antimicrobial agent in surrounding tissue. This property is especially important in early critical post-implantation period since it prevents initial adhesion of bacteria (Jamuna-Thevi et al. 2011). However, continuous silver ion release after this critical period is also desirable to prevent bacteria biofilm formation. The cumulative silver ion release from the non-sintered Ag/HAP/Lig with 1 wt.% Lig coating after ten days was measured to be 1.704 ppm (Eraković, Janković, Matić et al. 2013). Jamuna-Thevi et al. (Jamuna-Thevi et al. 2011) previously reported that minimum silver ion concentration is 0.1 ppb and the maximum cytotoxic concentration toward human cells is 10 ppm; therefore, the measured concentration was within this range.

Cytotoxicity of non-sintered Ag/HAP/Lig (1 wt. % Lig), Ag/HAP and Ag/HAP/Lig (10 wt. % Lig) coatings was determined by MTT test against PBMC and PHA-simulated PBMC cells (Table 3.4).

Examination of cytotoxic effects of Ag/HAP and Ag/HAP/Lig coatings showed mild decrease in survival of healthy immunocompetent PBMC, unstimulated and PHA-stimulated compared to the control cell sample ($S = 100$ %). According to classification found in literature (Sjögren, Sletten, and Dahl 2000), Ag/HAP coating and Ag/HAP/Lig coating with 1 wt. % Lig displayed as non-cytotoxic against PBMC, while Ag/HAP/Lig coating with 10 wt. % Lig is classified as slightly cytotoxic. The survival of PBMC was higher in the presence of Ag/HAP/Lig coating with 1 wt. % Lig than in the presence of Ag/HAP/Lig coating with 10 wt. % Lig, proving the optimum non-toxic lignin concentration of 1 wt. %.

3.1.3.3 Antibacterial Activity

Antibacterial effect of non-sintered Ag/HAP/Lig (1 wt.% Lig) coatings was investigated against pathogenic Gram-positive bacteria strain *S. aureus* TL in PB solution

TABLE 3.4
Survival of PBMC Cells and Stimulated PBMC with Addition of Mitogen Phytohaemagglutinin (PHA) in the Presence of Non-Sintered Ag/HAP and Ag/HAP/Lig Coatings (Reprinted from Eraković, Janković, Matić et al. 2013 with Permission from Elsevier)

Cell Type	**Peripheral Blood Mononuclear Cells (PBMC)**		
Coating	Ag/HAP	Ag/HAP/Lig (1 wt. % Lig)	Ag/HAP/Lig (10 wt. % Lig)
Cell Survival (*S*), %	94.6 ± 4.2	89.4 ± 3.5	76.0 ± 7.6
Classification	Non-cytotoxic	Non-cytotoxic	Slightly Cytotoxic
Cell Type	**PHA-Stimulated Peripheral Blood Mononuclear Cells (PBMC)**		
Cell Survival (*S*), %	92.1 ± 5.0	83.8 ± 6.3	79.6 ± 6.3
Classification	Non-cytotoxic	Non-cytotoxic	Slightly Cytotoxic

(Eraković, Janković, Matić et al. 2013). The titanium coated samples without silver (HAP and HAP/Lig coatings) were used as a control when comparing the antibacterial effect of Ag/HAP and Ag/HAP/Lig coatings (Figure 3.4). Pure HAP and HAP/Lig coatings did not show any antibacterial effect and inhibition was not observed even after 24 h. A slight decrease in the total number of cells after one hour of incubation with samples HAP and HAP/Lig probably occurs as a result of adhesion of cells to the particles of HAP. Antibacterial activity of the Ag/HAP and Ag/HAP/Lig coatings could be noticed immediately after inoculation of samples and further reduction of cells viability for two logarithm units was achieved after just one hour of incubation when compared to the initial number of cells in suspensions (percentage of cell reduction was 98.17% and 97.67%, respectively). Based on the silver ion released results, concentration of silver ion after one hour was 0.4493 ppm, which is a sufficiently small concentration to achieve antibacterial effect without causing cytotoxicity (Table 3.4). The antibacterial efficiency of non-sintered Ag/HAP and Ag/HAP/Lig coatings exhibited high reduction of bacteria strain *S. aureus* TL since after 24 hours analyzed samples did not contain any viable cell (Figure 3.4), providing good protection against infection. An immediate silver ion release provides for the imminent drop in CFU numbers even after one hour of exposure, which is bactericidal effect needed for prevention of biofilm formation (Jamuna-Thevi et al. 2011).

3.1.4 Hydroxyapatite/Graphene Coatings

3.1.4.1 Synthesis and Characterization

The extraordinary electrical, thermal, and mechanical properties of graphene (Gr) (e.g., tensile strength 130 GPa and Young's modulus 0.5–1 TPa) and high specific surface area (up to 2630 m^2g^{-1}) have drawn great attention as a reinforcement in the

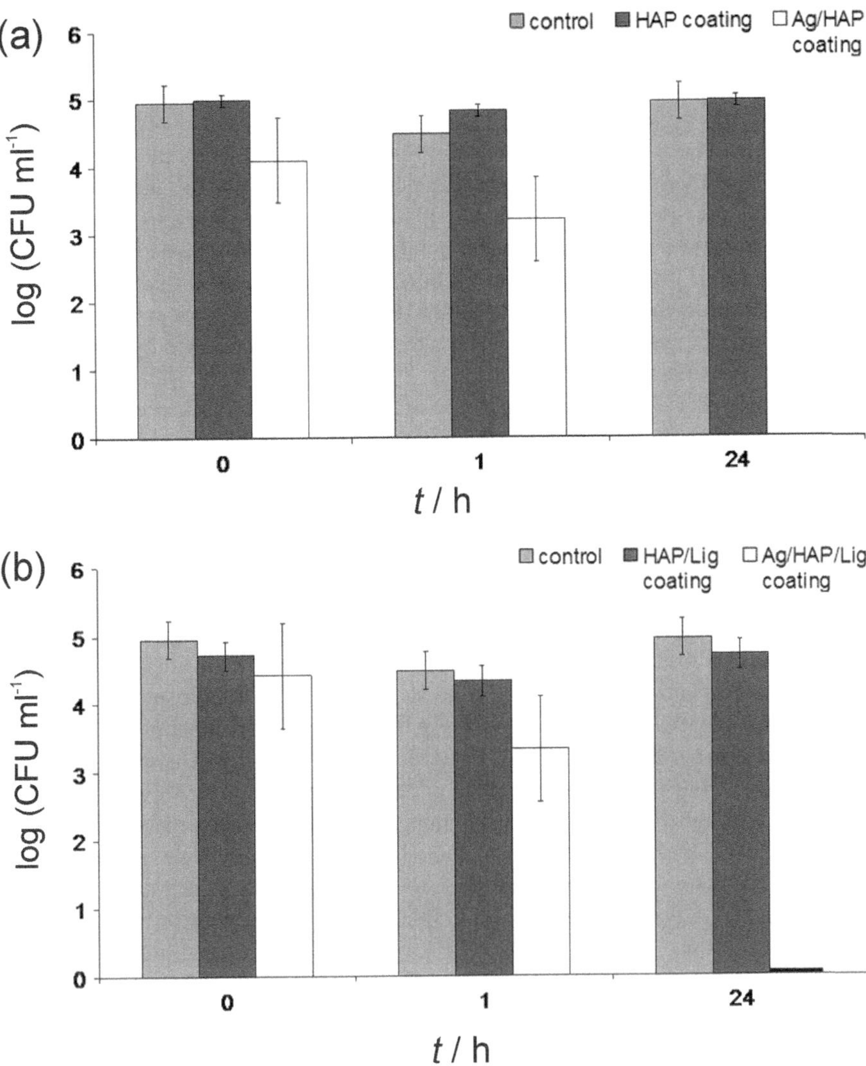

FIGURE 3.4 Reduction of viable cell number of *S. aureus* TL after contact with non-sintered (a) HAP and Ag/HAP coatings and (b) HAP/Lig and Ag/HAP/Lig coatings, for 0, 1 h, and 24 hours in PB as compared to the control w/o samples (reprinted from Eraković, Janković, Matić et al. 2013 with permission from Elsevier)

composite field of material science. Graphene materials possess physical properties identical to those of carbon nanotubes (CNTs) but have a larger surface area. It has been reported that inclusion of Gr into polymer or ceramic matrices leads to remarkable improvements in the properties of the host materials (Neelgund, Oki, and Luo 2013). Furthermore, graphene nanosheets (GNSs), formed by several layers of Gr with a thickness of up to 100 nm (Jian Liu et al. 2012), are much easier to produce than other graphene materials and successfully use as nanofillers for polymers (Kuilla et al. 2010), metals (Bartolucci et al. 2011), and ceramics (L. Zhang et al. 2013; Belmonte et al. 2013) to produce composites with exceptional mechanical properties.

Biomaterials used in orthopedic surgery usually encounter complex service environments and therefore require versatile performances from the materials (Witte 2010). HAP provides bioactivity, biocompatibility, and an ability to initiate osteogenesis, but on the other side it lacks good mechanical properties. Because of its poor mechanical properties, such as an intrinsic brittleness, low fracture toughness (0.8–1.2 MP), low flexural strength (<140 MPa), and wear resistance, the main focus of HAP research has been to improve its mechanical performance by combining it with various reinforcements.

The focus of the latest published research has been the fabrication of Gr or its derivatives to create reinforced HAP biocomposites because of the exciting findings regarding the biological performance of Gr. Nonetheless, the mechanical properties of hydroxyapatite limit its use in the regeneration of various parts of the bone systems, especially those under significant mechanical tension. The incorporation of Gr or its derivatives as reinforcing materials in HAP composites can be achieved using *in situ* synthesis, spark plasma sintering (SPS), biomimetic mineralization, chemical vapor deposition, and electrospinning. The general idea of using Gr as nanofiller is to minimize the brittleness of HAP and gain an improved composite. Any reinforcement material for HAP should not only significantly improve the mechanical properties, but also retain HAP's original biocompatibility. Graphene materials aimed to demonstrate that crack deflection is more effective for sheet-like reinforcement than for tubular-like reinforcement, suggesting that Gr exhibits a more pronounced toughening effect on brittle materials than do carbon nanotubes (CNTs). Unlike CNTs, Gr is synthesized in relatively pure ways and is therefore expected to show low cytotoxicity, since few metallic catalyst particles are associated with its production. Advantages of Gr and Gr-based composites are low toxicity toward human osteoblasts (Kalbacova et al. 2010), excellent antibacterial properties (Hu et al. 2010), and its potential to initialize apatite mineralization (H. Liu et al. 2012).

Electrophoretic deposition (EPD) was performed from ethanol suspension containing 1 wt. % nanosized HAP and 0.01 wt. % Gr at constant voltage method at 60 V and a deposition time of two minutes (Janković, Eraković, Mitrić et al. 2015). Compared to the pure HAP coating, the HAP/Gr composite coating had fewer cracks and no peeling off the Ti surface in the macroscopic observation. That is a solid indication that Gr effectively acts as a nano-reinforcement filler and prevents the creation and propagation of cracks by frictional pull out, crack deflection, and crack bridging as the major toughening mechanism that resists crack propagation. Namely, the high specific surface area of graphene nanosheets is capable of forming an increased contact area with matrix. As a result, the bonding strength between graphene and HAP grain could be significantly enhanced, and more energy would be required to make the nanofiller pull out from HAP matrix. As previously reported by Zhang et al. (L. Zhang et al. 2013), rough and wrinkled surface texture of the GNSs also plays an important role in enhancing mechanical interlocking, leading to an increased load-transfer efficiency between HAP matrix and GNSs. In addition, it was shown that the two ends of the GNS are well bonded to the adjacent HAP grains with GNS plane nearly parallel to the fracture surface. For ceramics, it is well known that the toughness of grain boundaries is lower than the grains. Thus, as a grain boundary toughening mechanism, it is hypothesized that the grain bridging by GNS plays a fundamental role in inhibiting crack propagation along the grain boundary.

Further evidence of bonding between Gr and HAP was observed by the FT-IR analysis (Janković, Eraković, Mitrić et al. 2015). Three absorption bands were clearly distinguished at 1089, 1024, and 962 cm^{-1} in the υ_3 and υ_1 phosphate mode region. The FT-IR spectra have distinct intensity vibrational bands at 601 and 560 cm^{-1}, corresponding to the υ_4 vibrational mode, as well as a weak intensity band at 470 cm^{-1} as a component of the υ_2 mode that corresponds to P-O bending. The characteristic band at 630 cm^{-1} can be attributed to structural OH^- groups in the HAP lattice. The low intensity band at 875 cm^{-1} indicates the acidic phosphate group HPO_4^{2-} due to the P-(OH) stretching vibration (Wu et al. 2010). The absorbance bands in the range of 1500–1400 cm^{-1} correspond to υ_3 asymmetrical stretching vibrations of the CO_3^{2-} ions. The position of the carbonate bands indicates predominately B-type HAP, which is the preferential substitution in human bones, known for its excellent bioactivity and osteoinductivity. Bands at ~1540 cm^{-1} correspond to the skeletal vibration of Gr (Lian et al. 2010; Xie et al. 2015) due to sp^2 hybridized C=C vibration stretching, confirming its presence in the HAP/Gr coating.

The surface elements of the HAP/Gr coating (14.20 % P2p, 11.90 % C1s, 15.16 % $Ca2p_{3/2}$, 7.33 % $Ca2p_{1/2}$, 51.32 % O1s) and the pure HAP coating (16.36 % P2p, 16.69 % $Ca2p_{3/2}$, 7.86 % $Ca2p_{1/2}$, 58.93 % O1s) were determined using XPS analysis (Janković, Eraković, Mitrić et al. 2015). In the XPS spectra, the Ca2p spectrum reveals a doublet with $Ca2p_{3/2}$ (BE=347.29 eV) and $Ca2p_{1/2}$ (BE=350.82eV), while the P2p spectrum reveals a single P2p peak at BE=133.33 eV, indicating the presence of HAP (Watling et al. 2011). The main O1s peak component at BE=531.27 eV for the HAP/Gr coating is attributed to PO_4^{3-} groups (Yao et al. 2010). Incorporation of Gr and the formation of the new composite are clearly evidenced by the presence of C1s in the HAP/Gr coating, whereas no trace of carbon is detected in the pure HAP coating. According to the literature, the C1s peak with BE = 285.0 eV is attributed to aromatic hydrocarbons (Watling et al. 2011), which is in excellent compliance with the single-sheet Gr structure of honeycomb six-membered rings. Calculated Ca/P ratio of 1.58 pointed to stable HAP phase since stable HAP phases have been found to exist over a range of Ca/P ratios from 1.3 to 1.8. The XPS results confirm the presence of Gr and stand in good agreement with the FT-IR analysis result.

Raman spectroscopy was performed to verify the Gr presence in the HAP/Gr composite coating (Janković, Eraković, Mitrić et al. 2015), revealing a distinct pattern of single-layer Gr. The first main feature is the G-peak, visible at 1594 cm^{-1}, which arises due to the in-plane vibration of sp^2 carbon atoms. The G-band corresponds to ordered sp^2-bonded carbon atoms. The second pronounced band is the D peak at 1320 cm^{-1} that represents defects originating from the disordered aromatic structure on the Gr edges.

The HAP/Gr composite coating was subjected to thermogravimetric analysis to explore their thermal stability in detail (Janković, Eraković, Mitrić et al. 2015). The thermogravimetric (TG) and differential TG (DTG) curves revealed the weight loss of the HAP/Gr coating in the observed temperature range (25 °C –1000 °C). The total weight loss for the HAP/Gr coating in the temperature range of 25 °C –1000 °C was 5.28 wt. %, indicating greater thermal stability of graphene-based HAP coating compared to pure HAP coating (7.16 wt. %). The HAP/Gr coating decomposed in a three-step weight loss process. The first stage occurred up to 150 °C, as observed by the sharp DTG peak at 68 °C. This stage is usually assigned to desorption of adsorbed water molecules on the crystallite surface. In the second stage, corresponding to the temperature range from 150 °C to 350 °C, a DTG peak appears at 241 °C that is attributed to the release of crystalline water that represents the beginning of HAP dehydroxylation (Eraković et al. 2012; Eraković, Janković, Veljović et al. 2013) and unstable carbon in the Gr structure (Liang et al. 2009). In the third stage, corresponding to the temperature range between 350 °C and 750 °C, a DTG peak appears at 445 °C that originates from decomposition of the remaining unstable carbon. The third stage can also be attributed to the dehydroxylation and early slow decomposition of HAP (Eraković et al. 2012). At temperatures between 750 °C and 1000 °C, HAP decomposition occurs. The pure HAP coating decomposed in a manner similar to its HAP/Gr counterpart. The first stage, up to 150 °C with a sharp DTG peak at 57 °C, is assigned to desorption of water molecules adsorbed on the crystallite surface. The second stage, from 150 °C to 350 °C with a DTG peak at 230 °C, corresponds to the release of crystalline water, i.e., the onset of HAP dehydroxylation. The third stage, between 350 °C and 750 °C, could be attributed to the complete dehydroxylation of HAP followed by its initial decomposition. Above 750°C, HAP decomposes. An important distinction in the thermal pattern is observed in DTG peak at 445 °C for the HAP/Gr coating, indicating the decomposition of the remaining Gr. That peak is not evident for the pure HAP coating, as expected.

All experimental results obtained from FT-IR, XPS, and TGA analyses confirmed the mechanism of HAP/Gr coating formation, as follows. According to Liu et al. (Yi Liu, Huang, and Li 2013a), there is no obvious evidence indicating the chemical reaction between HAP and graphene sheets at their interfaces. It is instead very likely that HAP and graphene sheets are connected by Van der Waals bonding. Nucleation of HAP crystals probably originates on either the graphene wall or the cross-section of graphene multisheets, followed by subsequent crystal growth along or perpendicular to the surface of the graphene sheet. They proved that the (300) plane of HAP crystals is very likely parallel to the surface of graphene walls. According to the atomic structure of HAP, its (300) plane contains Ca atoms at each corner of the rectangle and the distance between each pair of Ca atoms is 0.9418 nm and 0.6884 nm, whereas the distance between two neighboring Ca atoms in plane (100) is 0.9418 nm and 0.3442 nm, respectively. In addition, it was revealed that the distance between adjacent graphene sheets is 0.347 nm. In fact, single-layer graphene is constituted by carbon atoms arranged periodically in a hexagonal manner, and the nearest distance between two carbon atoms is 0.142 nm. Multilayer graphene sheets contain several graphene monolayers with the inter-wall distance of 0.34 nm. On the other hand, the lattice spacing of the (002) plane of HAP is 0.344 nm. Since (300) plane takes priority over the (100) plane to match with the surface of graphene sheets, and the open ends of graphene multisheets form relatively stronger interfaces with the (002) plane of HAP crystals than other planes like (211), it can be considered that the (300) plane of HA forms a naturally strong and coherent interfacial bond with the surface of the graphene wall and the cross-section of graphene builds with the (002) plane of HAP crystals a stronger interface due to the smaller lattice mismatch. As a consequence, the less cracked morphology and greater thermal stability of HAP/Gr coating were noticed in comparison to pure HAP coating.

3.1.4.2 Biomechanical Properties

The mechanical properties of the HAP/Gr and pure HAP coatings were examined using nanoindentation test and load-penetration depth curves (Janković, Eraković, Mitrić et al. 2015). The HAP/Gr coating was more resistant to indentation and had a higher load than HAP at the same indentation depth. For the HAP/Gr coating, the mean hardness, H, was 14.8±2.0 GPa, almost twice as high as the measured hardness values of pure HAP (7.4±3.3 GPa). The mean reduced elastic modulus, E_r, of the HAP/Gr coating was 190.9±18.0 GPa, an increase of almost 50% in respect to pure HAP coating (E_r = 132.2±25.5 GPa) (Table 3.5). The differences in the mechanical behavior of these two coatings could also be revealed from load-penetration depth curves. HAP/Gr coating with higher hardness has much lower penetration depth than that of the HAP coating. Moreover, the slope of the initial portion of the unloading curve for the HAP/Gr coating is higher than that for the HAP coating. These results are a definite demonstration that the introduction of graphene effectively improves the mechanical properties of HAP, even at a very low concentration. This can be attributed to the proposed toughening mechanism and grain bridging by graphene nanosheets that act by inhibiting crack propagation along the grain boundary. The E_r/H ratio for pure HAP and HAP/Gr coatings was 17.86 and 12.90, respectively, indicating that Gr reinforcement caused decrements in the value of E_r/H, implying that toughness increases with Gr addition as a result of crack bridging, deflection, and grain bridging by the Gr nanofiller.

TABLE 3.5
The Values of Mean Hardness, H, Mean Reduced Elastic Modulus, E_r, and E_r/H Ratio Obtained from the Nanoindentation Testing of HAP, HAP/Gr, Ag/HAP, and Ag/HAP/Gr Coatings

Coating	H / GPa	E_r / GPa	E_r/H
HAP	7.4±3.3	132.2±25.5	17.86
HAP/Gr	14.8±2.0	190.9±18.0	12.90
Ag/HAP	14.5±5.8	172.1±36.9	11.87
Ag/HAP/Gr	15.5±3.3	183.0±21.9	11.81

Although it is well known that the mechanical properties of the metals and alloys used for implantation are not well matched with those of bone, resulting in stress-shielding effects, and stress-shielding phenomenon can lead to severe clinical issues such as implant loosening and reduced stimulation of new bone growth (Niinomi and Nakai 2011), there are a few points that need to be considered especially for long-term implantation since the effect of biological compatibility has a greater bearing than the mechanical compatibility. The biological responses to implant materials strongly depend on the implant's surface properties since the interaction between the cells and biomaterials take place at the tissue–implant interface. Moreover, bio-ceramic coating should provide a Ti-based implant with not only the bioactivity and biocompability for facilitating chemical bonding with living bone tissues, but also a combination of high hardness and high modulus can enhance the wear resistance of the base material to prevent formation of wear debris from the implant surface.

3.1.4.3 *In Vitro* Bioactivity

The bioactivity of the HAP/Gr composite coating was assessed by immersion in SBF solution at 37 °C for seven days (Janković, Eraković, Mitrić et al. 2015). XRD patterns revealed high-intensity HAP peaks at crystal planes (002), (211), (112), and (300), 2θ = 25.8, 32.0, 32.9, and 34.1°, perfectly matching the HAP pattern. As predicted, the Ti substrate is mainly present in its pure form on the coating interface. According to a report by Sharma et al. (Sharma and Gosavi 2014), thermally reduced Gr showed a broad (002) peak at $2\theta = 23$–26°. However, HAP diffraction peaks mostly shielded that peak. In addition, the specific broad peak at $2\theta = 22°$ observed for pure Gr is also overlapped by diffraction peaks originating from HAP. Finally, the carbon peak at $2\theta = 26.6°$, as it appears in diffractograms, is attributed to starting carbon material. The XRD results along with FT-IR and Raman verified the successful incorporation of Gr along with HAP by EPD in the HAP/Gr coating. The formation of a bone-like apatite layer on the surface of bioactive materials has been reported after soaking those materials in a biomimetic system such as SBF. The shift of characteristic HAP peaks at crystal planes (002), (211), and (300) toward higher angles was evident after immersing the HAP/Gr coating in SBF for seven days. Those findings were attributed to carbonate ions in the crystal lattice and confirmed the growth of carbonated HAP. Therefore, the shifting of diffraction peaks is typical for weak crystalline carbonated HAP, as it is found in bone. Using the X-ray Line Profile Fitting Program (XFIT) with a fundamental parameters convolution approach for generating line profiles (Cheary and Coelho 1992), the coherent domain sizes and microstrain of the HAP/Gr composite coating were calculated using the (002), (211), (112), (300), (202), and (301) crystal planes. The crystallite domain size is calculated to be 18.9 nm and 33.7 nm, before and after immersion in SBF, respectively. The difference between the crystallite size before and after immersion is probably due to the incorporation of CO_3^{2-} ions into the apatite lattice by occupying the OH^- sites or the PO_4^{3-} position.

The FE-SEM microphotographs of the HAP/Gr coating before immersion in SBF displayed individual rod-like HAP grains, less than 50 nm in size. After soaking in SBF, the newly formed apatite layer containing plate-shaped HAP crystals was clearly visible (Janković, Eraković, Mitrić et al. 2015). The mineralization area ultimately penetrates the whole surface of the HAP/Gr composite. The morphology of the mineralization product varies dramatically with incorporation of Gr into the HAP matrix. Easily distinct are curled, plate-shaped apatite forms on the HAP/Gr composite coating. Also, the observed highly porous surface structure after soaking is beneficial for better cell adhesion, as it enables better connection between the implant and the bone.

The bioactivity of the HAP/Gr coating is confirmed by the formation of new apatite layer on the coating surface after just seven days soaking in SBF, as proven by XRD and FE-SEM analysis. According to the mechanism proposed by Zhang et al. (L. Zhang et al. 2013), the mineralization process proceeds in three stages: (1) dissolution controlled stage, (2) precipitation controlled stage, and (3) formation of bone-like apatite. In the first stage, dissolution of phosphate and calcium ions occurs. Calcium ion dissolution is governed by grain refinement and accelerates on the surface of the HAP/Gr coatings due to the suppression of HAP grain growth caused by adding Gr on the grain boundaries. As a result, the smaller grain size of the composite leads to increased specific area and improved interaction with SBF. In the second step, precipitation of an apatite layer occurs on the negative surface of the HAP/Gr coating as a consequence of the dissolution of calcium ions and subsequent emergence of nucleation sites. These events, elevated concentration of calcium ions in SBF, higher negative charge, and more available nucleation sites, allow the HAP/Gr coating to form a Ca-rich layer penetrating the whole sample surface. The third stage is the final formation of apatite as the Ca-rich layer attracts phosphate ions from the SBF and forms bonelike apatite clusters.

The bioactivity of HAP/Gr and HAP coatings was also evaluated by EIS measurements (Janković, Eraković, Mitrić et al. 2015), while the impedance spectra during different exposure times in SBF at 37 °C are presented in Figure 3.5.

Fitting of the Nyquist plots was accomplished using the equivalent electrical circuits (EECs) shown in Figures 3.2a and c. EECs consist of the electrolyte resistance, R_s, the coating pore resistance, R_p, and CPE_c and CPE_{ox}, constant phase elements that represent all the frequency-dependent electrochemical phenomena, such as the coating capacitance, C_c, and passive oxide film capacitance, C_{ox}. The obtained fitting values for each EEC parameter are presented in Table 3.6 for both the HAP/Gr and the HAP coatings. As clearly seen, the n_c and n_{ox} values are higher than 0.80 for both coatings; therefore, CPE_c can be considered the coating capacitance, C_c, and CPE_{ox} can be considered the capacitance of the oxide film on the Ti surface beneath the coating, C_{ox}. The EEC shown in Figure 3.2a was used for fitting the Nyquist plots of the HAP/Gr composite coating over 14 days, and the EEC in Figure 3.2c was used for fitting the Nyquist plot for the 15th day of SBF exposure, when coating adhesion loss had occurred. The R_p for the HAP/Gr coating decreased slightly during the first two days, indicating that the SBF solution diffused into the coating pores and filled it out during the initial 48 hours. After the third day, increasing values of R_p indicate the beginning of the biomineralization process to form a new apatite layer onto the HAP/Gr surface. Finally, the calculated value of R_p was 34.2 kΩ cm^2 (Table 3.6) after 14 days of immersion in SBF solution. The high value of the coating pore resistance, R_p, denotes improved bioactivity, which suggests that the HAP/Gr coating surface

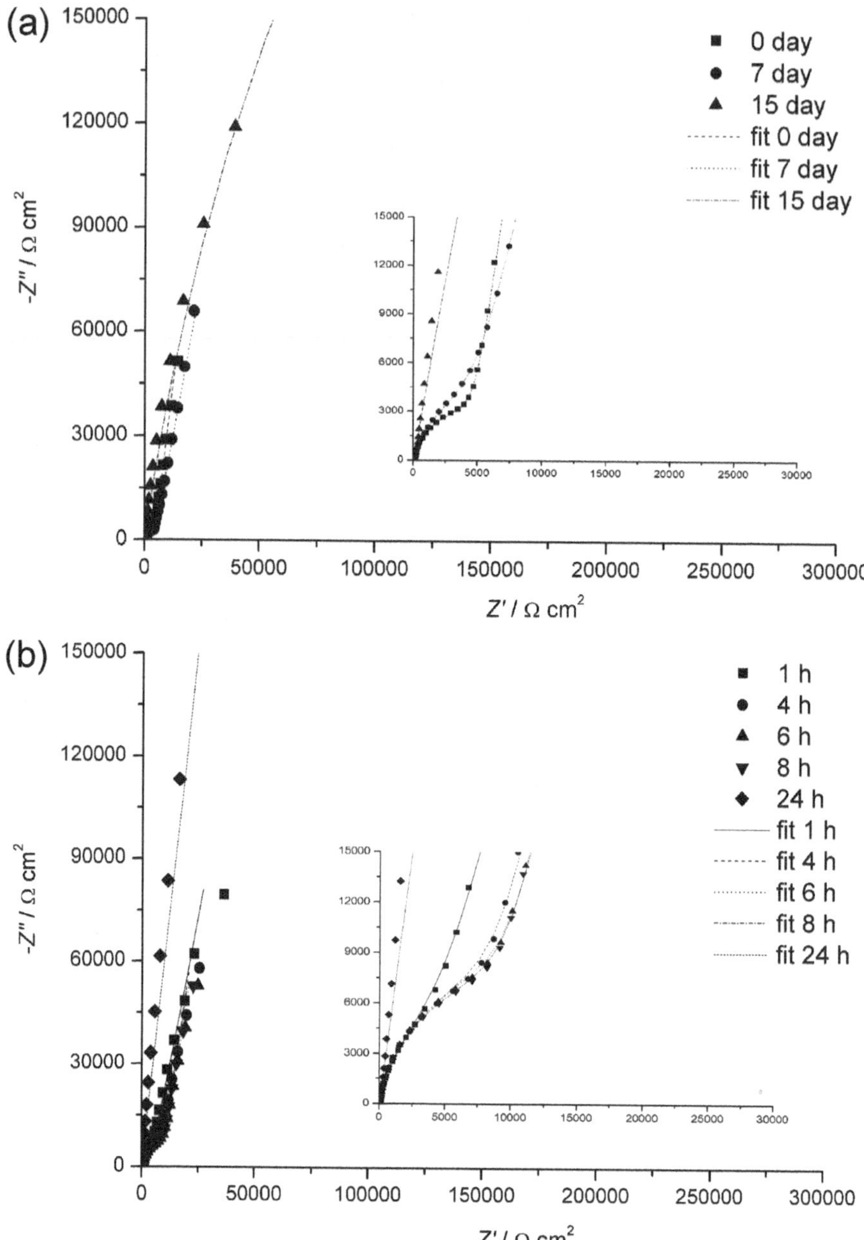

FIGURE 3.5 The Nyquist plots of HAP/Gr (a) and HAP coatings (b) after different immersion times in SBF at 37 °C (dash line – fitting) (reprinted from Janković, Eraković, Mitrić et al. 2015 with permission from Elsevier)

TABLE 3.6
Fitting Values of Equivalent Electrical Circuit Parameters and Goodness of Fit (GOF) for the HAP/Gr and HAP Coatings (Reprinted from Janković, Eraković, Mitrić et al. 2015 with Permission from Elsevier)

t / h	R_s / Ωcm^2	R_p/ $k\Omega cm^2$	CPE_c / μFcm^{-2}	n_c	CPE_{ox}/ μFcm^{-2}	n_{ox}	GOF
HAP/Gr							
1	20.6	12.5	60.4	0.80	131	0.87	$1.57e^{-4}$
3	21.7	11.5	58.4	0.81	209	0.93	$1.38e^{-4}$
5	21.7	9.3	56.0	0.81	213	0.91	$6.52e^{-5}$
7	22.7	7.6	53.2	0.82	215	0.90	$6.27e^{-5}$
24	36.1	3.9	47.8	0.85	227	0.90	$2.37e^{-5}$
48	38.2	3.7	48.7	0.84	194	0.90	$3.65e^{-4}$
72	21.6	5.0	49.8	0.84	180	0.86	$1.75e^{-4}$
120	42.2	6.5	53.8	0.83	146	0.85	$2.09e^{-4}$
168	45.8	9.3	58.2	0.82	117	0.84	$2.66e^{-4}$
216	66.6	15.1	58.1	0.82	96	0.85	$2.33e^{-4}$
264	18.9	27.5	57.9	0.81	65	0.87	$3.16e^{-4}$
312	48.9	34.2	57.7	0.82	58	0.85	$5.10e^{-4}$
HAP							
1	26.5	12.7	61.5	0.87	81	0.80	$5.21e^{-4}$
2	27.3	13.6	60.1	0.88	115	0.82	$4.32e^{-4}$
4	27.4	15.1	58.5	0.88	169	0.86	$4.00e^{-4}$
6	27.6	15.6	57.4	0.88	190	0.86	$2.88e^{-4}$
8	27.3	15.0	56.6	0.88	202	0.87	$2.14e^{-4}$
24	39.6	--	--	--	55.7	0.90	$2.84e^{-3}$

represented a site of nucleation and growth for a new apatite layer recognized as carbonated HAP, as confirmed by XRD and FE-SEM. According to the literature, the transformation of HAP to a bone-like apatite in the human body certainly induces stable bonding to natural bone (J.-H. Park et al. 2006). The Nyquist plots for the pure HAP coating during the initial exposure of eight hours in SBF were fitted by the EEC in Figure 3.2a. The values of R_p and C_c (Table 3.6) increased slightly during the initial eight hour period, indicating new apatite layer formation. However, after 24 hours, fitting could be done only with the EEC in Figure 3.2c that considers CPE_{ox}, indicating coating adhesion loss. Based on the EIS data, it is evident that HAP/Gr coating exhibited biomimetic mineralization superior to pure HAP coating.

3.1.4.4 Cytotoxicity and Antibacterial Activity

Cell survival in the presence of HAP/Gr coating on Ti was determined using a standard MTT test (Janković, Eraković, Mitrić et al. 2015). Cell survival of PBMCs was calculated to be 72.3±4.3%. Examination of the cytotoxic effects showed a mild decrease in the survival of healthy immunocompetent PBMC compared to the control cell sample. According to a classification found in the literature (Sjögren, Sletten, and Dahl 2000), HAP/Gr coating can be considered non-cytotoxic within the margin of error against target PBMC.

The antibacterial activity of HAP/Gr coating was tested against *S. aureus* TL and *E. coli* (ATCC 25922) in suspension using the spread-plate method (Janković, Eraković, Mitrić et al. 2015) and exhibited no reduction of *S. aureus* TL or *E. coli* after 24 hours. The same behavior of *S. aureus* TL was reported for a pure HAP coating (Eraković, Janković, Matić et al. 2013).

3.1.5 Silver/Hydroxyapatite/Graphene Coatings

3.1.5.1 Synthesis and Characterization

Biocomposite Ag/HAP/Gr coatings were electrodeposited on titanium using EPD from ethanol suspensions containing 1 wt.% nanosized Ag/HAP and 0.01wt.% Gr in order to obtain the bioactive coatings with antimicrobial activity aimed for hard tissue implants (Janković, Eraković, Vukašinović-Sekulić et al. 2015). A nanosized Ag/HAP powder was prepared utilizing a modified chemical precipitation method that involves reaction of calcium oxide, phosphoric acid, and silver nitrate (Eraković, Janković, Veljović et al. 2013; Eraković, Janković, Matić et al. 2013). Silver ion concentration was kept at 0.4 + 0.1 wt. % in the final powder.

Judging by FE-SEM analysis, addition of Gr, nano-reinforcement filler, strongly prohibits resurfacing and crack propagation. Graphene nanosheets are shown to prevent crack propagation by frictional pull out, crack deflection, and crack bridging. The less cracked morphology of graphene-based coating can be explained by the bonding mechanism between HAP lattice and graphene sheets, as was explained for HAP/Gr coating.

Raman spectroscopy was performed in order to confirm the incorporation of graphene in composite Ag/HAP/Gr coating. The D peak at 1260 cm^{-1} corresponding to edges, other defects, disordered sp^3-bonded carbon atoms and impurities, and G-peak at 1588 cm^{-1} corresponding to ordered sp^2-bonded carbon atoms confirmed the graphene structure in its pure form.

FT-IR analysis was employed to check the Gr presence in the composite coating and possible bonding within. The most prominent bands at the wave numbers 1089, 1024, 962, 601, 560, and 470 cm^{-1} are attributed to stretching and bending of phosphate groups in hydroxyapatite. The low intensity band at 875 cm^{-1} is assigned to acidic phosphate group, HPO_4^{2-} ions. The band at 630 cm^{-1} corresponds to structural OH^- groups of HAP lattice. The stretching vibrations of CO_3^{2-} ions in HAP are evidenced by the absorbance bands (1500–1200) cm^{-1} that correspond to $\upsilon\ _3CO_3^{2-}$. Analyzing this spectrum, the exact position of the CO_3^{2-}-bands indicates the prevalence of B-type hydroxyapatite advantageous in the human bone due to excellent bioactivity and osteoinductivity. Absorption bands located at ~1540 cm^{-1} in the FT-IR spectrum of the composite correspond to the skeletal vibration of Gr.

The thermogravimetric (TG) and differential TG (DTG) curves of Ag/HAP/Gr coating were obtained over temperature range of 25 °C –1000 °C (Janković, Eraković, Vukašinović-Sekulić et al. 2015). Similarly to HAP/Gr coating, from DTG curve can be clearly seen that thermal decomposition occurred in three steps. The first stage is evident from 25 °C to 150 °C, with 3.39 wt. % mass loss and sharp DTG peak at 46 °C and was assigned to desorption of adsorbed water from the crystallite surface. Second stage (150 °C –350 °C), with 2.62 wt. % mass loss and DTG peak at 239 °C, is attributed to the finalization of crystalline water release process and the beginning of HAP dehydroxylation and decomposing of unstable carbon in graphene structure. Finally, the third stage (350 °C –750 °C) with 1.11 wt. % mass loss and DTG peak at 584 °C, originated from decomposition of remaining unstable carbon. In addition, this stage can be attributed to early slow decomposition of HAP that continues above 750 °C . Total weight loss for the Ag/HAP/Gr coating in the temperature range of 25 °C –1000 °C was 7.12 wt. %, confirming the greater thermal stability of Ag/HAP/Gr compared to Ag/HAP coating with 7.90 wt.% weight loss (Janković et al. 2012).

The surface elements of the Ag/HAP/Gr coating (14.56 % P2p, 12.05 % C1s, 14.97 % $Ca2p_{3/2}$, 7.14 % $Ca2p_{1/2}$, 50.99 % O1s, 0.15% Ag3d) and Ag/HAP coating (16.70% P2p, 16.96 % $Ca2p_{3/2}$, 8.08 % $Ca2p_{1/2}$, 58.01 % O1s, 0.11% Ag3d) were determined using XPS (Janković, Eraković, Vukašinović-Sekulić et al. 2015). The XPS narrow scan spectra of Ag element is present in both Ag/HAP and Ag/HAP/Gr coatings. The peak for Ag3d peak (BE=369.5 eV) agrees well with the literature data (Ciobanu et al. 2013). Observation of main peak O1s at binding energy of 531.3 eV for Ag/HAP/Gr coating is attributed to the presence of PO_4^{3-} groups incorporated within apatite lattice. Survey spectra of the Ag/HAP/Gr coating revealed graphene incorporation, while no trace of C1s was detected for the Ag/HAP sample. The C1s peak corresponding to the binding energy of 285.0 eV could be attributed to aromatic hydrocarbons, actually C=C sp^2 bonds in the graphitic network. Based on the survey spectra the Ca/P ratio for the Ag/HAP/Gr coating was calculated to be 1.52. Since stable HAP phases have been found to exist over a range 1.3-1.8, graphene provided an optimal Ca/P ratio in the composite, thus enabling successful bone integration with biomaterial.

3.1.5.2 Biomechanical Properties

Nanoindentation testing was conducted to investigate the effect of added graphene to mechanical properties of the Ag/HAP/Gr coating (Janković, Eraković, Vukašinović-Sekulić et al. 2015). For the Ag/HAP/Gr composite coating, the mean hardness, H, was 15.5±3.3 GPa, approximately a 10 % increase compared to measured hardness values of Ag/HAP (14.5±5.8 GPa) (Table 3.5). The mean reduced elastic modulus, E_r, of the Ag/HAP/Gr composite was 183.0±21.9 GPa, an increase of almost 10 % (Ag/HAP, E_r = 172.1±36.9 GPa). Overall the mechanical properties of Ag/HAP/Gr are improved due to addition of Gr as nanofiller even at low concentration. The impact of Ag addition is revealed by comparing Ag/HAP and pure HAP coating, as observed Ag contributed to the increase of both E_r (172.1 GPa vs. 132.2 GPa) and H (14.5 GPa vs. 7.40 GPa) (Erakovic et al. 2014).

As already mentioned, evaluation of E_r/H value is a prerequisite for the evaluation of fracture toughness. In the case of pure HAP and Ag/HAP coatings, E_r/H ratios were 17.86 and 11.87, respectively, while in the case of HAP/Gr and Ag/HAP/Gr coatings E_r/H ratios were 12.90 and 11.81, respectively (Table 3.5), indicating that Ag reinforcement caused decrements in the value of E_r/H, implying that toughness increases with Ag addition (Erakovic et al. 2014). The Ag/HAP/Gr coating is more resistant to indentation and has higher hardness and much lower penetration depth than the Ag/HAP coating. Moreover, the higher reduced modulus of the Ag/HAP/Gr coating indicates that the slope of the initial portion of the unloading curve for the Ag/HAP/Gr coating is obviously higher than that for the Ag/HAP coating. The impact of graphene reflects on increased contact area with the surrounding HAP matrix and as a result, the bonding strength between graphene and HAP grains are significantly enhanced. Improved mechanical properties stem from increased energy required to pull the nanofiller out from the HAP matrix. Graphene as a two-dimensional component reduces the crack formation within the coating by bridging effect between adjacent HAP grains and also HAP and nanofiller Gr itself.

According to the proposed bonding mechanism between graphene and hydrohyapatite lattice, graphene nanosheets are well bonded to the nearby HAP grains, thus increasing the toughness along grain boundaries and inhibiting crack propagation along the grain boundary. Therefore, enhanced mechanical properties of the Ag/HAP/Gr coating are the result of crack bridging, deflection, and grain bridging by the graphene nanofiller.

3.1.5.3 *In Vitro* Bioactivity

The bioactivity of Ag/HAP/Gr coating was tested by immersion in SBF solution at 37 °C for seven days (Janković, Eraković, Vukašinović-Sekulić et al. 2015). XRD diffractogram revealed HAP, but incorporation of Ag in the crystal HAP lattice caused a shift of specific peaks to the left, confirming the silver substitution for calcium. In addition, Ag was also recognized by appearance of a characteristic peak at $2\theta = 43.9°$. High-intensity HAP peaks at (211), (112), and (300) crystal planes at $2\theta =$ 32.0, 32.9 and 34.1° are easily distinguished, as well as the presence of Ti substrate in its pure form on the coating interface. Thermally reduced graphene showed a broad (002) peak at $2\theta = 23–26°$, but strong HAP diffraction peaks at crystal plane (002) mostly shield graphene peak. In addition, the specific broad peak at $2\theta = 22°$ observed for pure graphene is also overlapped by HAP diffraction peaks. Finally, the carbon peak at $2\theta = 26.6°$ is evidenced. After immersion in SBF, a shift of characteristic peaks for Ag/HAP/Gr coating toward higher angles is evident. Carbonated HAP as it appears in diffractogram (shift in HAP diffraction peaks), mimicking bone mineral, is especially advantageous. The crystallite domain size is calculated to be 17.6 nm and 22.3 nm, before and after immersion in SBF, respectively. The difference between crystallite size before and after immersion is due to the CO_3^{2-} incorporation into the HAP lattice by occupying either the OH^- or the PO_4^{3-} sites.

Homogenous surface of Ag/HAP/Gr coating before immersion in SBF with rod-like HAP grains ($\leq$ 50 nm in size) was observed in FE-SEM microphotographs, while, after soaking in SBF, a newly formed highly porous apatite layer containing plate-shaped HAP crystals beneficial for better cell adhesion was observed (Janković, Eraković, Vukašinović-Sekulić et al. 2015). The high bioactivity of Ag/HAP/Gr coating is confirmed by forming an apatite layer after just seven days soaking in SBF.

The bioactivity of Ag/HAP/Gr coating was studied in SBF by EIS (Janković, Eraković, Vukašinović-Sekulić et al. 2015). The experimental impedance data of Ag/HAP/Gr and Ag/HAP coatings after different exposure times in SBF at 37 °C are presented as Nyquist plots (Figure 3.6). Fitting of Nyquist plots was accomplished by using the equivalent electrical circuits (EEC) shown in Figure 3.2. The fitted curves at different times of immersion in SBF are shown in Figure 3.6, while obtained fitting results are presented in Table 3.7.

In Table 3.7, n_c values are higher than 0.80, therefore CPE_c can be considered as coating capacitance C_c, while CPE_{ox} can be considered as capacitance of oxide film on titanium surface beneath Ag/HAP/Gr and Ag/HAP coatings, C_{ox}. EEC shown in Figure 3.2a was used for fitting the Nyquist plots for Ag/HAP/Gr coating during 21 days of exposure to SBF. According to these results, R_p slightly decreased during the first three days, indicating that coating pores were filled with SBF. However, after seven days R_p values started to increase, indicating the beginning of new apatite layer formation. Furthermore, after 21 days, the calculated value of R_p was 73.9 kΩ cm^2, indicating the deposition of a newly formed carbonated HAP, which was confirmed also by XRD and FE-SEM. This suggests that the Ag/HAP/Gr coating surface represented the site of nucleation and growth of new carbonated HAP. The Nyquist plots for Ag/HAP coating during exposure of 24 hours in SBF were also fitted by EEC in Figure 3.2a. After an initial eight hours period when R_p and C_c (Table 3.7) values were kept almost constant, substantial increase occurred at 24 hours, indicating the new apatite layer formation. However, after 72 hours, fitting could be done only with the EEC in Figure 3.2c that considers CPE_{ox}, indicating coating adhesion loss. Based on the EIS data, it is evident that Ag/HAP/Gr coating exhibited superior biomimetic mineralization compared to Ag/HAP coating.

3.1.5.4 Cytotoxicity and Antibacterial Activity

Cytotoxicity was determined by MTT test against healthy immunocompetent PBMC (Janković, Eraković, Vukašinović-Sekulić et al. 2015). Cell survival of PBMC was calculated to be 79.6±11.2%, indicating Ag/HAP/Gr coatings as non-cytotoxic against target PBMC.

The antibacterial activity of Ag/HAP/Gr coating was tested against *S. aureus* TL and *E. coli* (ATCC 25922) by test in suspension (Janković, Eraković, Vukašinović-Sekulić et al. 2015). As previously reported (Eraković, Janković, Matić et al. 2013), antibacterial activity of the graphene-free Ag/HAP coating against *S. aureus* TL was noticed immediately after inoculation and the same trend was clearly evidenced throughout the 24-hour duration of the experiment. Similar antimicrobial activity was noticed for the Ag/HAP/Gr coating. Namely, antimicrobial activity of the Ag/HAP/Gr coating (Figures 3.7a and b) could be noticed immediately after inoculation

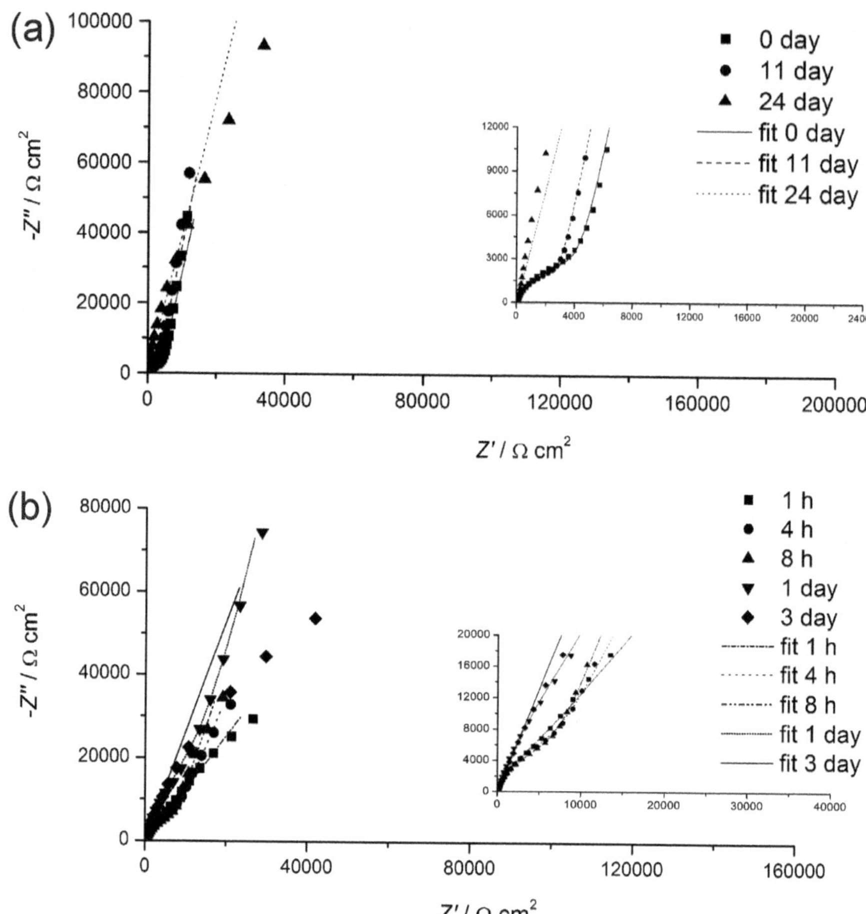

FIGURE 3.6 The Nyquist plots of the Ag/HAP/Gr (a) and Ag/HAP coatings (b) after different immersion times in SBF at 37 °C (dash line – fitting) (reprinted from Janković, Eraković, Vukašinović-Sekulić et al. 2015 with permission from Elsevier)

of samples and subsequently one logarithmic unit reduction of cell viability is achieved after only one hour of incubation. Calculations based on initial number of cells in suspensions and one hour post-incubation revealed that Ag/HAP/Gr coating exhibited reduction of both bacteria, *S. aureus* TL (72.9% percentage of cell reduction) and *E. coli* (68.4% percentage of cell reduction). Graphene-based coating exhibited strong antibacterial activity also after three hours of exposure, therefore suppressing harmful biofilm formation. Exactly as in the case of Ag/HAP coating, after 24 hours, analyzed Ag/HAP/Gr samples did not contain any viable cell and visible colony even when samples were taken directly from the suspensions. An immediate silver ion release for both Ag/HAP and Ag/HAP/Gr coatings provided for the imminent drop in CFU numbers, which fits well with bactericidal properties necessary for prevention of biofilm formation (Jamuna-Thevi et al. 2011).

TABLE 3.7
Fitting Values of Equivalent Electrical Circuit Parameters and Goodness of Fit (GOF) for the Ag/HAP/Gr and Ag/HAP Coatings (Reprinted from Janković, Eraković, Vukašinović-Sekulić et al. 2015 with Permission from Elsevier)

t / h	R_s / Ωcm²	R_p/ kΩcm²	CPE_c / μFcm⁻²	n_c	CPE_{ox}/ μFcm⁻²	n_{ox}	GOF
Ag/HAP/Gr							
1	38.83	6.12	55.1	0.804	241	0.882	5.84e⁻⁴
2	38.87	5.95	53.2	0.808	255	0.887	4.69e⁻⁴
4	39.13	5.83	57.7	0.813	264	0.888	3.89e⁻⁴
6	39.46	5.84	50.4	0.816	264	0.892	3.87e⁻⁴
8	39.63	5.69	49.3	0.819	271	0.898	3.12e⁻⁴
24	31.45	3.51	44.6	0.849	299	0.917	3.06e⁻⁵
72	15.30	2.48	38.6	0.871	303	0.879	3.08e⁻⁵
168	31.08	3.05	35.5	0.883	248	0.913	2.26e⁻⁵
264	25.88	4.17	43.6	0.850	197	0.884	3.45e⁻⁴
360	68.65	9.42	52.1	0.824	135	0.854	1.07e⁻⁴
504	133.2	73.9	51.1	0.816	82	0.823	5.31e⁻⁴
Ag/HAP							
1	30.1	9.50	92.3	0.83	119	0.70	3.90e⁻⁴
4	31.0	12.9	91.7	0.83	200	0.80	1.63e⁻⁴
8	31.7	12.0	88.6	0.83	223	0.80	1.38e⁻⁴
24	37.1	90.3	97.6	0.82	71	0.92	2.43e⁻⁴
72	54.7	-	-	-	153	0.80	3.84e⁻⁴

3.2 HYDROXYAPATITE-BASED COATINGS WITH GENTAMICIN AIMED FOR HARD TISSUE IMPLANTS

3.2.1 Bacterial Infections of Hard Tissue Implants

The application of bone cement dates from the mid-nineteenth century when it was introduced for total knee prosthesis fixing. Bone cement that was first applied consisted primarily of plaster and colophony. Almost a century later, in 1960, Sir John Charnley introduced polymethylmethacrylate (PMMA) as a new modern type of bone cement in total hip replacement surgery and PMMA was for years used as the golden standard in fixation of cemented total joint arthroplasty (Charnley 1960). Positive results obtained by modern surgical experiments regarding the suture and replacement of defects of superior tissue, as well as the utilization of reabsorbable and living tamponade in surgery, have been reported (Gluck 2011).

Different materials were investigated and used as bone replacement. A number of biomaterials for hard tissue implants, such as hips, knees, ankle, shoulder, elbow joints, and their application as drugs delivery systems, were investigated lately. During thc last 60 years, three different generations seem to be clearly marked: bioinert materials (first generation), bioactive and biodegradable materials (second generation), and materials designed to stimulate specific cellular responses at the molecular level (third generation). These applications require the use of biodegradable and/or bioerodible polymers in order to enable the permanent persistence of implanted drug carrier. The only requirement for the first generation materials was their minimal toxic effect: metals (stainless steel, cobalt–chrome molybdene, titanium, nickel-titanium), ceramics (alumina, bioglasses, biopex, glass ceramics, calcium phosphate cements), and polymers (polymethacrylic acid (PMMA), polyethylene (PE), polydimethylsulphoxide (PDMS), polyglycolic acid (PGA), polylactic acid (PLA), polycaprolactone (PCL), polydioxanone (PDS)) (Navarro et al. 2008; Ghalme, Mankar, and Bhalerao 2016).

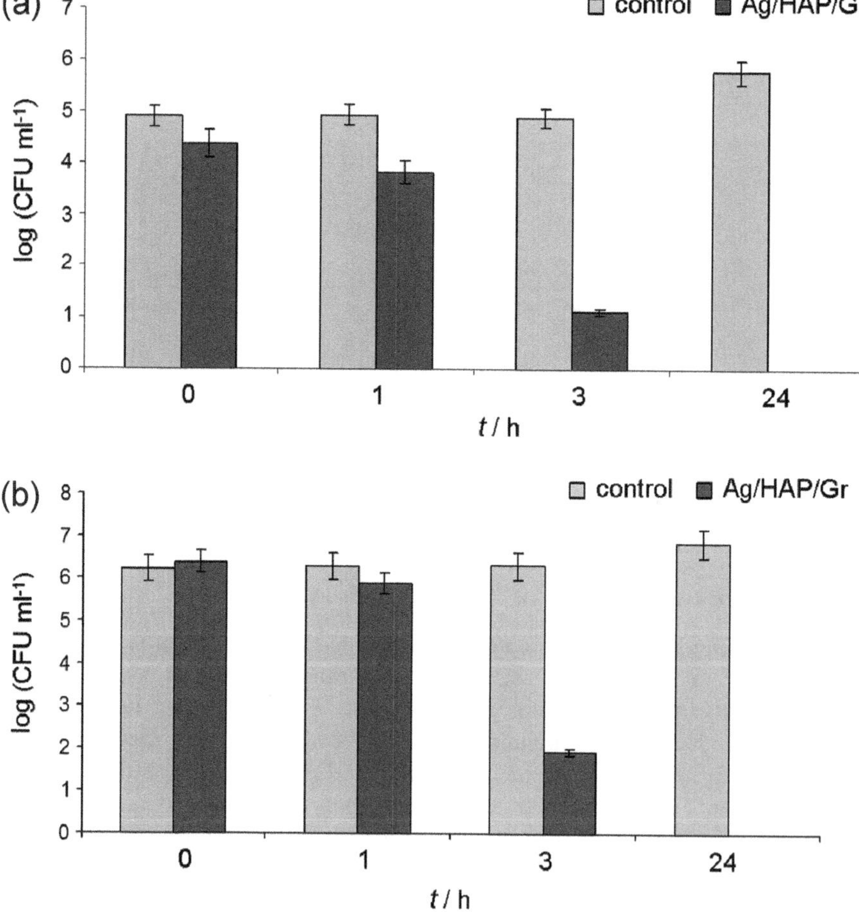

FIGURE 3.7 Reduction of viable cell number of *S. aureus* (a) and *E. coli* (b) after contact with the Ag/HAP/Gr coating for 0, 1, 3, and 24 hours in PB as compared to the control w/o samples (reprinted from Janković, Eraković, Vukašinović-Sekulić et al. 2015 with permission from Elsevier)

However, one of the most important problems in orthopedic surgery are bacterial infections, especially infections after total joints replacement. The infection after fracture fixation can be classified according to time of appearance into three groups: infections with early appearance (less than two weeks), delayed (between two and ten weeks), and late (more than ten weeks) (Metsemakers et al. 2018). Different bacteria may cause these infections, such as Gram-negative species, *Escherichia coli, Pseudomonas*, including *Enterobacteriaceae* or Gram-positive species such as *Staphylococcus aureus*; *Corynebacterium species and Streptococcus pyogenes*, including *Methicillin-resistant Staphylococcus aureus* (MRSA). MRSA infection is caused by a type of staph bacteria that has become resistant to many of the antibiotics used to treat ordinary staph infections. In many different studies, a number of antibiotics (gentamicin, vancomycin, tobramicin, clindamicin, erythromycin, ciprofloxacin, cephalosporins, tetracycline, and rifampicin) were investigated for application in antibiotic-loaded implants.

Antibiotics application is in relation to not only infective agents but also to implants chemical composition. Polymethylmethacrylate (PMMA), used as (acrylic) bone cement, was tested for local delivery of a number of different antibiotics in orthopedic treatment of bones or joints. The obtained results showed that gentamicin and vancomycin can cover a broad spectrum of pathogens, including MRSA (van Vugt, Arts, and Geurts 2019).

In open fractures or after surgical interventions, bone infection could occur, leading to significant complications (osteonecrosis, amputations, or sepsis), even implant loosening. The standard procedure after surgery includes systemically administered antibiotics, with the aim to prevent or cure bacterial infections. Those could be potentially harmful to the organism. The efficacy of antibiotics against implant-associated infections could be improved by localized administration of the drug, thus enabling high concentrations as well as a long-term antibiotic effect with few side effects. Localized administration of the drug at the site of the potential infection could be achieved using an antibiotic-loaded implant, bone void fillers, or cements. The most frequently used antibiotics for hard tissue implants are gentamicin (Pishbin et al. 2014; Stravinskas et al. 2018) and vancomycin (Cabrejos-Azama et al. 2016) in accordance with the severity of the bacterial infection that can occur during orthopedic surgery for hips, knees, and ankle replacement.

Gentamicin and vancomycin are antibiotics that exhibit bactericidal activity against a broad spectrum of microorganisms, such as *Pseudomonas aeruginosa*, *Escherichia coli*, and *Staphylococcus aureus*, but also MRSA bacteria since bacterial resistance to gentamicin and vancomycin are lower than to other group of antibiotics. The mixture of these antibiotics was prepared as bioabsorbable beads and used in operative revision of infected hip replacement. The vancomycin and gentamicin were both put into the femoral canal before closing the implant. There was no evidence of postoperative reinfection during the next five years. Also, no additional antibacterial drugs were necessary during the recovery period, demonstrating that antibiotic-impregnated bioabsorbable calcium sulfate beads can be very useful in veterinary orthopedics (Guthrie and Fitzpatrick 2019).

Different strategies for overcoming possible inflammatory processes and infections of the surgical site can be managed through the modification of the biomaterials' surface, e.g. doping materials with antimicrobial substances (AbouAitah et al. 2021; Mokabber 2020). The antibiotic-loaded implants' surface coatings enable a delivery of high drug concentrations directly at the infection site, reducing the possibility of side effects, which may occur during systemic antibiotic administration. Among the great number of techniques for biomaterials production (Harun et al. 2018), one of the most attractive is electrophoretic deposition (EPD) (Zielinski and Bartmanski 2020), due to the possibility to control the coatings' uniformity, morphology, and thickness by varying deposition parameters (Stevanović et al. 2021; Stevanović, Djošić, Janković, Kojić et al. 2020; Stevanović, Djošić, Janković, Nešović et al. 2020; M. Djošić, Janković, and Mišković-Stanković 2021; Laska and Bartmański 2020). According to the literature, successful incorporation of different drugs, e.g., ampicillin (Patel et al. 2012, 2014), vancomycin (Riahi, Seyedkhani, and Sadrnezhaad 2019; Bakhshandeh and Amin Yavari 2018), tetracycline and/or ibuprofen (Radda'a et al. 2017; Clifford and Zhitomirsky 2018), ciprofloxacin and gentamicin (Geuli et al. 2017), dexamethasone (Qiu et al. 2016), and gentamicin (Stevanović et al. 2021; Stevanović, Djošić, Janković, Kojić et al. 2020; Stevanović, Djošić, Janković, Nešović et al. 2020) using EPD was reported. In addition, poly(vinyl alcohol)/hydroxyapatite coatings for biomedical application were reported to be electrophoretically deposited on AZ91 Mg alloy (Aydin, İhsan Bahçepinar, and Gül 2020) and Ti6Al7Nb (Aydın et al. 2019) substrate from organic baths, as well as poly(vinyl alcohol)/hitozan coating with bioactive glass on AZ91D magnesium alloy and 316 stainless steel (Vafa et al. 2022).

The type of antibiotic is crucial in both prevention and treatment of bacterial infections (Bistolfi et al. 2011; Rathbone et al. 2011). Gentamicin (aminoglycoside antibiotic) is most often an antibiotic of choice for implants' coating incorporation (local administration), having broad-spectrum activity including *Escherichia coli*, *Klebsiella pneumonia*, *Enterobacter* spp., and *Pseudomonas aeruginosa*, rapid and dose-dependent activity and minimal host tissue toxicity. On the other side, if administered in a systemic therapy, gentamicin may be ototoxic (Grohmann et al. 2019). In clinical drug concentrations it exhibits good antibacterial activity against some coagulase-negative staphylococci and methicillin-susceptible *Staphylococcus aureus* isolates. Although gentamicin antibacterial effect is well known, the underlying mechanism is still a question mark. The most common hypothesis involves gentamicin binding for the 16S rRNA on the 30S ribosomal subunit, which disrupts mRNA translation leading to the formation of truncated or nonfunctional proteins and ultimately bacterial cells death. Moreover, gentamicin exhibits specific concentration-dependent efficacy, which is characteristic for aminoglycosides, meaning that its activity depends on peak concentration and higher concentrations are associated with better antibacterial effect (Batul et al. 2020). Furthermore, aminoglycosides, including gentamicin, have the ability to suppress bacteria cells regrowth a few hours after antibiotic concentration falls below the minimum inhibitory concentration (MIC), which is a key point in biofilm prevention that occurs in a short time period after implantation. As far as Gram (+) bacteria are concerned, synergistic effects of aminoglycosides with other medications against Gram (+) were observed, but the mechanism remained unknown (Shakil et al. 2008). It is noteworthy to mention that gentamicin is a thermostable antibiotic that sustains autoclaving while retaining its activity, which is a key feature from the biomedical applications perspective.

EPD of chitosan-based composite coatings containing gentamicin was reported in the literature, including various inorganic and/or polymer materials, e.g., chitosan/methyl-cellulose/gentamicin (Bonetti et al. 2023), gentamicin-loaded chitosan/gelatin/bioactive glass (Rehman and Batool 2022), cellulose/alginate/bioglass/gentamicin (Rahighi et al. 2021), chitosan/gelatin/silica-gentamicin/bioactive glass (Aydemir et al. 2021), Ce-doped nanobioactive glass/chitosan/gentamicin (Ibrahim et al. 2021), chitosan/gelatin/gentamicin (Jahanmard et al. 2020), gentamicin-loaded halloysite nanotubes/chitosan (Humayun, Luo, and Mills 2020), chitosan/gelatin/silica-gentamicin (Aydemir et al. 2020), silk fibroin/gentamicin (Han et al. 2017), gentamicin/hydroxyapatite (Geuli et al. 2017), calcium phosphate/chitosan/gentamicin-loaded carbon nanotubes (J. Zhang et al. 2016), chitosan/bioactive glass/gentamicin (Pishbin et al. 2014), hydroxyapatite/chitosan/graphene/gentamicin, and hydroxyapatite/chitosan/gentamicin (Stevanović, Djošić, Janković, Kojić et al. 2020; Stevanović et al. 2018). All of these coatings were prepared with the aim to improve bioactivity and biocompatibility of metallic implants for biomedical applications. The aforementioned composite coatings with gentamicin were prepared in the single-step process (Stevanović, Djošić, Janković, Kojić et al. 2020; Bonetti et al. 2023; Rehman and Batool 2022; Ibrahim et al. 2021; Jahanmard et al. 2020; Pishbin et al. 2014; Stevanović et al. 2018) or by gentamicin pre-loading (Geuli et al. 2017; Aydemir et al. 2021; Humayun, Luo, and Mills 2020; Aydemir et al. 2020; J. Zhang et al. 2016), from aqueous (Stevanović, Djošić, Janković, Kojić et al. 2020; Bonetti et al. 2023; Rahighi et al. 2021; Jahanmard et al. 2020; Han et al. 2017; Pishbin et al. 2014; Stevanović et al. 2018), mixed ethanol-water suspension (Rehman and Batool 2022; Aydemir et al. 2021; Ibrahim et al. 2021; Humayun, Luo, and Mills 2020; Aydemir et al. 2020; J. Zhang et al. 2016) or from organic solvent (Geuli et al. 2017), with final gentamicin concentration of 1mg/ml (Stevanović, Djošić, Janković, Kojić et al. 2020; Rahighi et al. 2021; Ibrahim et al. 2021; Jahanmard et al. 2020; Han et al. 2017; Stevanović et al. 2018) or 2mg/ml (Bonetti et al. 2023; Rehman and Batool 2022; Aydemir et al. 2021, 2020; Pishbin et al. 2014).

3.2.2 Hydroxyapatite/Chitosan and Hydroxyapatite/Chitosan/Graphene Coatings

3.2.2.1 Synthesis and Characterization

HAP/CS (1 wt. % HAP and 0.05 wt. % of CS) and HAP/CS/Gr coatings (1 wt. % HAP, 0.05 wt. % of CS and 0.01 wt. % of Gr) were obtained on titanium by EPD using a constant voltage method at an applied voltage of 60 V and deposition time of three minutes (Đošić et al. 2017). Chitosan is insoluble in water, and since intramolecular structure of CS consists of both hydrophilic and hydrophobic groups, CS can be dissolved in acid solutions. After dissolution, the protonated amines make

CS positively charged (C. Liu et al. 2014). Since HAP/CS suspension was obtained by adding HAP ethanol suspension into CS, previously dissolved in acetic acid, the positively charge CS molecules attracted HA particles, achieving electrostatic stabilization of HAP/CS suspension (Shi et al. 2016). When Gr dispersion was added to HAP/CS suspension, the interaction of Gr with CS occurs. Due to a large amount of *p* electrons in sp^2 hybrid orbital of carbon atom in Gr, negatively charged sheets would self-assemble with protonated amine groups in CS, making stable suspension for EPD process (C. Liu et al. 2014).

XRD analysis was performed for HAP/CS and HAP/CS/Gr coatings, as well as HAP coating as reference, before and after soaking in SBF solution at 37°C. The characteristic crystal planes for hydroxyapatite are denoted for HAP coating as (002), (211), (112), and (300), and their positions are listed in Table 3.8. Before soaking, the shifting of these diffraction maximums to higher 2θ angles, for HAP/CS coating and to lower 2θ angles for HAP/CS/Gr coating, clearly indicates the interactions of chitosan and graphene with HAP. As a consequence, corresponding *d*-spacing values for HAP/CS coating decreased in respect to HAP coating. The shifting of the characteristic crystal planes toward higher 2θ angles in the case of HAP/CS composite coating and decrease in *d*-spacing values is considered as the consequence of the compression from the contracting polymeric matrix through interfacial bonding, as well as of bonding between HAP and CS (Nikpour, Rabiee, and Jahanshahi 2012). The interaction of CS and HAP can be ascribed to the formation of intermolecular hydrogen bond and chelate interaction between the chitosan and HAP. There is a possible interaction between the NH_2 group and primary and secondary –OH group of CS with Ca^{2+} of HAP. Ca^{2+} ions appear on the surface of HAP crystals, having the coordination number of seven. So the coordination bonds between the -NH_2 of CS and Ca^{2+} of HAP can occur (Venkatesan and Kim 2010). Moreover, the crystallite domain sizes, calculated for (002) plane for HAP and HAP/CS coatings, amount to 485 Å and 209 Å, respectively. Similarly, the unit cell parameters *a* and *c*, as well as unit cell volume, decrease in HAP/CS coating with respect to the pure HAP coating. Overall, for HAP/CS composite coating the *d*-spacing values, cell parameters *a* and c, cell volume, and crystallite domain size decreased in respect to pure HAP coating as a consequence of the established interactions between HAP and CS.

Graphene is known as an excellent material for biopolymers modification because it acts as a reinforcing filler in the polymer-based composites (Sayyar et al. 2016; V. Geetha, Gomathi, and Sudha 2015; M. Li, Wang et al. 2013; Bustos-Ramírez et al. 2013). The diffraction peaks for characteristic hydroxyapatite crystal planes (002), (211), (112), and (300) have been shifted to the lower angles for HAP/CS/Gr coating compared to pure HAP coating (Table 3.8). As a consequence, corresponding *d*-spacing values increased. Namely, graphene is capable of forming strong bonds with polymer matrix (chitosan) due to a great specific surface area, which is the consequence of its structure (a single layer of carbon atoms in a closely packed honeycomb two-dimensional lattice) (Bustos-Ramírez et al. 2013). During the interaction with chitosan, graphene acts like a nanofiller throughout the polymer matrix. A reinforced polymer/graphene network enables HAP nanoparticles being impacted within, e.g., the intercalation of HAP occurs (Janković, Eraković, Vukašinović-Sekulić et al.

TABLE 3.8
The Characteristic Hydroxyapatite Crystal Planes, the Values of *d*-Spacing of Characteristic Crystal Planes, the Unit Cell Parameters *a* and *c*, Unit Cell Volume, and Crystallite Domain Size for HAP, HAP/CS, and HAP/CS/Gr Coatings Before and After Soaking in SBF at 37 °C for Seven Days (Reprinted from Đošić et al. 2017 with Permission from Elsevier)

Crystal Planes	HAP	HAP/CS	HAP/CS/Gr	
	2θ	2θ	2θ	
		Before Soaking in SBF		
(002)	25.6394	25.8376	25.3354	
(211)	31.5912	31.6704	31.2740	
(112)	31.9432	32.1234	31.7258	
(300)	32.7426	32.8686	32.3836	
		After Soaking in SBF		
(002)	25.8140	25.8596	25.9170	
(211)	31.7836	31.7686	31.7108	
(112)	31.1530	32.1874	31.1886	
(300)	32.9370	32.9010	32.8216	
Coating			**Crystal planes**	
	(002)	**(211)**	**(112)**	**(300)**
		***d*-Spacing, Å**		
		Before Soaking in SBF		
HAP	3.474	2.832	2.802	2.735
HAP/CS	3.448	2.825	2.786	2.725
HAP/CS/Gr	3.515	2.860	2.820	2.764
		After Soaking in SBF		
HAP	3.451	2.815	2.784	2.719
HAP/CS	3.445	2.817	2.781	2.722
HAP/CS/Gr	3.438	2.822	2.781	2.729
		Before Soaking in SBF		
Coating		**Parameter**		**Crystallite Domain Size, Å**
	***a*, Å**	***c*, Å**		***a*, Å**
HAP	9.475	6.949	HAP	9.475
HAP/CS	9.399	6.936	HAP/CS	9.399
HAP/CS/Gr	9.549	7.017	HAP/CS/Gr	9.549
		After Soaking in SBF		
HAP	9.420	6.902	HAP	9.420
HAP/CS	9.420	6.902	HAP/CS	9.420
HAP/CS/Gr	9.432	6.899	HAP/CS/Gr	9.432

2015; Janković, Eraković, Mitrić et al. 2015; M. Li, Wang et al. 2013). According to previous results (Janković, Eraković, Vukašinović-Sekulić et al. 2015; Janković, Eraković, Mitrić et al. 2015; Yi Liu, Huang, and Li 2013b), it is possible to assume that HAP and graphene sheets are connected by the Van der Waals bonding. The crystallite domain size calculated for (002) plane, for HAP and HAP/CS/Gr coatings, amounts to 485 Å and 511 Å, respectively. The increase in crystallite domain size in HAP/CS/Gr coating in respect to HAP coating confirms the interaction of HAP, CS, and Gr in composite coating. Similarly, the unit cell parameters *a* and *c*, as well as unit cell volume, increase in HAP/CS/Gr coating (Table 3.8). Overall, for HAP/CS/Gr coating the *d*-spacing values, cell parameters *a* and *c*, cell volume, and crystallite domain size increased in respect to pure HAP coating as a consequence of the established interactions among HAP, CS, and graphene sheets.

After soaking in SBF the formation of carbonated HAP, highly beneficial for bone tissue engineering was observed in the XRD pattern (Đošić et al. 2017). The peaks of carbonated (bone) HAP are broadened due to small crystallites size. The most broadening peaks were observed for the HAP/CS/Gr coating, confirming that the smallest crystallites of newly formed HAP (220 Å, calculated for (002) plane, Table 3.8). The contraction of the *c*-axis of unit cell for all investigated coatings in respect to the values of *c*-axis before immersion in SBF confirmed the formation of carbonated HAP. The *d*-spacing values, for all investigated coatings, decrease after soaking in SBF for seven days, with respect to the *d*-spacing values for pure HAP coating before soaking, confirming the growth of carbonated HAP through the incorporation of carbonate ions. The small crystallite domain size of newly formed HAP can be attributed to the strong electrostatic interactions between functional groups, enabling efficient interaction between the coating surface and mineral ions, and consequently promoted the nucleation of carbonated HAP on HAP, HAP/CS, and HAP/CS/Gr coatings. The biomineralization process, i.e., HAP growth on the coatings surface after immersion in SBF, in multicomponent system depends on the availability of functional groups and can be explained as follows. HAP surface become negative charged after soaking in SBF, by exposing hydroxyl and phosphate ions to the solution. As a consequence, the Ca^{2+} ions from SBF solution are attracted. The high consumption of calcium ions increases the local concentration, resulting in the precipitation of calcium phosphates. At the same time, the HAP dissolution occurs, increasing the calcium and phosphate ions concentration and, on the other hand, promoting the precipitation of HAP. Actually, the dissolution and precipitation of calcium phosphates in SBF is a reversible reaction (Marija S. Djošić, Mitrić, and Mišković-Stankovic 2015). Graphene could greatly promote deposition of HAP by attracting calcium ions, due to negatively charged surface, originated from the large amount of *p* electrons in sp^2 hybrid orbital of carbon atom in Gr. Additionally, the presence of amino and hydroxyl groups in CS influences the HAP nucleation and crystallization of HAP through electrostatic interaction with calcium ions (Depan, Pesacreta, and Misra 2014; Venkatesan and Kim 2010; Shi et al. 2016). On the basis of experimental results, it could be considered that both HAP/CS and HAP/CS/Gr coatings provided nucleation of HAP, showing the ability of promoting the bone bonding with the implant.

The FT-IR spectra of HAP/CS and HAP/CS/Gr coatings showed the entire characteristic band for HAP (Đošić et al. 2017). Bands at around 3380 cm^{-1} and 3381 cm^{-1} for HAP/CS and HAP/CS/Gr coatings, respectively, could be assigned to stretching vibration of hydroxyl groups. For pure HAP coating, band for stretching vibration of hydroxyl groups appeared at 3417 cm^{-1}. These slightly shifting toward lower wavenumbers, in the case of composite coatings with respect to pure HAP coating, could point out on the formation of hydrogen bonds between HAP and CS. Band that corresponds to deformation of β-glycosidic linkage in CS (891 cm^{-1}) disappeared in FT-IR spectra for both composite coatings, confirming the hydrogen interactions between HAP and CS. In addition, the disappearance of bond corresponding to pyranose ring in CS structure (1152 cm^{-1}) pointed to interconnection of HAP and CS (Szatkowski et al. 2015). Besides the characteristic band for HAP, a new band appeared in the spectrum of HAP/CS coating at 1640 cm^{-1} , assigned to the amide I band (stretching of the C=O group), and in the spectrum of HAP/CS/Gr coating at 1578 cm^{-1}, representing the band for skeletal vibration of Gr nanosheets (Surudžić et al. 2016; V. Mišković-Stanković et al. 2015; Lian et al. 2010; Janković, Eraković, Vukašinović-Sekulić et al. 2015). All these results proved the interactions between HAP and CS as well as among HAP, CS, and Gr in HAP/CS and HAP/CS/Gr composite coatings, respectively.

The thermal behavior of HAP/CS and HAP/CS/Gr coatings were investigated by using TG and DTG analysis (Đošić et al. 2017). The first stage of weight loss is in the temperature range from 30 °C to 170 °C, for HAP/CS and HAP/CS/Gr coating. The weight loss for both composite coatings is about 7 wt.%, while sharp peaks at 83 °C, for HAP/CS coating and at 82 °C for HAP/CS/Gr coating, obtained at DTG curves, correspond to the loss of adsorbed water on the coatings surface. The second stage of weight loss for the HAP/CS and HAP/CS/Gr coatings lies in the interval between 170 °C and 200 °C, with DTG peaks at 181 °C and 184 °C, respectively. The weight loss for both coatings is less than 1 wt.% and can be attributed to the release of crystalline water. The third stage of weight loss for the HAP/CS and HAP/CS/Gr coatings is in the interval between 200 °C and 336 °C (mass loss of 2.2 and 2.8 wt.%, respectively). A broad peak at DTG curves, observed at temperature of 273 °C and 271 °C for HAP/CS and HAP/CS/Gr coatings, respectively, can be attributed to the decomposition of CS. The next stage of weight loss is in the temperature range from 336 °C to 536 °C for the HAP/CS coating (mass loss of 1.53 wt.%) and from 336 °C to 572 °C for the HAP/CS/Gr coating (mass loss about 2.22 wt.%). In the DTG curve for HAP/CS coating a small peak at about 372 °C appeared due to the decomposition of the carbonate ions, also detected by IR spectroscopy of the HAP coating. For HAP/CS/Gr coating, the broad peak observed at DTG curve at ~540 °C can be attributed to the decomposition of Gr nanosheets (Neelgund, Oki, and Luo 2013). The final stage of weight loss of about 10.21 and 8.45 wt.%, for HAP/CS and HAP/CS/Gr coatings, respectively, at the temperature range from 536 °C to 740 °C for HAP/CS coating (with the sharp peak at 670 °C) and at the temperature range from 572 °C to 733 °C for HAP/CS/Gr coating (with the sharp peak at 678 °C), can be assigned to the decomposition of HAP. The further, small weight loss measured for both coatings in the temperature range from 800 °C to 1000 °C, was found to be about 0.5 wt.% corresponding to the dehydroxylation of HAP (Capanema et al. 2015; Janković, Eraković, Mitrić et al. 2015). Total mass loss in the temperature range from 30 °C to 1000 °C was 21.76 wt.% and 20.97 wt.% for the HAP/CS and HAP/CS/Gr coatings, respectively. This result proved the slightly increase in HAP/CS/Gr coating thermal stability by the addition of even a small amount of Gr in the composite.

FE-SEM micrograph of HAP/CS coating showed the sphere-like HAP particles embedded in CS polymer matrix (Đošić et al. 2017). The incorporation of Gr into waxy-looking CS matrix was observed, where graphene sheets, incorporated and well-dispersed thought the HAP/CS matrix, are represented by a wave-like sheet with slightly scrolled edges. Namely, with the aim to achieve the thermodynamic stability, corrugation, and scrolling of Gr nanosheet occurred during bending in composite coatings (Neelgund, Oki, and Luo 2013). This clearly indicates the existence of graphene sheets in HAP/CS/Gr composite coatings. In the case of HAP/CS coating, micro-cracks and porous structure were observed, while more compact coating surface was revealed when graphene was added. Denser structure of HAP/CS/Gr coating with respect to HAP/CS might be the consequence of bonding between CS and Gr, since Gr acts as reinforcement filler for polymer matrix, as well between HAP and Gr. So it is suggested that graphene inhibited crack formation and propagation through the crack deflection at the chitosan-graphene interface and crack bridging by Gr sheets (M. Li, Liu et al. 2013). As was explained earlier (Janković, Eraković, Mitrić et al. 2015), the HAP and Gr are connected by Van der Waals bonding. Nucleation of HAP crystals probably originates on either the graphene wall or the cross-section of graphene multisheets, followed by subsequent crystal growth along or perpendicular to the surface of the graphene sheet. The FE-SEM micrographs after soaking in SBF for seven days revealed the surface of the HAP/CS and HAP/CS/Gr coatings covered by sphere-like HAP agglomerates and confirmed the bioactivity of both coatings. These results are in accordance with XRD. The rapid formation of HAP in a relatively short time (after seven days) is of special interest, showing the ability to promote bone bonding with the implant.

Surface elements of HAP/CS (17.39 at.% Ca2p, 10.63 at.% P2p, 51.44 at.% O1s, 18.69 at.% C1s, 1.66 at.% N1s) and HAP/CS/Gr (14.50 at.% Ca2p, 8.33 at.% P2p, 43.58 at.% O1s, 32.50 at.% C1s, 1 at.% N1s) coatings were obtained by XPS (Đošić et al. 2017). The Ca2p spectrum reveals a peak at BE=346.57, 346.48, and 346.61 eV for HAP/CS/Gr, HAP/CS, and HAP coatings, respectively, while the P2p spectrum reveals a single P2p peak at BE=132 eV for all samples, verifying the presence of HAP. The main O1s peak component at BE=530 eV for all coatings is attributed to PO_4^{3-} groups incorporated within the apatite lattice. Incorporation of CS, and both CS and Gr in HAP network, and the formation of the new composite is clearly evidenced by the presence of C1s in the HAP/CS and HAP/CS/Gr coatings. C1s peak at around BE=285 eV, which could be attributed to aromatic hydrocarbons, is in excellent compliance with a single-sheet Gr structure of honeycomb six-membered rings. Since the reliable HAP phases have been found to exist over a range of Ca/P ratio between 1.3 to 1.8, both HAP/CS and HAP/CS/Gr coatings fit the stability requirements with the Ca/P ratio of 1.64 and 1.74, respectively.

3.2.2.2 *In Vitro* Bioactivity

In addition to the results obtained from XRD, FE-SEM, and FT-IR measurements after soaking in SBF solution at 37 °C, the *in vitro* bioactivity of HAP/CS and HAP/CS/Gr coatings was valuated electrochemical impedance spectroscopy (EIS) and potentiodynamic sweep (PDS) measurements were performed (Đošić et al. 2017). The EIS data in the complex plane for coated titanium with HAP/CS and HAP/CS/Gr coatings during different immersion times in SBF solution were fitted by using EEC shown in Figure 3.2b. Three basic criteria to evaluate the general accuracy of the fit were used: visual fit to Nyquist plots, low goodness of fit, and low relative standard errors for every circuit element (Orazem and Tribollet 2008) and suitably low goodness of fit ($<10^{-4}$), and the error associated with each element was lower than 10% were obtained. During the initial time of exposure to SBF solution the coating pore resistance, R_p, for both coatings decreased and achieved the minimum of 105 Ωcm^2 after 168 hours for HAP/CS coating, and 165 Ωcm^2 after 192 hours for HAP/CS/Gr coating, indicating that the SBF solution diffused into the coating pores. As a consequence, the dissolution of calcium phosphate on the coating surface occurred by ion exchange of calcium and phosphate ions in SBF solution. At the same time, the HAP dissolution increased the ions concentration that promoted the precipitation of a new apatite layer on the coating surface. Then, the slight increase in R_p after minimum values indicates the beginning of the biomineralization process and the formation of new apatite layer on the coating surface. Therefore, the R_p values increased after 28 days from 105 Ωcm^2 to 205 Ωcm^2 for HAP/CS, and from 165 Ωcm^2 to 484 Ωcm^2 for HAP/CS/Gr, indicating the growth of a newly formed carbonated apatite layer.

Potentiodynamic polarization curves of coated titanium with HAP/CS and HAP/CS/Gr coatings were monitored after 28 days in SBF solution at 37 °C. The corrosion potential, E_{corr}, and corrosion current density, j_{corr}, were determined according to Tafel extrapolation (Đošić et al. 2017). The E_{corr} value of HAP/CS/Gr coating (−0.149 V) was more positive than E_{corr} HAP/CS (−0.189 V) coating, while the j_{corr} of HAP/CS/Gr coating was lower (0.026 μAcm^{-2}) than j_{corr} of HAP/CS (0.067 μAcm^{-2}) coating, implying that graphene could effectively increase coating bioactivity, i.e., increased thickness of a new apatite layer formed on HAP/CS/Gr coating surface. Thus, the results of polarization measurements are in accordance with the impedance results, indicating that the HAP/CS/Gr coating has the highest corrosion resistance with the lowest corrosion current density, due to a biomimetic apatite layer on its surface. Therefore, the use of graphene-based composite HAP/CS/Gr coating could improve the bioactivity of bone implants, decrease metal ion release, and prevent tissue damage as a result of a surgically inserted implant inside the human/animal body.

3.2.2.3 Antibacterial Activity and Cytotoxicity

Antibacterial properties of HAP, HAP/CS, and HAP/CS/Gr coatings were tested against *S. aureus* TL and *E. coli* TL by monitoring changes in the viable number of bacterial cells in suspension (Figures 3.8a and b, respectively). Slight retention of

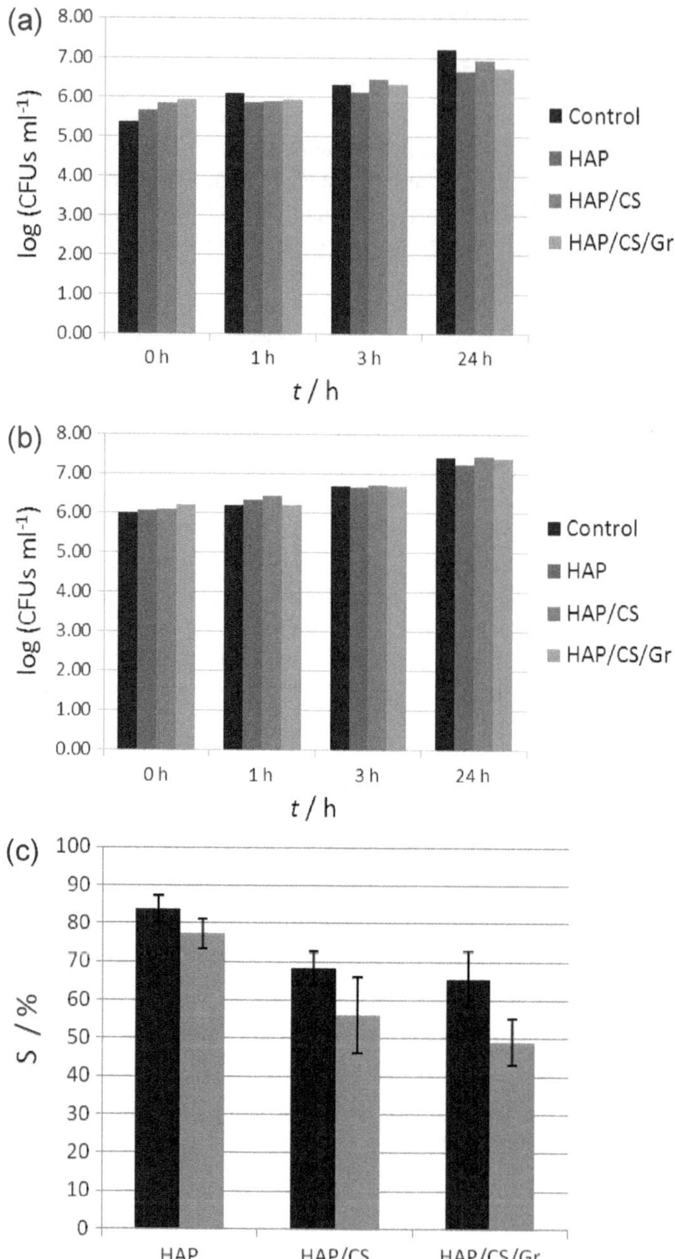

FIGURE 3.8 Survival of viable cell number of (a) *Staphylococcus aureus* and (b) *Escherichia coli* after contact with HAP, HAP/CS, and HAP/CS/Gr coated titanium for 0, 1, 3, and 24 hours in PB as compared to the control w/o samples, and (c) survival of PBMCs (reprinted from Đošić et al. 2017 with permission from Elsevier)

cell viability was observed even up to three hours post incubation when compared to the initial number of cells in suspensions for all samples. This effect is slightly more pronounced for the samples tested against *S. aureus* (Figure 3.8a) compared to behavior of *E. coli* (Figure 3.8b). However, after 24 hours all coatings exhibited no reduction of *S. aureus* TL and *E. coli.*

Cytotoxicity of HAP, HAP/CS, and HAP/CS/Gr coatings (Figure 3.8c) was determined by MTT test against PBMC cells. Examination of cytotoxic effects showed a mild decrease in survival of healthy immunocompetent PBMC compared to the control cell sample. According to classification, the HAP, HAP/CS, and HAP/CS/Gr coatings verified as non-cytotoxic within the margin of error against targeted PBMCs. However, when cells are stimulated for proliferation by PHA, there is a slight drop in viability noticed for all investigated coatings.

3.2.3 Hydroxyapatite/Chitosan/Gentamicin

3.2.3.1 Synthesis and Characterization

EPD was performed in aqueous suspensions containing 1wt% HAP and 0.05wt% chitosan for HAP/CS coating, and 1wt% HAP, 0.05wt% chitosan and 0.1 wt. % gentamicin sulfate for HAP/CS/Gent coating, at pH 4.4. HAP was added to previously prepared chitosan aqueous solution (1% acetic acid). Coatings were deposited at different values of constant voltage (1 to 10 V) for deposition times between 5 and 15 min (Stevanović et al. 2018).

Chitosan has pH-dependent solubility, due to its amino groups, that allowed processing from the aqueous suspension. The pKa value of chitosan is about 6.3. At pH values below pKa, chitosan becomes positively charged due to protonation of primary amino groups, so it becomes soluble in water, according to (Pishbin et al. 2014)

$$CS\text{-}NH_2 + H_3O^+ \leftrightarrow CS\text{-}NH_3^+ + H_2O \tag{3.4}$$

In the acidic aqueous solution, the surface of HAP consumed protons from the solution, leading to protonation of surface hydroxyl groups and making surface charge of HAP positive (Smičiklas et al. 2006). Gentamicin, aminoglycoside antibiotic, has high water solubility as well as high stability in the pH range from 2 to 10. At acidic pH, protonation of amino and hydroxyl groups makes gentamicin molecule positively charged (Pishbin et al. 2014). Additionally, hydrogen bonds are established between amino groups in chitosan and gentamicin with hydroxyl moieties, originated from hydroxyapatite, chitosan, and gentamicin.

EPD mechanism of HAP/CS and HAP/CS/Gent coatings deposition, under constant voltage could be explained as follows. In aqueous suspension, electrolysis of water and the electrochemical reactions of hydrogen and oxygen evolution occurred, leading to an increase in the local pH at cathode:

$$\text{cathode}: 2H_2O + 2e^- \rightarrow H_2 + 2OH \tag{3.5}$$

$$\text{anode}: 2H_2O \rightarrow 4H^+ + O_2 + 4e^- \tag{3.6}$$

Protonated chitosan molecules (Eq. 3.4) migrated toward the cathode and reacted with OH^- thus forming insoluble deposits on the cathode:

$$CS{-}NH_3^+ + OH^- \rightarrow CS{-}NH_2 + H_2O \tag{3.7}$$

HAP surface was positively charged in acidic solution, due to protonated surface, so HAP particles, driven by the electric field, moved to the cathode (Ti plate), deprotonated and formed deposits simultaneously with chitosan coagulation (Eq. 3.7). For HAP/CS/Gent coating deposition, positively charged gentamicin also migrated toward the cathode, deprotonated, and formed a composite coating with HAP and chitosan on Ti cathode.

Optimization of electrophoretic deposition parameters for HAP/CS coating was performed at constant voltages, between 1 and 10 V and for various deposition times between 5 and 15 min. At deposition voltages lower than 5 V, the mass of HAP/CS coating did not increase significantly with the prolongation of the deposition time, meaning that the applied electric field caused slow particle migration. At deposition voltage over 6 V, for all deposition times from 5 to 15 min, HAP/CS coatings with greater mass were deposited, but obtained coatings were porous and nonhomogeneous. Namely, for deposition voltages over 6 V, the coating deposition rate was greater due to the stronger applied electric field and more charged particles reached the cathode. Simultaneously, when higher deposition voltage is applied, the higher rate of hydrogen evolution reaction can be noticed. Consequently, evolved hydrogen left more pores in the deposited coating. The homogeneous HAP/CS coating of the greatest mass (0.67 mg/cm^2) was electrophoretically deposited at voltage of 5 V for a deposition time of 12 minutes. The HAP/CS/Gent homogeneous coating of the greatest mass (0.68 mg/cm^2) was deposited at the same deposition conditions (5 V, 12 min).

XRD analysis enabled the calculation of *d*-spacing values for characteristic HAP planes (002), (211), (112), and (300), unit cell parameters (*a* and *c*) and volume (*V*) as well as crystallite domain size. Incorporation of gentamicin in HAP/CS coating had no influence on *d*-spacing values or unit cell volume and parameters of hydroxyapatite. The crystallite domain size for HAP, calculated from the (002) diffraction maximum for HAP/CS and HAP/CS/Gent coatings, was 511 Å and 397 Å, respectively (Stevanović et al. 2018).The smaller crystallite domain size for HAP/CS/Gent coating could be explained as follows. Gentamicin incorporated in HAP/CS/Gent coating influenced the HAP crystallite domain size in two manners. Sulfate ions, originated from the gentamicin sulfate, might create a great number of nucleation sites during the drying process, limiting the HAP crystals growth rate. Additionally, the molecule of gentamicin is large, so it could be assumed that it suppressed further growth of HAP crystals, so smaller hydroxyapatite crystallites are formed in HAP/CS/Gent coating with respect to HAP/CS coating. HAP crystallites for biological application have to be very fine because a larger surface area contributes to better osseointegration, enhancing the adsorption of adhesive proteins as well as bone-like apatite formation (Marija S. Djošić, Mitrić, and Mišković-Stankovic 2015; Okada and Matsumoto 2015; Chiara et al. 2012), so gentamicin had a positive effect on HAP crystallite domain size in HAP/CS/Gent coating.

In FT-IR spectra of HAP/CS coating, in the region from 3000 cm^{-1} to 3500 cm^{-1} the broad band was observed corresponding to the stretching vibration of OH^- group originated from intermolecular and intramolecular hydrogen bonds, with wide band at around 3281 cm^{-1}. The HAP-chitosan interaction originated through the formation of intermolecular hydrogen bonds, e.g., -OH groups from HAP interacting with -OH and -NH_2 groups from chitosan. The intramolecular hydrogen bonds are related to H bonds that can be established between the oxygen atom and hydroxyl groups in chitosan. The pronounced 3570 cm^{-1} peak was attributed to OH^- stretching from HAP structure. The second band (630 cm^{-1}) could be assigned to the structural OH^- bending in HAP (Berzina-Cimdina and Borodajenko 2012). The presence of CO_3^{2-} functional group in HAP could be identified by characteristic bands that appear at 878 cm^{-1} (characteristic to the ν_2 vibration mode) and bands at 1412 cm^{-1} and 1457 cm^{-1} (attributed to CO_3^{2-} group stretching). The carbonate bands positions proved that "AB-type" substitution in the structure of HAP occurred, meaning that some phosphate and hydroxyl ions were substituted by CO_3^{2-} group (Lafon et al. 2003). Human bone mineral is always carbonate-substituted apatite, i.e., the "AB-type" apatite is the main constituent of the bone. The 472 cm^{-1} band corresponded to the phosphate group bending vibration in HAP (e.g., ν_2 O–P–O). Bands registered at 562 cm^{-1} and 601 cm^{-1} represented the evidence of asymmetric and symmetric deformation mode of phosphate group (e.g., ν_4 O–P–O). The band at 961 cm^{-1} originated from ν_1 symmetric stretching of P–O bond in PO_4^{3-}. Bands found at 1015 cm^{-1} and 1086 cm^{-1} were ascribed to the ν_3 vibration mode of phosphate group (Berzina-Cimdina and Borodajenko 2012). Additionally, the HAP/CS spectrum had fewer bands that proved the chitosan in composite coatings. The band at 1546 cm^{-1} could be ascribed to the N–H bending in chitosan (amide II). The amide I band (C=O stretching) was positioned at 1647 cm^{-1}. Bands at 2857 cm^{-1} and 2926 cm^{-1} represented typical C–H stretching in CS structure (Gebhardt et al. 2012). In the wavenumber range from 3000 cm^{-1} to 3500 cm^{-1}, the incorporation of gentamicin in HAP/CS/Gent coating caused the slight shift of wide band at 3281 cm^{-1} for HAP/CS toward a lower wavenumber (3278 cm^{-1}) for HAP/CS/Gent, indicating that hydrogen bonding of HAP and CS with gentamicin occurred as a consequence of gentamicin hydroxyl and amino groups interactions with hydroxyl groups of hydroxyapatite and hydroxyl and amino groups of CS.

TG and DTG analyses were performed in order to examine the thermal stability of HAP/CS and HAP/CS/Gent coatings (Stevanović et al. 2018). The first weight loss stage for both HAP/CS and HAP/CS/Gent coatings, corresponding to the water desorption, was in the temperature interval from 22 °C to 160 °C (mass loss of 2.8 wt.%) and from 22 °C to 170 °C (mass loss of 6.3 wt.%), respectively. Significant difference between mass losses in the first stage could be explained by smaller crystallite domain size for the coating HAP/CS/Gent. Therefore, the addition of gentamicin affected the increase in surface area of the coating, consequently creating a greater area for water adsorption. At the same time, gentamicin sulfate powder is hygroscopic, so an increase in water content adsorbed on the HAP/CS/Gent coating could be attributed to the antibiotic addition as well. The second weight loss stage occurred from 160 °C to 202 °C with mass loss of 0.6 wt.% for HAP/CS coating, and from 170 °C to 221 °C with mass loss of 0.7 wt.% for HAP/CS/Gent coating. For both coatings, maximums on DTG curves at 180 °C could be observed. In the case of both HAP/CS and HAP/CS/Gent coatings, weight loss was attributed to crystalline water release, e.g., the dehydroxylation process of HAP followed by the OH^- group loss (Đošić et al. 2017). The third weight loss stage for HAP/CS coating occurred in the temperature interval from 202 °C to 312 °C, with 1.3 wt.% mass loss and between 220 °C and 352 °C, with 2.0 wt.% mass loss in the case of HAP/CS/Gent. For both coatings, the well-defined peak at 293 °C was assigned to decomposition of chitosan. Thermal degradation of chitosan is a gradual process during which the decomposition of the chitosan chains to monomers occurs, followed by the dehydration and deamination processes that caused pyranose rings decomposition and, finally, lead to a ring-opening reaction mainly through a free radical mechanism. Spontaneous recombination of intermediate radical products led to formation of cross-linked structures (Zawadzki and Kaczmarek 2010). On the other hand, the melting point of pure gentamicin sulfate was reported to be in the temperature interval 200 °C–240 °C (Chaves et al. 2016; Dwivedi et al. 2018). The process of gentamicin sulfate melting occurred through the melting of the different isoforms and their fusion, leading to the formation of different compounds, which are degraded at higher temperatures. The difference in mass loss between HAP/CS coating (1.3 wt.%) and HAP/CS/Gent coating (2.0 wt.%) could be assigned to the thermal decomposition of gentamicin isoforms. The fourth weight loss stage for HAP/CS coating occurred in the temperature interval from 372 °C to 537 °C, with 1.2 wt.% mass loss and peak at 396 °C (DTG curve), and, ranging from 352 °C to 468 °C, with 1.6 wt.% mass loss (TG curve) and maximum at 405 °C (DTG curve) for HAP/CS/Gent coating. Mass loss of composite HAP/CS and HAP/CS/Gent coatings in this stage was assigned to the further CS and Gent degradation, along with the loss of carbonate ions from HAP structure as CO_2 molecules (McManamon et al. 2016). The difference between mass losses was due to the further decomposition of gentamicin. The next weight loss stage of ~ 0.7 wt.% for HAP/CS coating occurred between 537 °C and 683 °C, with maximum at DTG curve at 580 °C, and of about 4.6 wt.% for HAP/CS/Gent coating between 468 °C and 746 °C, with sharp maximum at DTG curve) at 640 °C. This mass loss for both coatings could be assigned to the decarbonation and dehydroxylation of HAP. Decarbonation of HAP occurred through the release of CO_2 (g), during structural rearrangement of crystal lattice of HAP, e.g., the carbonate loss from tetrahedral sites, while condensation of HPO_4^{2-} led to water release from the HAP structure. The greater mass loss for HAP/CS/Gent coating could be explained by decomposition of residual sulfates from gentamicin. Finally, the last stage of mass loss could be assigned to additional dehydroxylation and thermal decomposition of HAP (Meejoo, Maneeprakorn, and Winotai 2006). For HAP/CS coating, interval from 683 °C to 1000 °C, with broad maximum at 770 °C, exhibited 0.6 wt% mass loss. For HAP/CS/Gent coating, interval between temperatures 746 °C and 1000 °C, with broad maximum at 780 °C (DTG curve) exhibited 0.9 wt.% mass loss. In this temperature range, further dehydroxylation of HAP occurred, leading to the formation of oxyhydroxyapatite that could be transformed to β-tricalcium phosphate, calcium oxide, or tetracalcium phosphate at higher temperatures (Kamieniak et al. 2018). The total weight loss for the temperature interval between 22 °C and 1000 °C was 8.0 wt.% for HAP/CS coating and 16.1 wt.% for HAP/CS/Gent coating, which means the gentamicin addition caused lower thermal stability of HAP/CS/Gent.

The FE-SEM microphotographs of HAP/CS and HAP/CS/Gent coatings exhibited homogeneous, porous fracture-free surface that revealed strong interfacial interaction between HAP particles and the chitosan polymer matrix. Interfacial interactions could be explained by hydrogen bonding of hydroxyl groups of chitosan and HAP. Chitosan interacts via hydrogen bonding with OH^-, Ca^{2+}, and PO_4^{3-} groups of hydroxyapatite (El-Sayed et al. 2009; Stevanović et al. 2018).

The elemental composition of HAP/CS and HAP/CS/Gent samples was studied by XPS analysis (Stevanović et al. 2018). For HAP/CS coating, the high resolution C 1s peak was deconvoluted, and four components could be distinguished, positioned at 284.8, 286.4, 288.2, and 289.2 eV. Those peaks were ascribed to C-H/C-C (284.8 eV), C-N (286.4 eV), C-O (288.2 eV), C=O (289.2 eV) that originated from hydroxyl and acetamido groups from chitosan. The high resolution C 1s peak of HAP/CS/Gent was fitted, and five modes were found positioned at 284.8, 286.3, 286.7, 288, and 289.2 eV and were ascribed to C-H/C-C, C-N, O–C–O, O-C=N, and C=O, respectively. After introduction of gentamicin, peaks at 286.7 eV (O–C–O) and 288 eV (O-C=N) were noticed and assigned to the acetal bonds and methylamino groups carried by gentamicin, respectively. The percentage of these carbon interactions were 64.3 (C-H/C-C), 15.8 (C-N), 16.0 (C-O), and 3.8 % (C=O) for HAP/CS and 48.2 (C-H/C-C), 26.6 (C-N), 8.9 (O–C–O) 13.0 (O-C=N), and 3.2 % (C=O), for HAP/CS/Gent coating. Introduction of gentamicin in the composite coating caused an increase in the percentage of C-N interactions in HAP/CS/Gent (26.6 %) with respect to HAP/CS (15.8 %), as well as a decrease in the percentage of C=O interactions in HAP/CS/Gent (3.2 %) as opposed to HAP/CS (3.8 %).The interactions mentioned above were also confirmed by deconvolution of oxygen peaks. The high resolution O 1s peak was deconvoluted to three peaks at binding energies of 530.9, 532.2, and 533.1 eV for HAP/CS and at 530.8, 532.1, and 533.1 eV for HAP/CS/Gent coating, related to PO_4^{3-}, –OH, and C=O groups. The main O 1s peak component at ~ 531 eV for HAP/CS and HAP/CS/Gent coatings represented the contribution of PO_4^{3-} groups of HAP and second O 1s peak at ~ 532.2 eV might originate from –OH groups in HAP and chitosan. Third O 1s peak at ~ 533.1 eV was assigned to C=O, which originated from chitosan. The N 1s spectrum was deconvoluted into two peak components for both coatings, BE at 399.7, and 401.4 eV for HAP/CS, and 399.6 and 401.2 eV for HAP/CS/Gent coating, assigned to free and protonated amines, respectively. The increase of protonated amine content in HAP/CS/Gent coating (25.6 %), opposed to HAP/CS coating (23.3 %), indicated the gentamicin was actually incorporated in the composite. The reduction in amine content for HAP/CS/Gent coating (74.4 %) with respect to HAP/CS coating (76.7 %) was also observed. The HAP/CS XPS spectrum displayed the Ca 2p and P 2p high resolution spectra with Ca $2p_{1/2}$ (350.5 eV), Ca $2p_{3/2}$ (347 eV), and P $2p_{3/2}$ (133.1 eV) peak components indicating the presence of hydroxyapatite. For HAP/CS/Gent coating, Ca 2p spectra revealed Ca $2p_{1/2}$ (350.4 eV), Ca $2p_{3/2}$ (346.9 eV) peak components and P 2p spectrum with P

$2p_{3/2}$ at 133 eV. The S 2p high resolution spectrum with peak component at 168.1 eV indicated the gentamicin introduction into composite HAP/CS/Gent coating.

Based on the XPS results, the Ca/P atomic ratio for HAP/CS and HAP/CS/Gent coating was calculated to be 1.3 and 1.2, respectively. These surface analysis results are complemented with FT-IR data, confirming the presence of calcium-deficient hydroxyapatite (Ishikawa, Ducheyne, and Radin 1993). Calcium-deficient hydroxyapatite usually undergoes substitution with carbonate ions forming "AB-type" carbonate hydroxyapatite. These are promising results, since substituted hydroxyapatite is known for its outstanding bioactivity and osteoinductivity, compared to stoichiometric HAP.

3.2.3.2 Antibacterial Activity

Gentamicin is a prototypical aminoglycoside antibiotic and its mechanism of action involves inhibition of prion synthesis in bacteria. The drug actually binds irreversibly to host/bacterial 30S subunit leading to bacteria cells death (Kadurugamuwa, Clarke, and Beveridge 1993). A very potent antibiotic gentamicin is synthesized by microorganism *Micromonospora purpurea* and actually represents a mixture of components – gentamicin C1, C1a, and C2 being the three most prevalent. They have slightly different structure, but possess approximately the same antibiotic activity (Tangy et al. 1985). Aminoglycosides in general, and gentamicin in particular, irreversibly bind to the specific bacterial 30S subunit proteins and 16S rRNA, thus preventing the formation of the initiation complex with messenger RNA. Actually, small molecule-gentamicin binds to the four nucleotides of 16S rRNA and a single amino acid of S12 protein and thus formed complex interferes with the 30S subunit decoding site. Misreading of mRNA results in incorrect insertion of amino acids and therefore formation of nonfunctional or toxic peptides (Offermanns and Rosenthal 2008).

Figure 3.9 represents the effect of HAP/CS and HAP/CS/Gent coating against bacterial strains *S. aureus* TL and *E. coli* ATCC 25922 in PB medium. HAP/CS/Gent coating expressed strong bactericidal effect immediately after inoculation, supporting the "burst" release of antibiotic that reduced the initial count by two logarithmic units. The complete reduction of bacterial cells was achieved within one hour of exposure against *S. aureus* (Figure 3.9a). Antibacterial effect of HAP/CS/Gent coating against *E. coli* (Figure 3.9b) was much less pronounced, but there is a noticeable decline of surviving bacteria 24 hours post incubation opposed to the starting cell counts. However, since this reduction in bacterial cells is less than three logarithmic units, the effect could be classified as bacteriostatic rather than bactericidal (Pankey and Sabath 2004). The results for diminishing *S. aureus* cell count and bacteriostatic action toward *E. coli* could be recognized as significantly different ($p < 0.01$) compared to other samples and the control.

3.2.3.3 *In Vitro* Bioactivity

In vitro bioactivity of HAP/CS and HAP/CS/Gent coatings was investigated by immersion in SBF solution at 37 °C using XRD, FT-IR, F-SEM, and EIS (Stevanović, Djošić, Janković, Nešović et al. 2020). XRD diffraction maxima of biomimetic

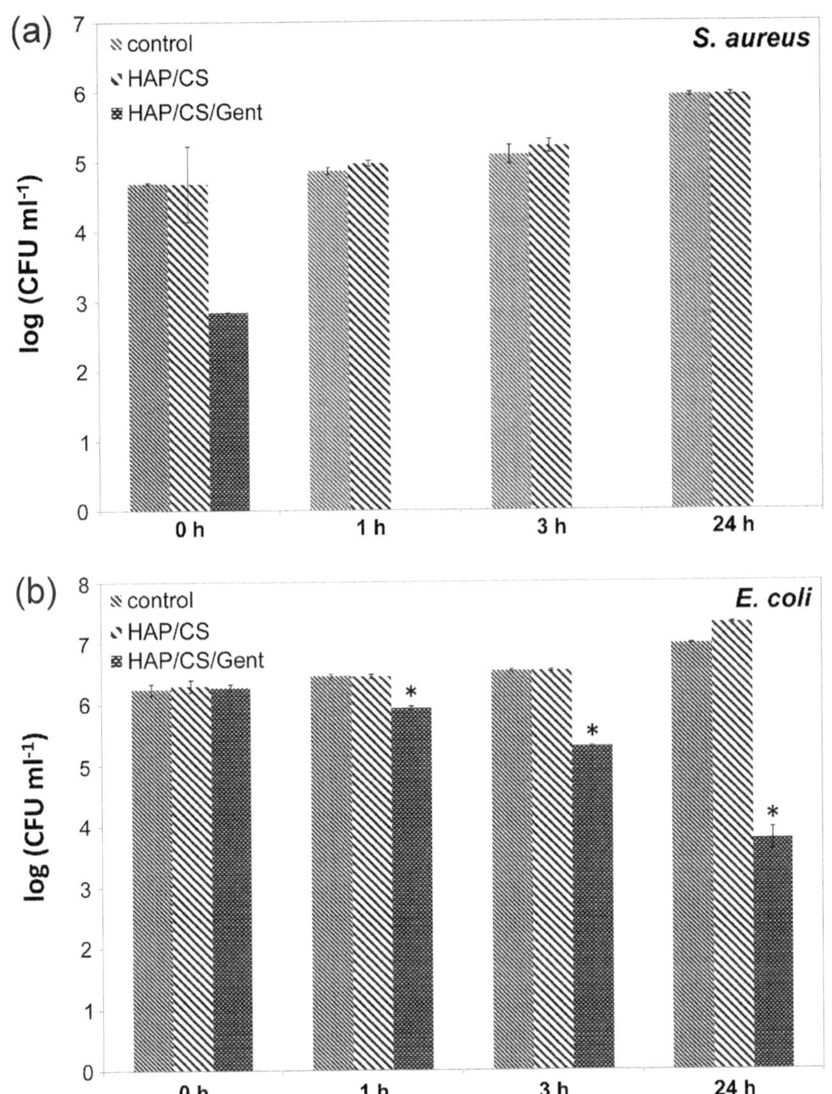

FIGURE 3.9 (a) *S. aureus* TL and (b) *E. coli* ATCC 25922 viable cell reduction after incubation in PB at 37 °C for 0, 1, 3, and 24 hours with HAP/CS/Gent and HAP/CS coatings * $p < 0.01$ (reprinted from Stevanović et al. 2018 with permission of the American Chemical Society)

coating, obtained on the top of both HAP/CS and HAP/CS/Gent coatings after soaking in SBF, were assigned to HAP (JCPDS 09-0432) and the underlying titanium substrate (JCPDS 89-2762). The HAP diffraction maxima broadening suggested fine crystallite size of the biomimetic coatings. The differences in the diffraction patterns of biomimetic HAP grown on HAP/CS and HAP/CS/Gent coatings at the 2θ values of 30° –40° can be explained by the differences between as-deposited HAP/CS and HAP/CS/Gent coatings, i.e., before soaking in SBF, that were caused by different mechanisms of their formation, as discussed earlier (Stevanović et al. 2018). Briefly, at suspension pH of 4.4 for both coatings deposition, primary amino groups of chitosan become protonated (CS-NH_3^+). At the same time, HAP acquires a positive charge due to the protonation of hydroxyl groups. During EPD, protonated CS and HAP molecules migrate toward the cathode (Ti) and react with OH^- ions evolved in the water electrolysis reaction, thus forming an insoluble HAP/CS deposit on the cathode. Additionally, hydrogen bonding occurs between the amino and hydroxyl groups from CS with hydroxyl groups from HAP. In the case of HAP/CS/Gent coating, gentamicin molecules are also positively charged due to protonation of hydroxyl and amino groups, enabling reaction of positively charged CS, HAP, and Gent molecules with OH^- ions at the cathode as explained above, thus forming an insoluble HAP/CS/Gent deposit on the cathode surface. The amino and hydroxyl groups in chitosan and gentamicin along with hydroxyl groups in HAP can form more hydrogen bonds compared to HAP/CS coating.

The calculated diffraction data, including crystallite domain size, cell volume, *V*, and unit cell parameters, *a* and *c*, as well as *d*-spacing for HAP (002), (211), (112), and (300) planes, are presented in Table 3.9. Slightly smaller crystallite domain size of biomimetic HAP on the HAP/CS/Gent coating (374 Å), compared to biomimetic HAP on the HAP/CS coating (387 Å), could be the consequence of smaller HAP/CS/Gent coating crystallite domain size before soaking (397 Å), with respect to HAP/CS coating before soaking (511 Å).

According to the presented unit cell parameters results, the biomimetic HAP (grown on both HAP/CS and HAP/CS/Gent coatings) exhibited a slight *a*-axes

TABLE 3.9
Calculated Values of *d*-Spacing, Unit Cell Parameters (*a* and *c*), Cell Volume (*V*), and Crystallite Domain Size, for Biomimetic HAP Formed on the HAP/CS and HAP/CS/Gent Coatings After Immersion in SBF for Seven Days (Reprinted from Stevanović, Djošić, Janković, Nešović et al. 2020 with Permission of the American Chemical Society)

Coating			HAP/CS	HAP/CS/Gent
Crystal Planes	**(002)**	***d*-Spacing, Å**	3.4247	3.4122
	(211)		2.8046	2.8125
	(112)		2.7642	2.7878
	(300)		2.7379	2.7504
Parameters		***a*, Å**	9.440	9.491
		***c*, Å**	6.881	6.820
		***V*, Å^3**	531.1	532.1
Crystallite Domain Size, Å			387	374

increase (9.440 Å and 9.491 Å, respectively) compared to the theoretically reported value of 9.418 Å for HAP hexagonal crystal structure with a $P6_3/m$ space group (Ragu, Senthilarasan, and Sakthivel 2015). On the other hand, a slight *c*-axes decrease (6.881 Å and 6.820 Å, respectively, compared to the literature value of 6.884 Å (Ragu, Senthilarasan, and Sakthivel 2015)) suggested carbonate group incorporation in the hydroxyapatite structure. Hydroxyl and phosphate ion sites in the biological apatites can be substituted by various anions. When the OH^- or PO_4^{3-} sites become occupied by carbonate ions, A- or B-type carbonated hydroxyapatites, respectively, can be achieved (Rincón-López et al. 2018). Replacing the linear OH^- or tetrahedral PO_4^{3-} ions with planar CO_3^{2-} ions causes unit cell parameters changes (expansion or contraction of *a* or *c*-axes) (Peng et al. 2012). Biological apatites, e.g., bone mineral, usually belong to the so-called AB-type mineral, meaning that simultaneous carbonate substitution of OH^- and PO_4^{3-} sites occurs, while greater lattice parameters changes can point to a higher carbonate substitution degree in the hydroxyapatite structure (Yang et al. 2013). The unit cell parameters changes (Table 3.9) suggested that biomimetically grown HAP on the top of HAP/CS and HAP/CS/Gent coatings is in fact carbonate-substituted hydroxyapatite. Greater *a* and *c* parameter changes with respect to the theoretical ones (Ragu, Senthilarasan, and Sakthivel 2015) were observed in the case of biomimetic HAP on HAP/CS/Gent coating, suggesting that more OH^- and PO_4^{3-} ions were substituted by CO_3^{2-}, compared to biomimetic HAP on HAP/CS coating.

Having in mind that apatites with Ca/P ratio lower than 1.67 are usually considered as carbonate-substituted (Ishikawa, Ducheyne, and Radin 1993), EDS analysis additionally proved that biomimetic HAP grown on the top of both HAP/CS and HAP/CS/Gent coatings is carbonate-substituted HAP, since the Ca/P ratios were calculated to be 1.64 and 1.46, respectively. The obtained results are encouraging since substituted HAP is known to improve the bioactivity and osteoconductivity and increase adhesion, growth, and differentiation of osteoblast cells compared to the HAP that retains stoichiometric ratio (Cacciotti 2016; Gibson and Bonfield 2002).

FT-IR intense bands in the 960 cm^{-1} to 1200 cm^{-1} region (960 cm^{-1}, 1014 cm^{-1}, and 1087 cm^{-1} for HAP/CS coating and 959 cm^{-1}, 985 cm^{-1}, and 1087 cm^{-1} for HAP/CS/Gent coating) were assigned to (P–O) stretching vibrations of the PO_4^{3-} group (Stevanović, Djošić, Janković, Nešović et al. 2020). The phosphate group band position shifts can be explained by the phosphate ions deviation from their ideal tetrahedral structure (Müller and Müller 2006). The O–P–O bending modes were detected as bands at 558 cm^{-1} and 600 cm^{-1} for both coatings, confirming the formation of calcium phosphate phases (Müller and Müller 2006; Cromme et al. 2007). Usually, in HAP structure, a sharp band at about 3570 cm^{-1} can be detected and assigned to the OH^- stretching from HAP structure (Berzina-Cimdina and Borodajenko 2012). However, this band was absent from the FT-IR spectra for both HAP/CS and HAP/CS/Gent coatings, suggesting the existence of substituted, i.e., carbonated biomimetic HAP, occurring through the carbonate groups occupying the OH^- sites. There are also several bands whose positions indicated the AB-type nature of carbonate substitution in biomimetic HAP (Ren, Ding, and Leng 2014). Various vibrational modes of the CO_3^{2-} group were detected in the FT-IR spectra of both coatings: 878 cm^{-1} (O–C–O), at 1415 cm^{-1} and 1456 cm^{-1} (O-C), "shoulder" at 1466 cm^{-1} (HAP/CS) and at ~1470 cm^{-1} (HAP/CS/Gent), and finally ~1546 cm^{-1} (HAP/CS) and ~1548 cm^{-1} (HAP/CS/Gent). These carbonate bands locations suggested that the structure of biomimetically obtained HAP was similar to the structure of all biological apatites (Ren, Ding, and Leng 2014). For both biomimetic coatings, XRD and EDS results are in accordance with the FT-IR analysis, confirming that biomimetic HAP corresponds to carbonate-substituted hydroxyapatite.

FE-SEM microphotographs of HAP/CS and HAP/CS/Gent coatings on Ti pointed out that gentamicin encapsulation did not change the coating's morphology. Spherical agglomerates of different sizes were observed at both coatings' surfaces before (Figures 3.10a and b) and after seven-day soaking in SBF at 37 °C (Figures 3.10c and d).

The electrochemical measurements were performed in order to investigate the bioactivity of HAP/CS and HAP/CS/Gent coatings during immersion in SBF at 37 °C. Bode modulus plots indicated increased overall impedance for both HAP/CS and HAP/CS/Gent coatings that confirmed the formation and growth of a new apatite

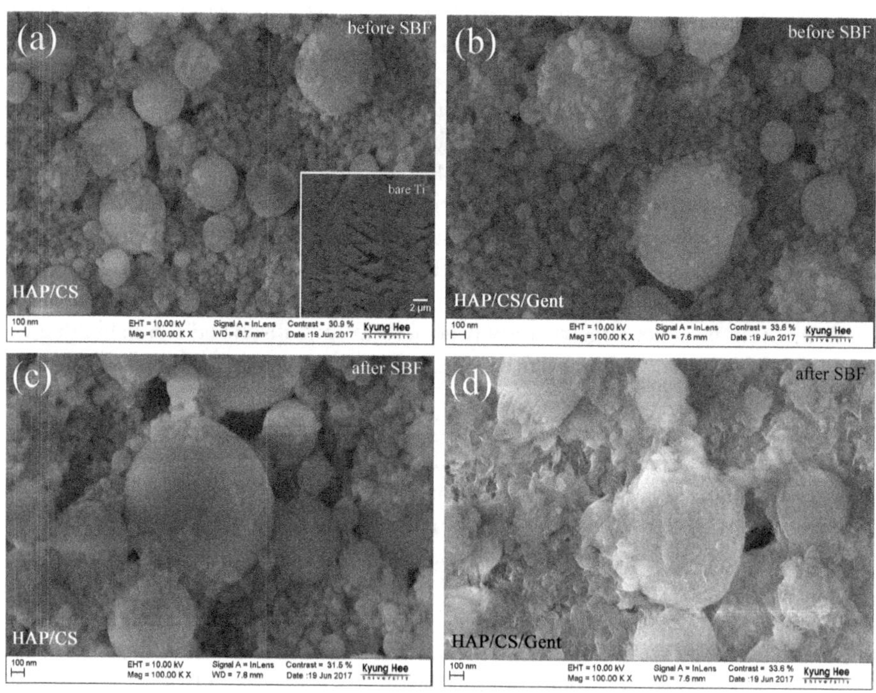

FIGURE 3.10 SEM microphotographs of: (a, c) HAP/CS and (b, d) HAP/CS/Gent coatings on titanium (a, b) before and (c, d) after soaking in SBF at 37 °C, respectively. Inset in (a): bare Ti (reprinted from Stevanović, Djošić, Janković, Nešović et al. 2020 with permission of the American Chemical Society)

layer (Stevanović, Djošić, Janković, Nešović et al. 2020). The biomineralization process is a reversible one, where the dissolution of the coating and apatite precipitation occur simultaneously and the dominant reaction depends on Ca^{2+} and PO_4^{3-} ions concentration. However, mechanisms for dissolution and precipitation are different – ion exchange governs the dissolution process while the concentration gradient and particle solubility influence the precipitation (Q. Zhang et al. 2003). The quick impedance increase during the first four days indicated that the predominant reaction was precipitation of calcium phosphate and the formation of a new HAP layer. Further apatite growth could slow down upon reaching equilibrium since the impedance increase was much slower between days 11 and 28. Impedance spectra were fitted with an equivalent electrical circuit (EEC) presented in Figure 3.11c. The EEC contained ohmic resistance, R_Ω, coupled in series with a parallel RC circuit depicting the coating behavior (with CPE_c – coating capacitance and R_p – coating pore resistance). The constant phase element, CPE, was used instead of a pure capacitor to account for deviations from ideal dielectric behavior. Another parallel RC circuit was coupled in series with R_p and contained double layer capacitance, CPE_{dl}, and charge transfer resistance, R_{ct}. This second time constant described charge transfer processes and electrochemical reactions on the metal/electrolyte interface and was present due to the high porosity of the coating, which enabled the electrolyte to enter the pores and reach the metal underneath. The impedance of a CPE element, Z_{CPE} can be expressed using Eq. 3.3, while the capacitance value can be calculated using equation

$$C_{CPE} = Y_0 \left(\omega_{max}\right)^{\alpha-1} \tag{3.8}$$

where the ω_{max} is the angular frequency at which the imaginary component of the impedance reaches its maximum (Hsu and Mansfeld 2001). It is obvious that for α values close to unity, $C_{CPE} = Y_0$. As in the case of HAP/CS and HAP/CS/Gent α was always higher than 0.8, Y_0 values obtained from the fit were used as the coating capacitance, C_c, and double layer capacitances, C_{dl}. The goodness of fit values (χ^2) were always in the 10^{-6}–10^{-4} range (Stevanović, Djošić, Janković, Nešović et al. 2020). Both C_c and C_{dl} exhibited decreasing trends over the investigated 28-day period (Figure 3.11), which is in line with an increase in impedance, indicating the formation of a new apatite layer. Similar behavior was observed in time dependences of coating pore resistance, R_p. The R_p values increased for both coatings after four days (27.8 kΩ cm^2 for HAP/CS and 33.1 kΩ cm^2 for HAP/CS/Gent), compared to initial immersion (17.6 kΩ cm^2 for HAP/CS and 25.9 kΩ cm^2 for HAP/CS/Gent), indicating the coating thickness increase due to the precipitation of the newly formed HAP layer. After this initial four-day phase, further increase was slower, reaching 38.7 kΩ cm^2 for HAP/CS and 32.4 kΩ cm^2 for HAP/CS/Gent after 28 days. As discussed above, HAP dissolution and precipitation are parallel processes and their simultaneous occurrence was expected during exposure to SBF. The coatings with smaller crystallites are more prone to dissolution as the specific contact area with the solution is higher in this case (Q. Zhang et al. 2003). Thus, the smaller R_p values

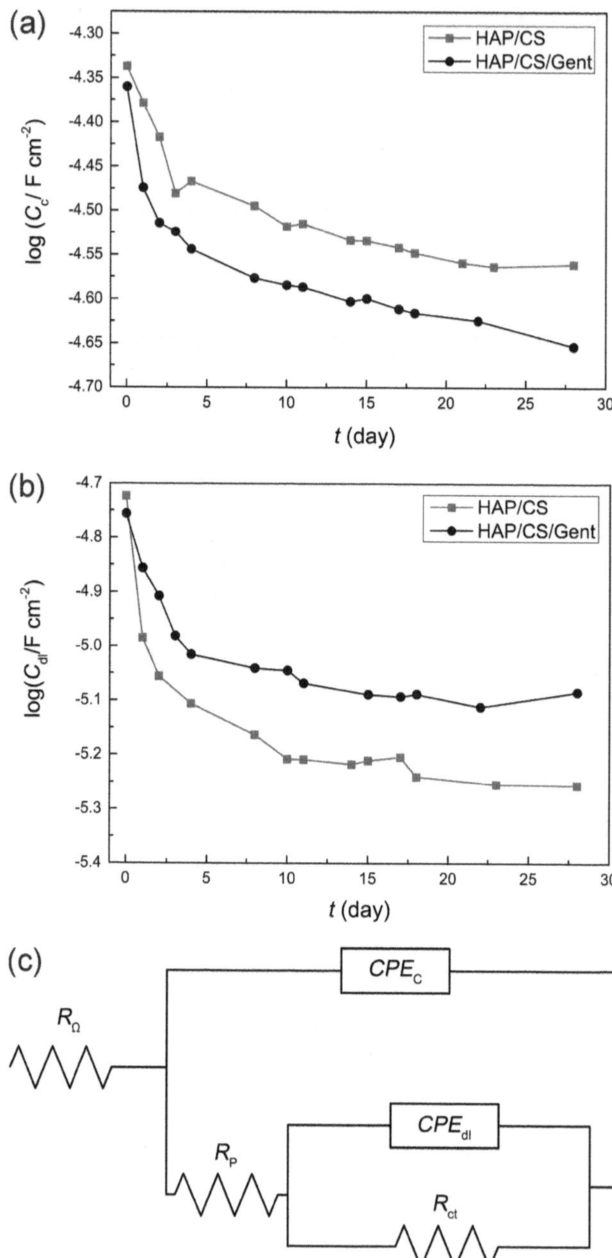

FIGURE 3.11 Time dependence of (a) coating capacitances, C_c, and (b) double layer capacitances, C_{dl}, for HAP/CS and HAP/CS/Gent coatings, obtained from EIS measurements during 28-day exposure to SBF at 37 °C, (c) the equivalent electrical circuit used for EIS spectra fitting (reprinted from Stevanović, Djošić, Janković, Nešović et al. 2020 with permission of the American Chemical Society)

of HAP/CS/Gent coating could be attributed to the smaller crystallite domain size before soaking, as determined from XRD (397 Å for HAP/CS/Gent compared to 511 Å for HAP/CS) (Stevanović et al. 2018).

Polarization measurements were conducted in order to evaluate the bioactivity of HAP/CS and HAP/CS/Gent coatings, after predetermined periods (0, 7, and 28 days) of exposure to SBF. The shifting of polarization curves toward lower values of current density with exposure time indicated biomimetic HAP formation. The corrosion current densities, j_{corr}, were calculated by extrapolating the cathodic curves, which were linear over at least a decade of current, to corrosion potential, E_{corr}. A steady decrease in j_{corr} values was observed for HAP/CS (0.061, 0.012, and 0.011 μA cm^{-2}) and HAP/CS/Gent coatings (0.52, 0.035, and 0.017 μA cm^{-2}) after 0, 7, and 28 days, respectively, confirming the improved resistance as a consequence of the newly formed apatite layer (Stevanović, Djošić, Janković, Nešović et al. 2020). The PDS results agreed well with EIS data suggesting bioactivity of both HAP/CS and HAP/CS/Gent coatings and growth of biomimetic hydroxyapatite layer that should greatly improve the osseointegration process of hard tissue implants.

3.2.3.4 Gentamicin Release

Gentamicin release from HAP/CS/Gent coating was studied during a 21-day immersion in deionized water as a model system, using high-performance liquid chromatography coupled with mass spectrometry (HPLC-MS). The cumulative release profile for HAP/CS/Gent coating with time) verified the initial burst release effect of gentamicin from the composite coating, i.e., more than 50 % of the loaded antibiotic was released within seven days. A pronounced burst release effect (~21 %) was also observed in the first 48 hours, which could be very useful in preventing biofilm formation. This initial seven-day period was followed by a slower release pattern, where only 13 % of the drug was released until day 21 (Stevanović, Djošić, Janković, Nešović et al. 2020). Considering the gentamicin release profiles, the obtained composite coatings could have a potential use as prolonged drug delivery systems for treating orthopedic infections.

To investigate the governing mechanism and diffusion coefficient of release, experimental data fitting was performed. The first model used was the Korsmeyer-Peppas model (Korsmeyer et al. 1983), described by Eq. 3.9, where c_t represents the concentration of gentamicin released at time t, c_0 represents the initial concentration of gentamicin in the coating, k_{KP} is the Korsmeyer-Peppas constant that encompasses the particular carrier system properties, and n is a coefficient that depends on the diffusion type ($n < 0.5$ for Fickian and $n > 0.5$ for non-Fickian diffusion) and is supposed to imply the mechanism of mass transport during the release process. The Korsmeyer-Peppas model was applied in its linear form, where the data were transformed to the logarithmic scale (Korsmeyer et al. 1983)

$$\frac{C_t}{C_0} = k_{KP} \cdot t^n \tag{3.9}$$

and n was calculated to be 0.528, indicating that the mechanism of gentamicin release from HAP/CS/Gent was governed by theFick's diffusion law. Using the early time approximation (ETA) model proposed by Ritger and Peppas (Ritger and Peppas 1987) the value of diffusion coefficient, *D*, of gentamicin was calculated to be 2.4×10^{-14} cm^2 s^{-1}. The ETA model assumes the linear correlation of c_t/c_o ratio and square root of time (Eq. 3.10) appropriate for the one-dimensional release from thin coating, where δ is the thickness of the coating

$$\frac{C_t}{C_0} = 4 \times \left(\frac{Dt}{\pi \delta^2} \right)^{1/2} \tag{3.10}$$

3.2.3.5 Cytotoxicity and ALP Activity

Trypan blue DET testing is a commonly used method for estimating the proportion of viable cells (Phillips 1973). Tested cells are simply mixed with a solution of a dye and stained cells are assumed to be damaged and those unstained to be undamaged. The percent of stained/unstained cells or inhibition of growth (% K) was expressed as a percent of the control. The results of the DET test for MRC-5 (human fibroblasts) and L929 (mice fibroblasts) when tested in the presence of HAP/CS and HAP/CS/Gent coatings on Ti are given in Figure 3.12a. There was no inhibition of growth in the case of either cell line, MRC-5 and L929, for HAP/CS coating on Ti since values were ≈100 %. Gentamicin release resulted in decreased cell growth in the presence of HAP/CS/Gent coated Ti samples, but percent viabilities were above 85 % for both cell lines. According to the one-way analysis of variance statistical test, the differences in viability of both MRC-5 and L929 cell lines were statistically negligible ($p>0.01$) between the two samples when DET testing was considered. Therefore, DET provided strong evidence to support the non-cytotoxic effect for both HAP/CS and HAP/CS/Gent coatings, which could be thus considered a safe material for biomedical use.

Alkaline phosphatase (ALP) is the most widely recognized biochemical marker for osteoblast activity. Although its precise function is poorly understood, it is believed to play a role in skeletal mineralization. Alkaline phosphatase catalyzes the hydrolysis of phosphate esters in the alkaline buffer and produces an organic radical and inorganic phosphate. Changes in alkaline phosphatase level and activity are associated with various bone disease states. The differentiation of osteoblast-like cells is important in the healing process, and inducing biomineralization is required for a biomaterial to be considered bioactive. ALP is a membrane-bound biochemical marker of bone turnover that is secreted from osteoblasts. Usually, ALP assay is performed on osteoblast cells or other cell lines that can differentiate into osteoblasts; however, it could confirm the basic biomineralization potential of HAP/CS and HAP/CS/Gent coatings before moving on to more tissue-specific cells such as osteoblasts. Moreover, it was shown that MRC-5 fibroblasts respond to differentiating factors that promote osteoblastic phenotype in bone-derived cell cultures (Almeida et al. 2001). Both HAP/CS and HAP/CS/Gent coatings had significantly increased ALP activity compared with the control (three and four times increase in ALP expression levels

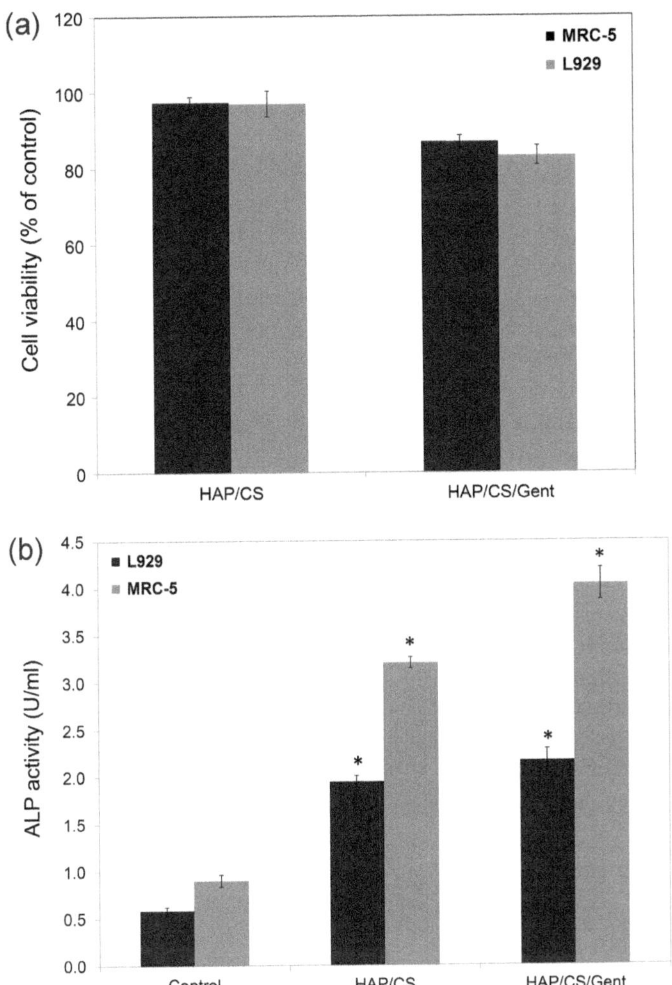

FIGURE 3.12 Cell viability (expressed as percent of control) of MRC-5 and L929 cell cultures (a) and ALP activity in the MRC-5 and L929 cell extract (b) in the presence of HAP/CS and HAP/CS/Gent coatings (reprinted from Stevanović, Djošić, Janković, Nešović et al. 2020 with permission of the American Chemical Society)

for MRC-5 cell line, respectively). However, HAP/CS/Gent (4.039 U/mL) coating increased ALP expression levels of MRC-5 cells more than HAP/CS (3.206 U/mL), suggesting improved biomineralization potential of the gentamicin-loaded coating (Figure 3.12b). Due to cell compatibility, there was no surprise that the MRC-5 cell line overall performed better in this assay. The ALP assay results indicated that both of these materials could induce biomineralization and are therefore strong candidates for further studies with tissue-specific (i.e. osteoblasts) or stem cells, and they could be considered as prospective bone implant coatings.

3.2.4 Hydroxyapatite/Chitosan/Graphene/Gentamicin Coatings

3.2.4.1 Synthesis and Characterization

Aqueous suspensions containing 1 wt. % HAP nanopowder, 0.05 wt. % chitosan, 0.01 wt. % graphene, and 0.1 wt. % gentamicin sulfate were used for EPD process in order to obtain HAP/CS/Gr and HAP/CS/Gr/Gent composite coatings. Cataphoretic deposition was performed on pure Ti plate, serving as working electrode (cathode), at constant voltage of 5 V for deposition time of 12 min (Stevanović, Djošić, Janković, Kojić et al. 2020). Deposited coatings were highly porous due to the electrolysis of water (Eqs. 3.5 and 3.6). From a bioactivity point of view, this can be very convenient, since a porous structure would allow bone ingrowths. Chitosan is soluble in aqueous solutions, at lower pH values (slightly acidified environment, pH 4.4), due to the protonation of amine groups, e.g., CS-NH_3^+ (I. Zhitomirsky and Hashambhoy 2007). Protonated amine groups of the CS molecule in acidic media facilitate electrostatic interactions between individual CS chains, increasing the overall suspension stability. The deposition of insoluble chitosan CS-NH_2 coating occurred due to CS-NH_3^+ and OH^- ions interacting on the cathode (Eq. 3.7) since OH^- ions are being formed as a result of electrochemical water decomposition (Eq. 3.5). When HAP inorganic particles were added in slightly acidic solution, the protonation of hydroxyapatite surface occurred.

Special attention should be paid to the addition of graphene, aimed to serve as reinforcement filler (Shi et al. 2016; Ordikhani et al. 2015). Gr is known to form a strong bond with chitosan matrix as a consequence of its characteristic surface architecture, i.e., great number of p electrons in sp^2 hybrid orbitals inducing the negative charge on the Gr sheet surface. A negatively charged surface of Gr could interact with protonated amino groups of chitosan, forming a stable suspension for the coating deposition process (Đošić et al. 2017). On the other hand, Van der Waals interaction between graphene sheets and HAP, through the calcium ions, occurred as well (Janković, Eraković, Vukašinović-Sekulić et al. 2015; V. Geetha, Gomathi, and Sudha 2015). Therefore, all particles (chitosan, graphene, and hydroxyapatite) interact between each other, making a well-dispersed suspension suitable for composite coating deposition. For HAP/CS/Gr coating loaded with gentamicin, positively charged Gent (due to the protonation of amino and hydroxyl groups (Pishbin et al. 2014)) migrated toward the cathode and formed a four-component coating along with HAP, CS, and Gr.

The composition of electrodeposited HAP/CS/Gr and HAP/CS/Gr/Gent coatings on Ti was investigated by FT-IR (Stevanović, Djošić, Janković, Kojić et al. 2020). Spectral carbonate bands for HAP/CS/Gr composite coating were observed in the regions from 800 to 900 cm^{-1} and from 1350 to 1600 cm^{-1} (Brangule and Gross 2015; Ren, Ding, and Leng 2014; Berzina-Cimdina and Borodajenko 2012). Carbonate ions can substitute hydroxyl and/or phosphate groups, leading to the formation of carbonate-substituted hydroxyapatite. When the replacement of OH^- groups by CO_3^{2-} groups occurs, the change in HAP structure is known as A-type substituted HAP. When PO_4^{3-} groups are substituted by CO_3^{2-} groups, then such substitution is denoted as B-type hydroxyapatite. The carbonate band at 878 cm^{-1} represented the vibration mode of O–C–O group (Ren, Ding, and Leng 2014). For more precise analysis of FTIR spectra of electrodeposited composite coatings, e.g., determination of the type of carbonate substitution in HAP (A-, B- or AB-type), deconvolution of carbonate peak in the region 800–900 cm^{-1} was performed. Deconvolution of carbonate band at 878 cm^{-1} revealed three different peaks. The peak at 879 cm^{-1} can be assigned to the A-type carbonate substitution, the peak at 872 cm^{-1} suggested the presence of B-type substitution, while the peak at 865 cm^{-1} represented the non-apatite carbonate (Brangule and Gross 2015). After the deconvolution of FT-IR peaks in the region from 1350 to 1600 cm^{-1} the presence of A- and B-type of substitution in HAP structure was confirmed. The bands at 1421 and 1470 cm^{-1}, as well as a doublet at 1407 and 1441 cm^{-1}, can be assigned to B-type of carbonate-substituted HAP (Ren, Ding, and Leng 2014; Yang et al. 2013; Xu et al. 2005; K. Zhang et al. 2011; Surudžić et al. 2016; Berzina-Cimdina and Borodajenko 2012; Rapacz-Kmita et al. 2015). The presence of A substituted HAP can be confirmed by the presence of band at 1528 cm^{-1}, while band at 1456 cm^{-1} can be assigned to the both A- and B-type of carbonate-substituted HAP. Based on the positions of carbonate bands, it could be concluded that "AB-type" substitution occurred through the substitution of hydroxyl and phosphate groups with the CO_3^{2-} group. Two distinctive bands at 1654 cm^{-1} (amide I band) and 1546 cm^{-1} (amide II band) for HAP/CS/Gr coating were assigned to the C=O stretching vibration of –NHCO– group and the N–H bending in $-NH_2$ group of CS, respectively. The chitosan in HAP/CS/Gr coating was also verified by bands at 2857 cm^{-1} and 2926 cm^{-1}, originating from C-H stretching in the CS structure (Nikpour, Rabiee, and Jahanshahi 2012; Marija S. Djošić, Mitrić, and Mišković-Stankovic 2015). At 1388 cm^{-1} the band for CH_3 symmetrical deformation in chitosan structure can be distinguished. Bands at 473, 563, 600, 952, 1020, and 1085 cm^{-1} undoubtedly confirmed the hydroxyapatite presence in the HAP/CS/Gr composite coating. All these bands were ascribed to the different vibration modes of the PO_4^{3-} group. The band at 1560 cm^{-1} can be assigned to the skeletal vibration of Gr, confirming the successful incorporation of graphene in HAP/CS/Gr coating. The band at 1640 cm^{-1} can be assigned to the N-H bending vibration of primary aromatic amines (Fan et al. 2013), confirming incorporation of gentamicin in HAP/CS/Gr/Gent. The slight shift from 3279 cm^{-1} (for HAP/CS/Gr) to 3261 cm^{-1} (for HAP/CS/Gr/Gent) was noticed after gentamicin introduction. These bands were attributed to the valence vibrations of hydroxyl groups, sensitive to hydrogen bonding. Therefore it can be assumed that hydrogen bonding between hydroxyl groups of HAP and amino and hydroxyl groups of CS with gentamicin hydroxyl and amino groups occurred.

Using the HAP characteristic crystal planes (002), (211), (112), and (300), the values of *d*-spacing (3.4537, 2.8271, 2.7899, and 2.7326, respectively), unit cell volume, V (523 Å^3), and parameters a (9.383 Å), c (6.863 Å), and crystallite domain size (311 Å) were calculated for HAP/CS/Gr/Gent coating. As a consequence of gentamicin incorporation, a decrease in the *d*-spacing values for HAP/CS/Gr/Gent with respect to the HAP/CS/Gr coating could be observed. Additionally, bonding can occur through the mutual interaction of hydroxyl and amino groups from CS and Gent. All of these interactions are accompanied by the intermolecular bonding, causing contracting in the chitosan matrix and, consequently, decreasing in *d*-spacing value of HAP (Nikpour, Rabiee, and Jahanshahi 2012). As a consequence, the unit cell parameters *a* and *c* and the unit cell volume, as well as the crystallite domain size, have smaller values than for the HAP/CS/Gr coating (9.446 Å, 6.907 Å, 536 Å^3, and 435 Å). Many factors influence the crystallization process (temperature, aging, and environment) and crystallite domain size is also the result of the crystallization rate and the rate of crystal growth. During the coating drying process, sulfate ions (from the gentamicin sulfate) influence the formation of a large number of nucleation sites. At the same time, as gentamicin is a bulky molecule, there is also a possibility that it prevents further crystal growth. Both of these effects lead to finer crystallite structure and smaller size in the case of HAP/CS/Gr/Gent composite coating, which is important for biological applications contributing to better osteointegration due to bone-like apatite formation.

XPS C 1s peak was fitted into five different modes with binding energy (BE) values of 284.6, 285.5, 286.9, 288.65, and 290.2 eV (Stevanović, Djošić, Janković, Kojić et al. 2020). These peaks were assigned to C–H/C–C (284.6 eV), C-O/C-N (285.5 eV), O–C–O (286.9 eV), O–C=N (288.65 eV), and C=O (290.2 eV) originates from Gr, and acetyl and amide groups characteristic for chitosan (M. Li, Wang et al. 2013). Similar BE for C1s peaks were also found in case of HAP/CS/Gr/Gent where five peaks were distinguished at 284.8, 285.85, 287.2, 288.8, and 290.3 eV and were ascribed to C–H/C–C, C–O/C-N, O–C–O, O–C=N, and C=O, respectively. Due to the similarity of gentamicin structure with chitosan, and due to the small amount of gentamicin in the coatings, similar peaks were obtained for both coatings. Characteristic peaks for gentamicin at 287.2 eV (O–C–O) and 288.8 eV (O–C=N), originating from acetal bonds and methylamino groups from gentamicin, overlapped with acetal and amide groups from chitosan (Yang Liu et al. 2017). Carbon interactions were evaluated in order to estimate the type of bonding. In the case of HAP/CS/Gr, the percentages of carbon interactions were 24.3 % (C–H/C–C), 26.0 % (C-O/C–N), 34.5 % (O-C–O), 12.2 % (O–C=N), and 3.0 % (C=O), while HAP/CS/Gr/Gent exhibited 29.1 % (C–H/C–C), 27.6 % (C-O/C–N), 28.0 % (O–C–O), 12.0 % (O–C=N), and 3.3 % (C=O). The ratio of the absorptive peaks area corresponding to C-O/C-N interactions was increased after gentamicin introduction for HAP/CS/Gr/Gent (27.6 %) with respect to HAP/CS/Gr (26.0 %) due to an increase in the number of amino groups. The increase in the percentage of C=O interactions for HAP/CS/Gr/Gent (3.3 %) compared to HAP/CS/Gr (3.0 %) was caused by the larger number of acetyl groups.

The high-resolution O1s peak was fitted into three different modes with BE at 531.4, 532.7, and 533.6 eV for HAP/CS/Gr and at 531.7, 532.7, and 533.8 eV for HAP/CS/Gr/Gent coating. The obtained peaks confirmed the interactions obtained from C 1 high resolution and were ascribed to PO_4^{3-}, –OH and C=O groups (Maachou et al. 2013). The peaks at 531.4 and 531.7 eV for HAP/CS/Gr and HAP/CS/Gr/Gent, respectively, could be assigned to the PO_4^{3-} groups of HAP, while peaks at 532.7 eV for both samples could represent the contribution from hydroxyl groups from HAP, chitosan, and gentamicin. The peaks at 533.6 and 533.8 eV could be assigned to the C=O interactions, originating from chitosan and gentamicin (Stevanović et al. 2018). For both coatings N 1s spectra were fitted into two different modes at 400.2

and 401.7 eV for HAP/CS/Gr, and at 400.5, 401.7 eV for HAP/CS/Gr/Gent coating. The peaks at 400.2 and 400.5 eV, for HAP/CS/Gr and HAP/CS/Gr/Gent, respectively, were assigned to C-NH_2 interactions (free amines), while peaks at 401.7 eV for both spectra could be assigned to the C-NH_3^+ interactions (protonated amines). For HAP/CS/Gr spectrum, Ca2p revealed two peak components $Ca2p_{1/2}$ at 350.5 eV, and $Ca2p_{3/2}$ at 347 eV, Ca2p of HAP/CS/Gr/Gent exhibited $Ca2p_{1/2}$ at 351 eV and $Ca2p_{3/2}$ at 347.9 eV. P2p spectra with $P2p_{3/2}$ at 133.1 eV and 133.9 eV for HAP/CS/Gr and HAP/CS/Gr/Gent, respectively, were also observed. Since gentamicin sulfate solution was used, XPS spectrum of HAP/CS/Gr/Gent composite displayed the S2p peak at 170 eV, clearly confirming the gentamicin incorporation. The C, O, N, P, and Ca elemental compositions, calculated from XPS, were quite similar for both coatings: 21.0, 51.6, 1.3, 11.6, and 14.6 at %, respectively, for HAP/CS/Gr and 21.5, 51.3, 1.2, 11.1, and 14.1at %, respectively, for HAP/CS/Gr/Gent. The only difference that undoubtedly confirmed the gentamicin incorporation was sulfur content in the HAP/CS/Gr/Gent coating (0.7 at %). The calculated values of Ca/P ratio of 1.26 and 1.27 for HAP/CS/Gr and HAP/CS/Gr/Gent coatings, respectively, confirmed the FT-IR conclusion on calcium-deficient hydroxyapatite. It is known that bioactivity and osseoinductivity are improved in the case of substituted HAP compared to the HAP that retains a stoichiometric ratio.

Due to a similar morphology of HAP/CS/Gr and HAP/CS/Gr/Gent coatings, it was evident that the incorporation of gentamicin did not significantly affect surfaces on the micro-level, consisting of HAP spherical particles that are mostly agglomerated. In some cases, agglomerates large surface was covered with small HAP spherical particles. At the same time, agglomeration of particles could occur due to interface interaction between HAP and polymer matrix and attributed to the high specific surface energy of HAP particles. Even at higher magnification, the surface of both coatings seems highly porous and homogeneous. This well-dispersed network is reinforced by graphene since graphene is known to act as a "bonding" material, making bridges through the polymer matrix and preventing the crack formation in the coatings.

From Raman spectra of HAP/CS/Gr/Gent coating the significant difference could be observed after gentamicin introduction. The first difference was spotted in the band position, which refers to γ_1 stretching vibrations of PO_4^{3-} group from HAP. Obviously, both the wavenumber and the intensity of the band corresponding to PO_4^{3-} groups were decreased in HAP/CS/Gr/Gent coating (920 cm^{-1}) with respect to HAP/CS/Gr coating (959 cm^{-1}). This could be explained by the change in the vibrational mode of PO_4^{3-} caused by gentamicin introduction through establishing chemical bonds between hydroxyl groups of HAP with OH^- groups from CS and gentamicin. Further, the band at 1566 cm^{-1} was evident in the HAP/CS/Gr spectrum, whereas in the case of HAP/CS/Gr/Gent this band was not observed. This band at 1566 cm^{-1} was assigned to the G-band characteristic for graphene overlapping with in-plane bending vibrations of –NH_2 bonds from chitosan. At the same time, the absence of this band in the HAP/CS/Gr/Gent spectrum could be explained by the interactions between amino groups of CS and gentamicin, as well as the low initial graphene content in the samples. Regardless of the G-band absence in HAP/CS/

Gr/Gent spectrum, bands at 1358 cm^{-1} and 1372 cm^{-1} for HAP/CS/Gr and HAP/CS/Gr/Gent, respectively, originating from D-band (associated with the disorder in graphene structure), indicated the graphene incorporation. Moreover, characteristic 2D-band for graphene presence was noticed at 2704 cm^{-1} for HAP/CS/Gr and at 2728 cm^{-1} for HAP/CS/Gr/Gent. The range from 2800 to 3000 cm^{-1} could be assigned to stretching vibrations of -CH and $-CH_2$ groups. Therefore, the bands found at 2936 cm^{-1} and 2912 cm^{-1} in the case of HAP/CS/Gr and HAP/CS/Gr/Gent, respectively, were assigned to the symmetric stretching of the C-H bond from the $-CH_2$ group in the CS. After the introduction of gentamicin, the band at 2912 cm^{-1} became more pronounced in comparison to the peak at 2936 cm^{-1} probably because of the change in vibration modes of –CH and $-CH_2$ groups after gentamicin introduction. In the case of HAP/CS/Gr coating, this peak is of lower intensity and it is shifted to larger wavenumbers, pointing to the interactions between CS and oxygen-containing groups in graphene (commercially available graphene always contains a certain amount of impurities and oxidized groups). The band at 1441 cm^{-1} for HAP/CS/Gr/Gent could be explained by the in-plane bending of CH_2 and OH bond from CS and gentamicin.

HAP/CS/Gr and HAP/CS/Gr/Gent coatings expressed gradual weight loss through several steps in TG curves. Initial weight loss, ascribed to the water desorption, appeared in the temperature interval from 16 °C to 118 °C (mass loss of 2.6 wt. %) for HAP/CS/Gr and in the temperature interval from 18 °C to 158 °C (mass loss of 6.5 wt. %) for HAP/CS/Gr/Gent coating. Addition of gentamicin caused the significant increase in mass loss due to reduced crystallite domain size, i.e., larger specific surface area of HAP/CS/Gr/Gent coating compared to HAP/CS/Gr coating, as it was shown by XRD results. The next stage of weight loss was observed in the intervals from 166 °C to 212 °C (mass loss of 0.6 wt. %) with a sharp maximum in DTG curve at 180 °C for HAP/CS/Gr coating. Maximum at 187 °C, in the temperature interval from 117 °C to 238 °C, with 1.2 wt. % mass loss was observed for HAP/CS/Gr/Gent coating. This stage was assigned to the crystalline water release and the beginning of HAP dehydroxylation. The third weight loss stage, observed in the temperature interval from 240 °C to 345 °C for HAP/CS/Gr with 1.4 wt. % mass loss and from 213 °C to 365 °C with 2.4 wt. % mass loss in the case of HAP/CS/Gr/Gent coating, suggesting the thermal decomposition of chitosan (Yoshizawa, Fourmy, and Puglisi 1998; Tangy et al. 1985). However, the prominent peak that appeared at 294 °C in the case of HAP/CS/Gr coating (DTG curve) indicating CS degradation, was shifted to 305 °C in the case of HAP/CS/Gr/Gent coating (DTG curve). According to the literature, the significant weight loss for the gentamicin sulfate is reported in the range 225 °C–330 °C. So the greater mass loss obtained in the case of HAP/CS/Gr/Gent coating with respect to the mass loss of HAP/CS/Gr coating can be assigned to the gentamicin decomposition. Next stage of weight loss for HAP/CS/Gr coating of about 1.2 wt. % occurred in the temperature interval from 345 °C to 433 °C with two maximums at 378 °C and 401 °C (DTG curve). For HAP/CS/Gr/Gent coating, 0.7 wt. % mass loss was detected in the temperature range from 364 °C to 425 °C with two distinguished maximums at 379 °C and 405 °C (DTG curve). Bearing in mind that HAP in both coatings is carbonate substituted, as confirmed by the FT-IR analysis, decrease in mass for both coatings was due to the loss of carbonate ions as

CO_2 as well as to the further degradation of chitosan (for HAP/CS/Gr coating) and chitosan and gentamicin (for HAP/CS/Gr/Gent coating), as was found also in literature (Pishbin et al. 2014; Dwivedi et al. 2018; Patel et al. 2012). The next stage of weight loss can be observed in the temperature interval from 433 °C to 509 °C with 0.5 wt. % mass loss for HAP/CS/Gr coating and between 425 °C and 580 °C with 1.4 wt. % mass loss for HAP/CS/Gr/Gent coating. Two maximums can be observed in this temperature interval, e.g., at 443 °C for HAP/CS/Gr coating (DTG curve) and at 450 °C for HAP/CS/Gr/Gent coating (DTG curve). These two peaks can be attributed to the decomposition of Gr (Janković, Eraković, Mitrić et al. 2015), remaining components from CS and residual functional groups of gentamicin (Dwivedi et al. 2015; Ivanova et al. 2001). The last stage of weight loss occurs in the range from 514 °C to 685 °C with 1.8 wt. % mass loss for HAP/CS/Gr coating, and between 582 °C and 662 °C with 0.8 wt. % mass loss for HAP/CS/Gr/Gent coating can be attributed to the decarbonation and dehydroxylation processes of HAP (Ivanova et al. 2001). In this stage, at DTG curves peak at 630 °C for HAP/CS/Gr coating and at 625 °C for HAP/CS/Gr/Gent coating can be observed. According to the literature (Meejoo, Maneeprakorn, and Winotai 2006; Capanema et al. 2015), carbonate-substituted HAP has the tendency to transform into a stoichiometric hydroxyapatite and tricalcium phosphate in the temperature range below 700 °C, through the decarbonation (the CO_3^{2-} release from the hydroxide or phosphate sites in the form of CO_2) and dehydroxylation processes (OH^- groups loss through the water release from the hydroxyapatite structure). In the temperature interval from 17 °C to 1000 °C, the total weight loss for HAP/CS/Gr and HAP/CS/Gr/Gent coatings was calculated to be 10.5 wt. % and 14.8 wt. %, respectively, pointing to lower thermal stability of HAP/CS/Gr/Gent coating.

3.2.4.2 Antibacterial Activity and Cytotoxicity

Figure 3.13 depicts the effect of HAP/CS/Gr and HAP/CS/Gr/Gent coating against *S. aureus* TL and *E. coli* ATCC 25922 in PB medium, respectively (Stevanović, Djošić, Janković, Kojić et al. 2020). Statistical evaluation for samples done in triplicate was performed using one-way ANOVA, with a multiple comparisons post hoc analysis. If the p-value was lower than 0.01, results were considered statistically significant. After the initial contact, the adhered molecules of gentamicin are readily released and reduce the initial bacteria count by two logarithmic units. However, in the first hour, drug release seems to be delayed, indicating the strong hydrogen bonding reinforced through non-specific interaction of gentamicin to chitosan and graphene. Diminishing of *S. aureus* bacterial growth occurred within three hours of exposure (Figure 3.13a). Based on the results of HAP/CS/Gr/Gent composite coating against *S. aureus*, the effect is highly bactericidal.

Retained antibacterial effect of HAP/CS/Gr/Gent coating was clearly seen against *E. coli* (Figure 3.13b). In the initial period after inoculation the release of the drug hardly affected the bacteria, i.e., their sensitivity toward antibiotic was low. For the duration of the experiment (24 hours post-incubation), a substantial decline of surviving *E. coli* cells was observed. Comparing the effects of composite HAP/CS/Gr and HAP/CS/Gr/Gent coatings and based on the kinetics testing against *E. coli*, since the

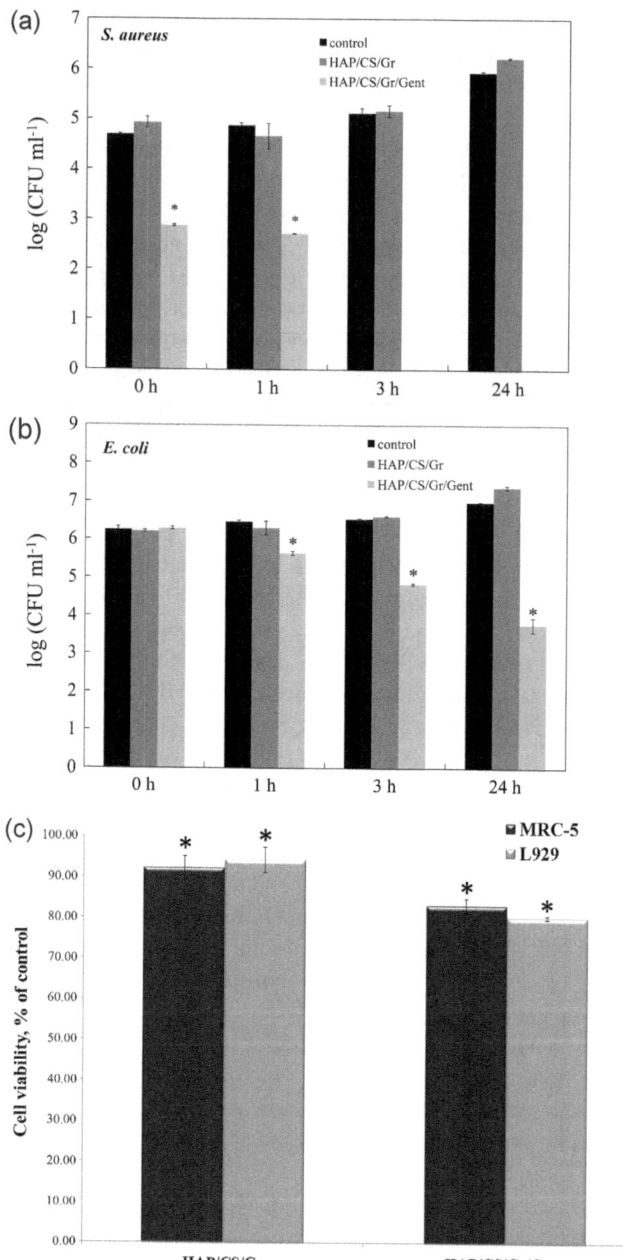

FIGURE 3.13 Reduction of viable cell number of: (a) *S. aureus* and (b) *E. coli* after contact with HAP/CS/Gr and HAP/CS/Gr/Gent coatings in PB as compared to the control samples coatings (* $p < 0.01$ for the respective bacteria strain) (reprinted from Stevanović, Djošić, Janković, Kojić et al. 2020 with permission from John Wiley and Sons) and (c) DET test cytotoxicity against MRC-5 and L929 cell (* $p < 0.01$ within the cell line (reprinted from Stevanović et al. 2021 with permission from Elsevier)

reduction in bacterial cells was less than three logarithmic units, HAP/CS/Gr/Gent coating was classified as bacteriostatic. For the duration of the experiment (24 hours post-incubation), a substantial decline of surviving *E. coli* was observed. Comparing the effects of composite HAP/CS/Gr and HAP/CS/Gr/Gent coatings, based on the in suspension test against *E. coli*, since the reduction in bacterial cells was less than three logarithmic units, HAP/CS/Gr/Gent coating was classified as bacteriostatic.

The evaluation of cell growth (% K) in trypan blue DET test was expressed as a percent of control and further estimated based on the ratio of stained and unstained cells since damaged cells were stained as opposed to undamaged that were unstained. HAP/CS/Gr coating provoked the inhibition of growth neither in the case of MRC-5 (92.2 %) nor for L929 (96.4 %). After the gentamicin introduction, the cell growth appeared to decrease slightly for both MRC-5 (83.1 %) and L929 (79.7 %) cell lines, so the HAP/CS/Gr/Gent coating is non-cytotoxic (Figure 3.13c). A slight drop in the survival rate was attributed to the antibiotic presence, as well documented in a recent study when high concentrations of therapeutic agent – gentamicin (250–270 μg/mL) – that was reached during the immersion of the gentamicin containing films affected osteoblastic proliferation (MC3T3-E1 cells) when compared to the control (Permyakova et al. 2021). One-way analysis of variance statistical tests, when applied to the DET test, pointed out that the differences in the cell growth for both MRC-5 and L929 cell lines between the two samples were statistically significant ($p < 0.05$).

3.2.4.3 *In Vitro* Bioactivity

To investigate the bioactivity of HAP/CS/Gr and HAP/CS/Gr/Gent coatings on titanium the FT-IR, XRD, FE-SEM and electrochemical measurements (EIS and PDS) have been performed (Stevanović et al. 2021). Differences in FT-IR bands position, for both HAP/CS/Gr and HAP/CS/Gr/Gent coatings before and after immersion, indicated the new biomimetic HAP layer formation in SBF at 37 °C. Bands in the 450–600 cm^{-1} region represent the (O–P–O) bending modes in the phosphate group, while characteristic bands of the (P–O) stretching vibrations of the PO_4^{3-} group can be observed in the 900–1200 cm^{-1} region. In HAP structure, hydroxyl and/or phosphate ions can be substituted by carbonate ions, leading to the formation A-, B-, or AB-type of carbonate-substituted HAP. Based on the position of carbonate bands in the FT-IR spectra for both HAP/CS/Gr and HAP/CS/Gr/Gent coatings after immersion in SBF at 37 °C for seven days, vibrational modes of O–C–O (878 cm^{-1}) and O-C groups (region 1400-1500 cm^{-1}) can be distinguished. The position of these carbonate bands confirmed that the AB-type substitution in newly formed HAP occurred. Bands assigned to the structural OH– bending also confirmed HAP structure. The presence of carbonate-substituted HAP on the top of the investigated coatings is preferred for numerous reasons. The fact that carbonate-substituted HAP is already found in the natural bone and dentine tissue can stand out as the most important reason (Madupalli, Pavan, and Tecklenburg 2017).

XRD analysis confirmed the formation of carbonate-substituted HAP after seven-day immersion in SBF, supporting the FT-IR results. Diffraction maxima were identified by standard JCPDS file no. 09-0432 for HAP and standard JCPDS file no. 89-2762 for titanium. The crystallite domain size for as-deposited HAP/CS/Gr and

HAP/CS/Gr/Gent coatings was calculated to be 43.5 and 31.1 nm, and after immersion in SBF 16.6 and 36.0 nm, respectively (M. Djošić, Janković, and Mišković-Stanković 2021).

Carbonate ions can substitute OH^- (A-type), PO_4^{3-} (B-type), or both OH^- and PO_4^{3-} (AB-type substitution, found in biological apatites) (Rincón-López et al. 2018) ions in HAP lattice, causing the changes in unit cell parameters and crystallinity. A-type substitution is known to cause *a*-axes expansion and *c*-axes contraction as opposed to B-type substitution that causes a contraction in *a*-axes and expansion in *c*-axes. It was calculated that newly formed HAP on HAP/CS/Gr coating, obtained after immersion in SBF, exhibited the changes in both *a* (9.390 Å) and *c* (6.871 Å) axes in respect to the values of *a* (9.446 Å) and *c* (6.907 Å) for HAP/CS/Gr coating before immersion in SBF. In the case of newly formed HAP on the HAP/CS/Gr/Gent coating, the changes in both unit cell parameters *a* (9.451 Å) and *c* (6.912 Å) were observed in respect to the HAP/CS/Gr/Gent coating before immersion (*a*-9.383 Å, *c*-6.863 Å), suggesting the presence of AB-type carbonate substitution in the newly formed HAP. According to the literature (Sakthivel, Ragu, and Senthilarasan 2015), values of HAP unit cell parameters are as follows: a=9.418 Å, c=6.884 Å, (JCPDS 09-0432). The difference between theoretical and experimental values in the *a*- and *c*- axis is greater in the case of newly formed HAP on the top of the HAP/CS/Gr/Gent coating, suggesting that more hydroxyl and phosphate ions were substituted by carbonate ions compared to newly grown HAP on the antibiotic-free coating (HAP/CS/Gr).

The Ca/P ratio according to the energy dispersive spectrometry (EDS) analysis was calculated to be 1.61 and 1.36 for HAP/CS/Gr and HAP/CS/Gr/Gent coatings before immersion in SBF, respectively. After immersion in SBF, Ca/P ratio has a lower value for both coatings, 1.52 and 1.24 for HAP/CS/Gr and HAP/CS/Gr/Gent, respectively, confirming the formation of a new biomimetic HAP layer on the top of both coatings. Since the value of Ca/P ratio in stoichiometric HAP is 1.67, the lower obtained values of Ca/P ratio proved that newly formed HAP on both coatings is carbonate substituted (Ishikawa, Ducheyne, and Radin 1993; Wopenka and Pasteris 2005). Due to the lower Ca/P ratio in the case of HAP grown on the top of the HAP/CS/Gr/Gent coating (1.24) with respect to the HAP on the top of the coating without antibiotic (1.52), the additional confirmation of the greater carbonate substitution in the HAP crystallite formed on the top of the coating with antibiotic was achieved. These results are quite promising as it is known that carbonate-substituted HAP can improve the biological performances of prosthetic implant materials (bioactivity, osteoconductivity, growth, and differentiation of osteoblast cells) with respect to the stoichiometric HAP (Cacciotti 2016) due to the presence of carbonate ions in HAP structure, which contribute to the increased HAP solubility and simultaneously reduce HAP crystallinity (Borkowski et al. 2016). The presence of newly formed HAP consisting of characteristic spherical agglomerates could be clearly distinguished from FE-SEM micrographs (Stevanović et al. 2021).

Both HAP/CS/Gr and HAP/CS/Gr/Gent coatings exhibited an increase in impedance obtained from EIS during a 28-day exposure to SBF at 37 °C due to the growth of a new biomimetic HAP layer, in accordance with the results of FT-IR, XRD, and

FE-SEM. The rapid increase in pore resistance, R_p, and decrease in coating capacitance, C_c, obtained from impedance plots in complex plane were observed during the first couple of days, indicating the coating thickness increase due to the precipitation and growth of the newly formed HAP layer (Figure 3.14a and b, respectively). After the first four days, the R_p increase and C_c decrease became slower. The bioactive nature of HAP/CS/Gr and HAP/CS/Gr/Gent coatings was also assessed using polarization measurements that gave insight into valuable corrosion parameters (Figure 3.14c). The cathodic curves were linear over one decade of current, so they were extrapolated in order to determine the values of the corrosion current density, j_{corr}, and the cathodic Tafel slopes, b_c, were calculated from their slopes. On the other hand, the anodic parts of the polarization curves did not exhibit sufficiently linear behavior due to the changing nature of the anodic reactions, and they could be used neither for j_{corr} calculation nor for obtaining the anodic Tafel slope. The corrosion current density significantly decreased for both samples after 28-day exposure – a tenfold decrease for HAP/CS/Gr (from 0.17 to 0.016 $\mu A\ cm^{-2}$) and HAP/CS/Gr/Gent (from 0.14 to 0.043 $\mu A\ cm^{-2}$), denoting the growth of newly formed biomimetic HAP layer. The cathodic Tafel slopes, b_c, did not change significantly from 0 to 28 days for both coatings; in the case of HAP/CS/Gr from -220 to -215 mV dec^{-1} , and for HAP/CS/Gr/Gent from -276 to -264 mV dec^{-1}, meaning that the reaction mechanism did not change during prolonged exposure to SBF. Carefully considering all the electrochemical results obtained from EIS and PDS, i.e., increase in R_p and decrease in C_c and j_{corr}, it can be concluded that both HAP/CS/Gr and HAP/CS/Gr/Gent coatings showed a tendency to promote the growth of new HAP layer growth after exposure to physiological solute-ions.

3.2.4.4 Gentamicin Release

The highly desired effect of the initial burst release of gentamicin was manifested during the first seven days (~ 60 %) followed by a slower release rate reaching up to 74 % after 21 days. Experimental data (Figure 3.15) were fitted with the Korsmeyer–Peppas and early time approximation (ETA) kinetic models. From Korsmeyer–Peppas model (Eq. 3.9) and its linear form the value of exponent n was calculated to be 0.392, pointing out that the gentamicin release process followed the Fick's diffusion law. Using early time approximation (ETA) model (Eq. 3.10) the diffusion coefficient, *D*, for gentamicin release from HAP/CS/Gr/Gent coating was calculated to be $4.5 \times 10^{-14}\ cm^2\ s^{-1}$. The use of graphene as a drug carrier is the subject of much research owing to its high surface area enabling the drug loading on both sides of the Gr sheet (Jinzhao Liu et al. 2018).

3.2.4.5 ALP Activity

When comparing the results of ALP activity of HAP/CS/Gr and HAP/CS/Gr/Gent coatings for MRC-5 and L929 cell extracts with control, the statistically significant ($p<0.05$) increase for both coatings was noticed (Figure 3.16). MRC-5 fibroblast cell line exhibited higher ALP values contrary to the L929 cell line in the presence of both samples. The HAP/CS/Gr/Gent coating expressed higher ALP potential (2.449 U/mL for MRC-5 and 0.805 U/mL for L929) as opposed to HAP/CS/Gr coating

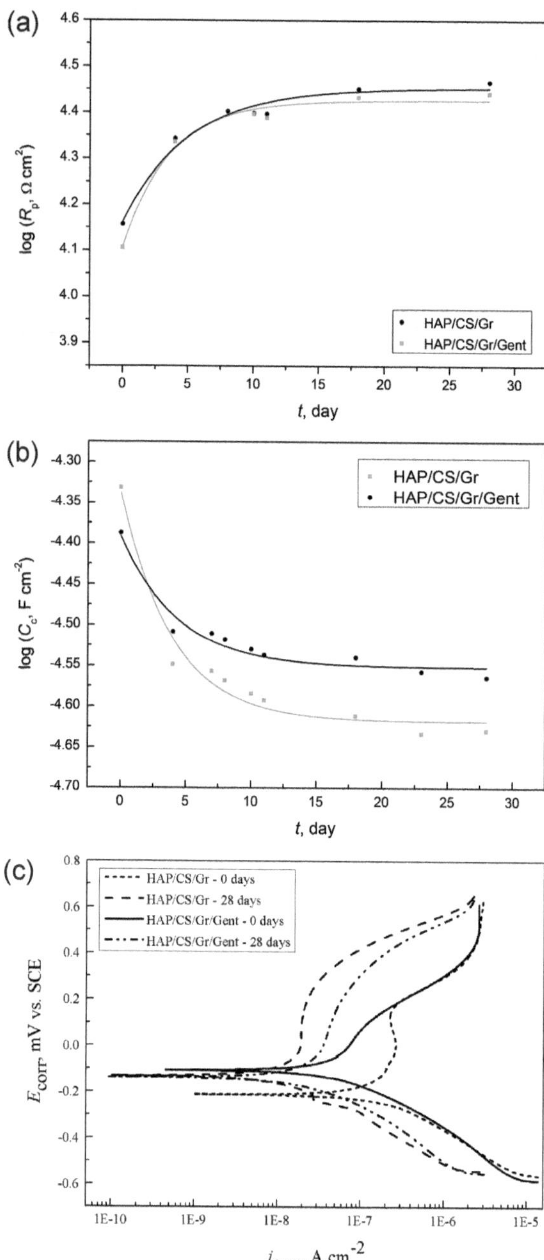

FIGURE 3.14 Time dependence of: (a) coating pore resistance, R_p, (b) coating capacitance, C_c and (c) potentiodynamic polarization curves for HAP/CS/Gr and HAP/CS/Gr/Gent coatings during a 28-day exposure to SBF at 37°C (reprinted from Stevanović et al. 2021 with permission from Elsevier)

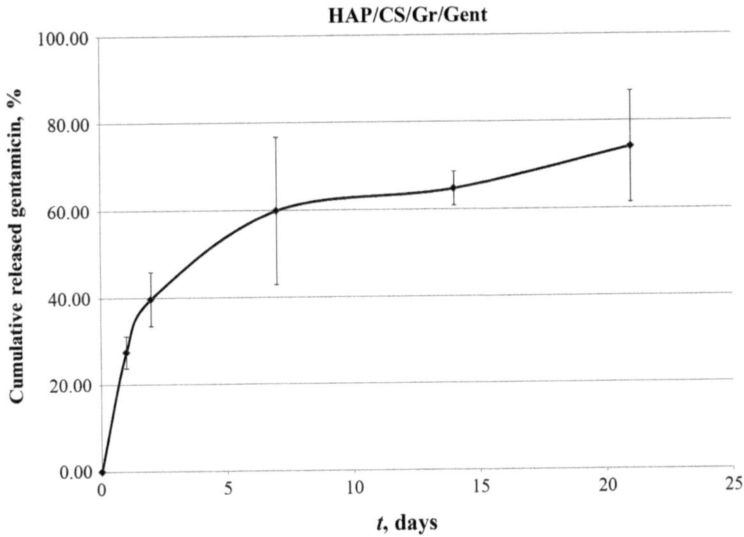

FIGURE 3.15 The average cumulative release profile of gentamicin from HAP/CS/Gr/Gent coating (reprinted from Stevanović et al. 2021 with permission from Elsevier)

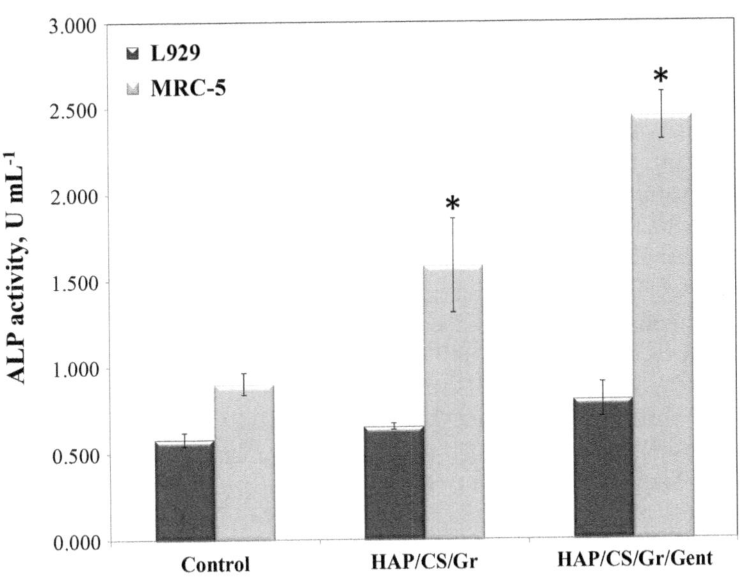

FIGURE 3.16 ALP levels in MRC-5 in L929 cell extracts in the presence of HAP/CS/Gr and HAP/CS/Gr/Gent coatings. * $p < 0.05$ for the respective cell line (reprinted from Stevanović et al. 2021 with permission from Elsevier)

(1.584 U/mL for MRC-5 and 0.654 U/mL for L929). Based on the presented ALP data, both coatings possess high biomineralization potential even in the case of non-specific fibroblast cell lines. High ALP levels in cell extracts represent encouraging prospects of the HAP/CS/Gr and HAP/CS/Gr/Gent coatings for further investigation toward tissue-specific cell lines.

3.2.5 Hydroxyapatite/Polyvinyl Alcohol/Chitosan/Gentamicin

3.2.5.1 Synthesis and Characterization

The bath composition for electrophoretic deposition of HAP/PVA/CS coating was 1 wt.% HAP, 0.1 wt.% PVA and 0.05 wt.% CS, while in the bath for deposition of HAP/PVA/CS/Gent coatings with antibiotic, 0.1 wt.% of gentamicin sulfate was added. EPD was performed at a constant voltage of 7 V, and for deposition time of 12 minutes (M. Djošić et al. 2023).

In FT-IR spectrum of HAP/PVA/CS coating small band attributed to the –OH stretching vibration in HAP structure was detected at 3568 cm^{-1}. The broad band, detected at around 3283 cm^{-1}, can be assigned to the –OH stretching vibration in HAP structure, sensitive to hydrogen bonding. In the region from 3000 to 2800 cm^{-1}, bands detected at 2988, 2971, 2921, 2910, and 2900 cm^{-1} can be assigned to the PVA and CS. Small band at 1654 cm^{-1} confirms the presence of C=O group that originated from the CS structure (amide I band). From wide and strong band in the region 1600–1300 cm^{-1}, small band at 1559 cm^{-1}, originated from the –OH bending vibration can be distinguished. Other bands at this region can be attributed to the vibration in carbonate group, which position suggesting the existence of carbonate-substituted HAP. Small band at 1465 cm^{-1} and the strong one at 1407 cm^{-1} can be attributed to the B-type carbonate substitution-related signals, while small band at 1458 cm^{-1} can be attributed to the AB-type substitution-related signal. In the region 1200–450 cm^{-1}, detected bands corresponded to the vibration mode in typical groups in HAP structure. Bands positioned at 1087, 1035, and 961 cm^{-1} represents the P-O stretching vibration in PO_4^{3-} group. The band at 866 cm^{-1} indicated the presence of CO_3^{2-} functional groups in HAP, while the band at 631 cm^{-1} can be assigned to the -OH bending vibration in HAP structure. Bending modes of (O–P–O) in PO_4^{3-} group can be distinguished at 601 and 568 cm^{-1}.

In the FT-IR spectrum of HAP/PVA/CS/Gent coating small band detected at 3571 cm^{-1} can be assigned to the –OH stretching vibration in HAP structure. The slight shift of the broad band, at around 3291 cm^{-1} in HAP/PVA/CS/Gent, with respect to the band position in HAP/PVA/CS (3283 cm^{-1}) represents the –OH stretching vibration in HAP structure, sensitive to hydrogen bonding. Bands shifting to the higher wavenumbers points to hydrogen bonds between HAP (-OH groups), PVA (-OH groups), CS (-OH and $–NH_2$ groups), and Gent (-OH and $–NH_2$ groups). The weak band at 1456 cm^{-1} (AB- type substitution) and the stronger one at 1417 cm^{-1} (B-type), as well as the band at 866 cm^{-1}, are recognized as carbonate-related signals, suggesting the carbonate-substituted HAP. After the gentamicin introduction, the small band assigned to the amide (N-H) bending vibration of amino group from gentamicin structure appeared at 1540 cm^{-1}, confirming the successful loading of antibiotic

TABLE 3.10
Unit Cell Parameters (*a, c,* and *V*), Crystallite Domain Size and *d*-Spacing of HAP/PVA/CS and HAP/PVA/CS/Gent Coatings (Reprinted from M. Djošić et al. 2023 with Permission from Elsevier)

	Parameter				Crystallite
Coating	a/Å		c/Å	V/Å^3	Domain Size/A
HAP/PVA/CS	9.3754		6.8549	521.82	172
HAP/PVA/CS/Gent	9.3637		6.8400	519.38	165
	Crystal Planes (*hkl*)				
	(002)	(211)	(112)	(300)	(202)
	d-Spacing, Å				
HAP/PVA/CS	3.4228	2.8009	2.7744	2.7065	2.6189
HAP/PVA/CS/Gent	3.4069	2.7970	2.7644	2.7031	2.6142

in composite coating. The gentamicin in HAP/PVA/CS/Gent coating did not alter the HAP structure and the characteristic band positions of phosphate group vibrations are almost the same as for the coating without gentamicin, at 1087, 1027, and 962 cm^{-1}. Despite the position of the bands remained almost unchanged, the bands intensity increased after the gentamicin introduction, indicating also that gentamicin was successfully loaded into the composite coating (Hamdan, Darnis, and Khodir 2021). At 600 and 567 cm^{-1} O–P–O bending modes were detected, while -OH bending vibration in HAP structure is represented by the band positioned at 630 cm^{-1}.

XRD calculations of unit cell parameters, unit cell volume (*a, c* and *V*), and crystallite domain size, considered parameters of hydroxyapatite characteristic crystal plane (002), are represented in Table 3.10.

The unit cell parameters changed as a consequence of ions replacement. Comparing the theoretical values of unit cell parameters for HAP hexagonal crystal structure ($P6_3/m$ space group, a=9.418 Å and c=6.884 Å (Sakthivel, Ragu, and Senthilarasan 2015)), with calculated values for hydroxyapatite detected in HAP/PVA/CS and HAP/PVA/CS/Gent coatings, a slight deviation was observed. These differences in unit cell parameters values are the consequence of incorporation of carbonate ions in the HAP structure, leading to formation of carbonate-substituted HAP in both coatings. The carbonate substitution (AB- and B-type) in both coatings was confirmed by FT-IR. In the case of HAP/PVC/CS coating, additional diffraction maximum of carbonate-substituted HAP can be distinguished, corresponding to JCPDS 19-0272 card, classified as B-type substituted hydroxyapatite, $Ca_{10}(PO_4)_3(CO_3)_3(OH)_2$. Introduction of gentamicin (HAP/PVA/CS/Gent) caused a slight decrease in the unit cell parameters (including unit cell volume), and crystallite domain size of HAP. Briefly, a smaller dimension of HAP crystallites in HAP/PVA/CS/Gent coating (165 Å) with respect to HAP/PVA/CS coating (172 Å) could be explain as follows: large molecules of gentamicin are able to suppress the growth of HAP crystallites, while sulfate ions influence the formation of a great number of nucleation sites. As a result of these two parallel processes, smaller hydroxyapatite crystallites of HAP/PVA/CS/Gent coating with respect to HAP/PVA/CS coating were observed. Smaller crystallite domain size causes the larger surface area, having a beneficial impact on the bone-like apatite formation. Values for *d*-spacing for both coatings remain almost unchanged with antibiotic addition.

Thermal stability of HAP/PVA/CS and HAP/PVA/CS/Gent coatings was examined by TG/DTG analysis. The first weight loss stage, corresponding to water desorption was observed up to 170 °C with weight loss of 4.6 wt.% and sharp peak at 103 °C (DTG curve) for HAP/PVA/CS coating and up to 184 °C with weight loss of 6.3 wt.% and sharp peak at 101 °C (DTG curve) for HAP/PVA/CS/Gent coating. Based on XRD analysis, smaller crystallite domain size of HAP/PVA/CS/Gent coating was determined (165 Å) compared to HAP/PVA/CS coating (172 Å), suggesting higher surface area for water adsorption.

The second weight loss was observed below 350 °C, with sharp maximums on DTG curves at 250 °C and 259 °C for HAP/PVA/CS and HAP/PVA/CS/Gent coatings, respectively. In the case of HAP/PVA/CS coating, weight loss in stage II can be attributed to the partial degradation and dehydratation of PVA accompanied by polyene formation (Budrugeac 2008) along with chitosan degradation through the decomposition of the CS chains. Weight loss for HAP/PVA/CS/Gent coating can be assigned to the PVA and CS decomposition as already mentioned, along with gentamicin degradation. Having in mind that gentamicin sulfates' decomposition occurs through the transformation of different isoforms, it is reported that pure gentamicin sulfate decomposed in the temperature interval 240 °C –300 °C (Purcar et al. 2021). Increase in weight loss for HAP/PVA/CS/Gent coating (4.5 wt.%) with respect to the coating without antibiotic (2.5 wt.%) can be attributed to the decomposition of gentamicin.

The third weight loss stage for HAP/PVA/CS coating occurred in the temperature interval from 334 °C to 427 °C with 1.4 wt. % weight loss, and in the temperature interval from 347 °C to 440 °C with 2.0 wt. % weight loss for HAP/PVA/CS/Gent coating. For both coatings, maximum on DTG curves appeared at 394 °C. Weight loss in stage III can be attributed to the further CS and PVA degradation (polyene decomposition) (Budrugeac 2008) or CS, PVA, and gentamicin degradation of composite HAP/PVA/CS and HAP/PVA/CS/Gent coatings, respectively, along with decomposition of carbonate ions originated from HAP structure. Additionally, further decomposition of gentamicin causing the greater weight loss for HAP/PVA/CS/Gent coating (2.0 wt.%) compared to the weight loss for HAP/PVA/CS coating (1.4 wt.%,).

Next weight loss interval, stage IV, occurred between 427 °C and 531 °C with weight loss of 2.3 wt.% for HAP/PVA/CS coating, and between 440 °C and 515 °C with weight loss of about 1.3 wt. % for HAP/PVA/CS/Gent coating, with sharp maximum at 464 °C for both coatings (DTG curve). Weight loss could be assigned to the thermo-oxidation of carbonized residue of PVA (Budrugeac 2008) along with dehydroxylation and decarbonation of HAP, e.g., release of water and CO_2 from HAP lattice. The final interval of weight loss up to 800 °C, stage V, corresponds to the further dehydroxylation of HAP leading to formation of oxyhydroxyapatite (Kamieniak et al. 2018) along with decarbonation of B-sites in HAP lattice. Weight loss for HAP/PVA/CS coating was determined to be 13 wt.%, while significant lower weight loss of 6.9 wt.% was determined for HAP/PVA/CS/Gent coating. Maximum on DTG curves was detected at 736 °C and 707 °C for HAP/PVA/CS and HAP/PVA/CS/Gent coatings, respectively. Significant difference in weight loss between antibiotic-free coating and coating with antibiotic can be explained by decarbonation process of B-sites. Namely, in HAP/PVA/CS coating, XRD analysis revealed a high amount of B-type substituted HAP as separate phase, while no distinct diffraction maximums for B-type substituted HAP were recognized in the case of HAP/PVA/CS/Gent coating. Total weight loss in the temperature range 25 °C –800 °C for HAP/PVA/CS and HAP/PVA/CS/Gent coatings was 23.8 wt.% and 20.9 wt.%, respectively. Higher amount of carbonate-substituted HAP caused lower thermal stability in the case of HAP/PVA/CS coating.

From FE-SEM microphotographs the porous surface with homogeneously distributed spherical HAP agglomerates embedded in wax-like polymers' matrix of PVA and CS were observed for both HAP/PVA/CS and HAP/PVA/CS/Gent coatings, while gentamicin incorporation did not influence the coating's morphology.

3.2.5.2 Antibacterial Activity and Cytotoxicity

Antibacterial activity of HAP/PVA/CS and HAP/PVA/CS/Gent coatings against *S. aureus* TL and *E. coli* ATCC 25922 in PB medium showed a powerful antibiotic effect against both bacteria species, leading to a rapid complete reduction in the bacteria cell numbers. *S. aureus* viable cells (Figure 3.17a) were completely diminished immediately after inoculation of PB media, during the first initial contact, which proved the high efficacy of gentamicin and reduced the initial bacteria cell count by five logarithmic units. The antibacterial effect of HAP/PVA/CS/Gent was also evident against *E. coli* (Figure 3.17b), causing a swift bacteria cells reduction (three logarithmic units) in the first 15 minutes of exposure. Given the rapid and effective reduction of both bacteria species, HAP/PVA/CS/Gent could be classified as bactericidal material, convenient for possible future applications.

Figure 3.17c shows the results of the MTT test for the HAP/PVA/CS and HAP/PVA/CS/Gent coatings. Both cell lines (MRC-5 and L929) showed high cell viability in the presence of the tested samples >90%, indicating a non-cytotoxic effect. Even in the case of HAP/PVA/CS/Gent coating, the cell viability was above 97 % for both investigated cell lines, indicating that the gentamicin addition had no effect on cells. Results of one-way analysis of variance statistical tests for cytotoxicity testing, pointed out that the differences in the cell growth for both MRC-5 and L929 cell lines between the HAP/PVA/CS and HAP/PVA/CS/Gent were not statistically significant ($p < 0.05$).

3.2.5.3 Alkaline Phosphatase Activity

Bone mineralization is a complex process that involves two steps: formation of hydroxyapatite crystals within matrix vesicles (produced from the plasma membrane of osteoblasts, chondroblasts, and odontoblasts) and its propagation in the extracellular matrix and deposition between collagen fibrils (Orimo 2010). HAP deposition

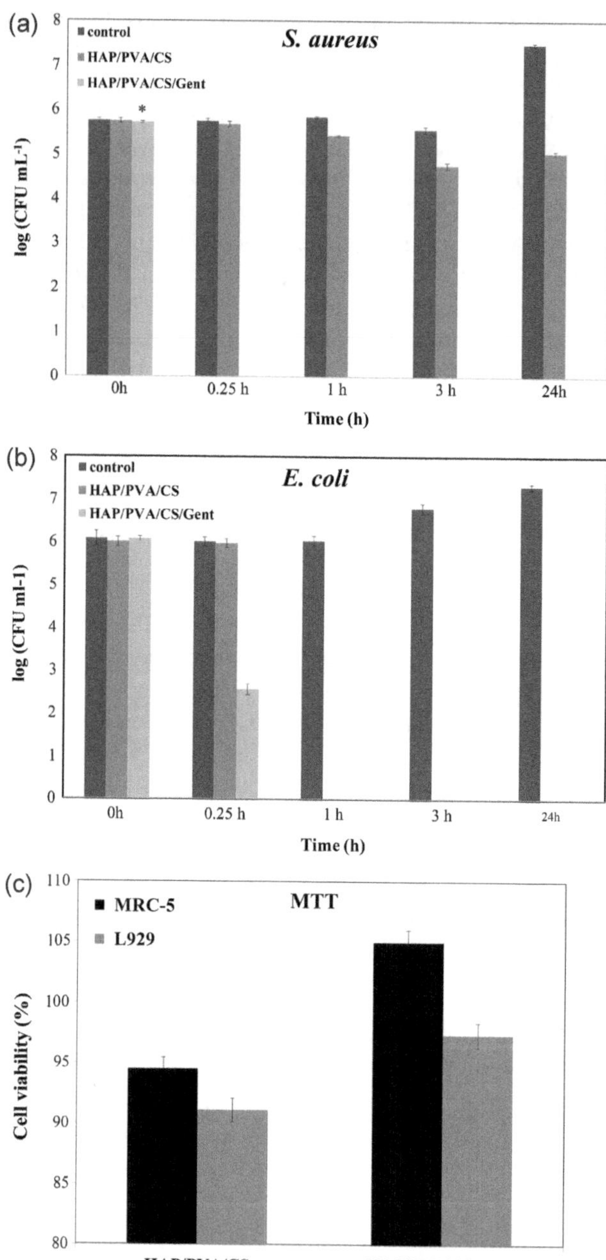

FIGURE 3.17 Antibacterial activity of HAP/PVA/CS and HAP/PVA/CS/Gent coatings against *S. aureus* (a) and *E. coli* (b), MRC-5 and L929 cells viability determined by MTT test (c) (reprinted from M. Djošić et al. 2023 with permission from Elsevier)

is highly affected by the concentration of calcium and phosphate ions in extracellular matrix, meaning that only sufficient ions concentrations will lead to the HAP crystal elongation and, consequently, HAP deposition. Alkaline phosphatase, precisely tissue non-specific alkaline phosphatase (TNAP), plays a significant role in the mineralization process, providing phosphate ions and destabilizing the amorphous phase of the mineral. Furthermore, TNAP, expressed by osteoblasts, reduces the pyrophosphate (PPi) levels (since PPi inhibits HAP formation) and provides inorganic phosphate (Pi) for hydroxyapatite formation while maintaining the Pi/PPi ratio within the required ranges (Ansari, Ito, and Hofmann 2022; Sekaran, Vimalraj, and Thangavelu 2021). Alkaline phosphatase activity determination proved to be a very useful indicator of biomaterials' ability to induce biomineralization. In this study, the ALP assay was performed on MRC-5 and L929 cell lines in order to test the baseline potential of ALP expression in the presence of the tested HAP/PVA/CS and HAP/PVA/CS/Gent coatings and their ability to induce the biomineralization process, as well as to ensure the consistency of the two biological assays using the same cell lines (MRC-5 and L929) used in the biocompatibility study (i.e., the cytotoxicity assay). Obtained results would be a good basis for further investigations into tissue-specific osteoblasts cells.

Figure 3.18 presents the results of ALP activity as a potential marker of biomineralization when tested on MRC-5 and L929 cell lines. MRC-5 cell line showed twofold higher ALP expression levels (1.424 U/ml for HAP/PVA/CS and 1.699 U/ml for HAP/PVA/CS/Gent) compared to the control (0.678 U/ml for HAP/PVA/CS and 0.897 U/ml for HAP/PVA/CS/Gent). In the case of L929 mice, fibroblast cell

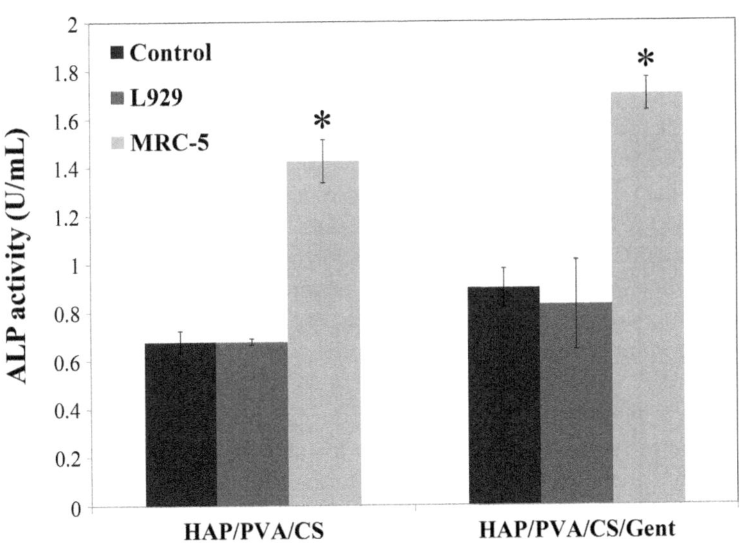

FIGURE 3.18 ALP activity of MRC-5 and L929 cells when exposed to HAP/PVA/CS and HAP/PVA/CS/Gent coatings. *$p < 0.05$ for the respective cell line (reprinted from M. Djošić et al. 2023 with permission from Elsevier)

line ALP levels remained within the same range as the control (0.678 U/ml for HAP/PVA/CS and 0.828 U/ml for HAP/PVA/CS/Gent). Based on these results, it is obvious that both materials HAP/PVA/CS and HAP/PVA/CS/Gent coatings have strong potential for future applications in the field of hard tissue implants.

One-way analysis of variance statistical tests when applied to ALP activity test revealed the differences in ALP levels between MRC-5 and L929 cell lines for both samples were statistically significant ($p < 0.05$).

3.2.5.4 *In Vitro* Bioactivity

In vitro bioactivity of HAP/PVA/CS and HAP/PVA/CS/Gent coatings has been investigated by FT-IR, XRD, and FE-SEM analysis (Jaćimović et al. 2023).

Characteristic FT-IR bands, confirming the presence of PO_4^{3-} groups, can be detected in two regions: 450–620 cm^{-1} region (O–P–O bending modes in the phosphate group) and 900–1200 cm^{-1} region (P-O stretching vibrations of the phosphate group). Structural hydroxyl groups in HAP structure can be detected at 630 cm^{-1} (OH^- bending) and at 3568 cm^{-1} (OH^- stretching) for both HAP/PVA/CS and HAP/PVA/CS/Gent coatings. Wide band at around 3300 cm^{-1} (for HAP/PVA/CS) and 3350 cm^{-1} (for HAP/PVA/CS/Gent) can be assigned to the adsorbed water. The substitution occurred between hydroxyl and phosphate groups from HAP, with carbonate groups, leading to formation of A- and B-type substituted HAP, respectively, or combined AB-type substitution (M. Djošić, Janković, and Mišković-Stanković 2021). The carbonate bands in HAP grown on the top of both HAP/PVA/CS and HAP/PVA/CS/Gent coatings after immersion in SBF at 37 °C for 7 and 14 days were found at around 873 cm^{-1} (vibrational mode of O–C–O) and in the region 1400–1500 cm^{-1} (vibrational mode of O-C) indicating B-type substitution. More precisely, bands at around 1413 and 1420 cm^{-1}, along with band positioned at 1465 cm^{-1} known as the "signature" band for B-type substitution, confirmed this statement.

XRD patterns for biomimetic HAP grown on the top of HAP/PVA/CS and HAP/PVA/CS/Gent coatings after 14 days immersion in SBF at 37 °C corresponded to hydroxyapatite (HAP, JCPDS 09-0432) and carbonate-substituted hydroxyapatite (C-HAP, JCPDS 19-0272). The values of *d*-spacing have been calculated from the characteristic HAP crystal planes (002), (211), (112), (300), and (202) (Table 3.11). Crystal plane (002) was used for the calculation of unit cell parameters (*a* and *c*) and unit cell volume (*V*), as well as the crystallite domain size. Values of *d*-spacing, cell parameters (*a* and *c*), and unit cell volume (*V*) are almost the same for both coatings, but gentamicin incorporation induced a decrease in crystallite domain size of HAP/PVA/CS/Gent.

Growth of biomimetic HAP occurred through the parallel processes of precipitation and dissolution during exposure to the SBF solution (biomineralization process). After the coatings were exposed to the SBF, negatively charged hydroxyl and phosphate ions from the coatings' surface attracted calcium ions from the SBF solution, leading to formation of supersaturated solution toward apatite, and consequently nucleation and growth of biomimetic HAP. Along with biomimetic HAP precipitation, its dissolution occurred, leading to an increase in Ca^{2+} and PO_4^{3-} ion

TABLE 3.11
The *d*-Spacing Values, Unit Cell Parameters (*a* and *c*), Unit Cell Volume (*V*), and Crystallite Domain Size of Hydroxyapatite Layer on the Top of HAP/PVA/CS and HAP/PVA/CS/Gent Coatings After 14 Days Immersion in SBF at 37 °C (Reprinted from Jaćimović et al. 2023 with Permission from the Society of Chemists and Technologists of Macedonia)

Coating	Time in SBF, Days	Crystal Planes				
		(002)	(211)	(112)	(300)	(202)
		d-Spacing, Å				
HAP/PVA/CS	14	3.4514	2.8100	2.7811	2.7183	2.6300
HAP/PVA/CS/Gent	14	3.4487	2.8115	2.8051	2.7184	2.6300
Coating	**Time in SBF, Days**	**Parameter *a*, Å**	***c*, Å**	***V*, Å³**	**Crystallite Domain Size, Å**	
HAP/PVA/CS	14	9.4585	6.8962	534.30	421	
HAP/PVA/CS/Gent	14	9.4449	6.8929	532.51	305	

concentrations on the coating surface. The precipitation rate dominated over the dissolution rate of HAP, leading to the formation of biomimetic coatings. After drug-loaded coating (HAP/PVA/CS/Gent) exposure to the SBF, release of antibiotic occurred simultaneously as the biomimetic HAP precipitation/dissolution. The release of antibiotic from biodegradable systems could be described through the diffusion, dissolution, and erosion mechanism, or a combination thereof (Macha et al. 2015; Kamaly et al. 2016). As a consequence of all processes mentioned above, the difference in crystallite domain size could be observed after 14 days exposure to the SBF. It can be assumed that the large molecule of gentamicin could suppress further growth of biomimetic HAP crystals, leading to the formation of finer crystallites in the case of biomimetic HAP coating formed on the top of gentamicin-loaded coating (305 Å) with respect to the antibiotic-free coating (421 Å). Based on these data, both HAP/PVA/CS and HAP/PVA/CS/Gent coatings are able to induce the nucleation and growth of biomimetic HAP and therefore could be considered as potential biomaterials for improving implant and natural bone integration. Additionally, carbonate-substituted HAP (JCPDS 19-0272) detected in all biomimetic coatings is known to be B-type substituted ($Ca_{10}(PO_4)_3(CO_3)_3(OH)_2$) (Bhattacharjee et al. 2019). Based on the literature data, all carbonate substitutions in bone minerals are primarily B-type substitutions (Madupalli, Pavan, and Tecklenburg 2017); therefore, both HAP/PVA/CS and HAP/PVA/CS/Gent coatings are promising biomaterials for osseointegration. FE-SEM micrographs also suggested the formation of new biomimetic HAP agglomerates of needle-like shape (Jaćimović et al. 2023) and, along with XRD and FT-IR results, confirmed bioactivity of both HAP/PVA/CS and HAP/PVA/CS/Gent.

3.2.5.5 Gentamicin Release

The concentration of released gentamicin from HAP/PVA/CS/Gent hydrogel was determined using a high-performance liquid chromatography (HPLC) coupled with ion trap as a mass spectrometer (MS), according to procedure published earlier (Stevanović et al. 2021). Briefly, gentamicin release studies were carried out during 21-day immersion in deionized water, at 37 °C, as a model system. All the measurements were done in triplicate. HPLC was utilized for gentamicin components separation and the detection and quantitative analysis was done in an ion trap mass spectrometer with an electrospray ionizer. Methanol (A), deionized water (B), and 10 % acetic acid (C) comprised the mobile phase. The optimized HPLC and MS operating parameters (mobile-phase gradient, analytes' precursor ions, fragmentation reactions used for quantification, and optimal collision energies) for the determination of gentamicin compounds were published previously (Stevanović, Djošić, Janković, Nešović et al. 2020). The gentamicin mass spectra were collected in the *m/z* range of 50–1000. As expected, the MS spectrum revealed the three most abundant ions since gentamicin is composed of three compounds – gentamicin C1a, C2, and C1. These ions were further chosen as the precursor ions for each compound. Their most sensitive transitions were selected for quantification purposes. The presented gentamicin concentrations represented sums of the three determined gentamicin compounds.

The experimental gentamicin release profiles for HAP/PVA/CS/Gent coating are shown in Figure 3.19, where c_0 is the initial concentration of gentamicin in the deposited coating, c_t is the concentration of released gentamicin after certain time t, and $c_{coat,t}$ is the concentration of gentamicin remained in coating after certain time, t. Release profiles verified the initial burst release effect of gentamicin from the coating (30 % within first 48 hours), which could be very useful in preventing biofilm formation, followed by slow release of gentamicin in a later time period. This behavior is in favor of both application requirements; namely, for effective bone implant with antibacterial properties, initial burst release can be favorable to quickly suppress the

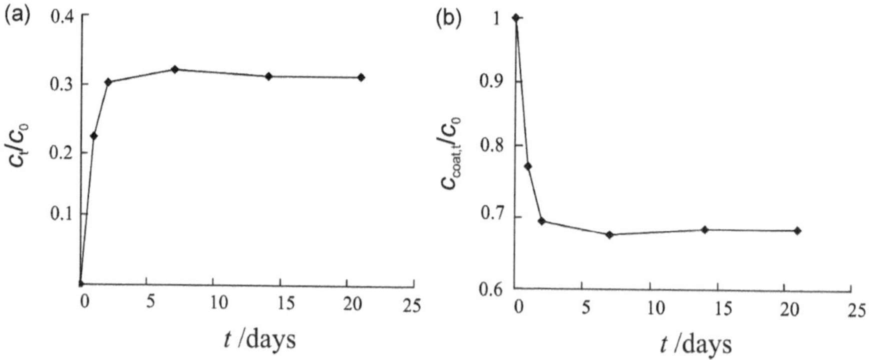

FIGURE 3.19 (a) Increase in concentration of released gentamicin from HAP/PVA/CS/Gent coating, c_t, and (b) decrease in concentration of gentamicin remained in HAP/PVA/CS/Gent coating, $c_{coat,t}$, with time in deionized water at 37 °C during 21 days

bacterial adhesion and biofilm formation in the implant environment, whereas the sustained release over longer period would ensure maintained sterility of implanted bone. This behavior is a consequence of gentamicin molecules entrapped in the cross-linked HAP/polymer matrix.

To determine the mechanism of gentamicin release and diffusion coefficient, experimental data were fitted by Korsmeyer-Peppas model described by (Eq. 3.9) in its linear form. Coefficient n was calculated to be 0.0808, indicating that the gentamicin release from HAP/PVA/CS/Gent coating is governed by the Fick's diffusion law. The value of diffusion coefficient, *D*, of gentamicin was calculated from early time approximation (ETA) model (Eq. 3.10), appropriate for the one-dimensional release from thin coating. The diffusion coefficient, *D*, was calculated to be 9.6×10^{-10} cm^2 s^{-1}. Detailed pharmacokinetics analysis of gentamicin release using Makoid-Banakar, Korsmeyer-Peppas, and Kopcha models in comparison with novel General fractional derivative (GFD) model is presented in Section 4.4.3.

REFERENCES

AbouAitah, Khaled, Monika Bil, Elzbieta Pietrzykowska, Urszula Szałaj, Damian Fudala, Bartosz Woźniak, Justyna Nasiłowska, et al. 2021. "Drug-Releasing Antibacterial Coating Made from Nano-Hydroxyapatite Using the Sonocoating Method." *Nanomaterials*. https://doi.org/10.3390/nano11071690.

Almeida, Maria José, Lucilia Pereira, Christian Milet, Josiane Haigle, Mário Barbosa, and Evelyne Lopez. 2001. "Comparative Effects of Nacre Water-Soluble Matrix and Dexamethasone on the Alkaline Phosphatase Activity of MRC-5 Fibroblasts." *Journal of Biomedical Materials Research* 57 (2): 306–12. https://doi.org/10.1002/1097-4636(200111)57:2<306::AID-JBM1172>3.0.CO;2-H.

Alves Cardoso, D, JA Jansen, and SCG Leeuwenburgh. 2012. "Synthesis and Application of Nanostructured Calcium Phosphate Ceramics for Bone Regeneration." *Journal of Biomedical Materials Research Part B: Applied Biomaterials* 100B (8): 2316–26. https://doi.org/10.1002/jbm.b.32794.

Ansari, Sana, Keita Ito, and Sandra Hofmann. 2022. "Alkaline Phosphatase Activity of Serum Affects Osteogenic Differentiation Cultures." *ACS Omega* 7 (15): 12724–33. https://doi.org/10.1021/acsomega.1c07225.

Aydin, İbrahim, Ali İhsan Bahçepinar, and Canser Gül. 2020. "Surface Characterization of EPD Coating on AZ91 Mg Alloy Produced by Powder Metallurgy." *Revista de Metalurgia* 56 (3 SE-Articles): e176. https://doi.org/10.3989/revmetalm.176.

Aydın, İbrahim, Ali İhsan Bahçepınar, Mustafa Kırman, and Mustafa A Çipiloğlu. 2019. "HA Coating on Ti6Al7Nb Alloy Using an Electrophoretic Deposition Method and Surface Properties Examination of the Resulting Coatings." *Coatings*. https://doi.org/10.3390/coatings9060402.

Aydemir, Tuba, Liliana Liverani, Juan I Pastore, Silvia M Ceré, Wolfgang H Goldmann, Aldo R Boccaccini, and Josefina Ballarre. 2020. "Functional Behavior of Chitosan/Gelatin/Silica-Gentamicin Coatings by Electrophoretic Deposition on Surgical Grade Stainless Steel." *Materials Science and Engineering: C* 115: 111062. https://doi.org/10.1016/j.msec.2020.111062.

Aydemir, Tuba, Juan I Pastore, Emilio Jimenez-Pique, Joan Josep Roa, Aldo R Boccaccini, and Josefina Ballarre. 2021. "Morphological and Mechanical Characterization of Chitosan/Gelatin/Silica-Gentamicin/Bioactive Glass Coatings on Orthopaedic Metallic Implant Materials." *Thin Solid Films* 732: 138780. https://doi.org/10.1016/j.tsf.2021.138780.

Bai, Xiao, Stefan Sandukas, Mark R Appleford, Joo L Ong, and Afsaneh Rabiei. 2009. "Deposition and Investigation of Functionally Graded Calcium Phosphate Coatings on Titanium." *Acta Biomaterialia* 5 (9): 3563–72. https://doi.org/10.1016/j.actbio.2009.05.013.

Bakhshandeh, Sadra, and Saber Amin Yavari. 2018. "Electrophoretic Deposition: A Versatile Tool against Biomaterial Associated Infections." *Journal of Materials Chemistry B* 6 (8): 1128–48. https://doi.org/10.1039/c7tb02445b.

Bartolucci, Stephen F, Joseph Paras, Mohammad A Rafiee, Javad Rafiee, Sabrina Lee, Deepak Kapoor, and Nikhil Koratkar. 2011. "Graphene–Aluminum Nanocomposites." *Materials Science and Engineering: A* 528 (27): 7933–37. https://doi.org/10.1016/j.msea.2011.07.043.

Batmanghelich, Farhad, and Mohammad Ghorbani. 2013. "Effect of PH and Carbon Nanotube Content on the Corrosion Behavior of Electrophoretically Deposited Chitosan–Hydroxyapatite–Carbon Nanotube Composite Coatings." *Ceramics International* 39 (5): 5393–402. https://doi.org/10.1016/j.ceramint.2012.12.046.

Battistoni, C, MP Casaletto, GM Ingo, S Kaciulis, G Mattogno, and L Pandolfi. 2000. "Surface Characterization of Biocompatible Hydroxyapatite Coatings†." *Surface and Interface Analysis* 29 (11): 773–81. https://doi.org/10.1002/1096-9918(200011)29:11<773::AID-SIA928>3.0.CO;2-2.

Batul, Rahila, Mrinal Bhave, Peter J Mahon, and Aimin Yu. 2020. "Polydopamine Nanosphere with In-Situ Loaded Gentamicin and Its Antimicrobial Activity." *Molecules*. https://doi.org/10.3390/molecules25092090.

Belmonte, Manuel, Cristina Ramírez, Jesús González-Julián, Johannes Schneider, Pilar Miranzo, and María Isabel Osendi. 2013. "The Beneficial Effect of Graphene Nanofillers on the Tribological Performance of Ceramics." *Carbon* 61: 431–35. https://doi.org/10.1016/j.carbon.2013.04.102.

Berzina-Cimdina, Liga, and Natalija Borodajenko. 2012. "Research of Calcium Phosphates Using Fourier Transform Infrared Spectroscopy." In *Infrared Spectroscopy - Materials Science, Engineering and Technology*, edited by Theophile Theophanides, 123–48. Rijeka: IntechOpen. https://doi.org/10.5772/36942.

Bhattacharjee, Birendra Nath, Vijay Kumar Mishra, Shyam Bahadur Rai, Om Parkash, and Devendra Kumar. 2019. "Structure of Apatite Nanoparticles Derived from Marine Animal (Crab) Shells: An Environment-Friendly and Cost-Effective Novel Approach to Recycle Seafood Waste." *ACS Omega* 4 (7): 12753–58. https://doi.org/10.1021/acsomega.9b00134.

Biest, O Van der, and LJ Vandeperre. 1999. "Electrophoretic Deposition of Materials." *Annual Review of Materials Science* 9: 327–52. https://doi.org/10.1146/annurev.matsci.29.1.327.

Bistolfi, Alessandro, Giuseppe Massazza, Enrica Verné, Alessandro Massè, Davide Deledda, Sara Ferraris, Marta Miola, Fabrizio Galetto, and Maurizio Crova. 2011. "Antibiotic-Loaded Cement in Orthopedic Surgery: A Review." *ISRN Orthopedics* 2011: 290851. https://doi.org/10.5402/2011/290851.

Boccaccini, AR, J Cho, T Subhani, C Kaya, and F Kaya. 2010. "Electrophoretic Deposition of Carbon Nanotube–Ceramic Nanocomposites." *Journal of the European Ceramic Society* 30 (5): 1115–29. https://doi.org/10.1016/j.jeurceramsoc.2009.03.016.

Boccaccini, AR, S Keim, R Ma, Y Li, and I Zhitomirsky. 2010. "Electrophoretic Deposition of Biomaterials." *Journal of The Royal Society Interface* 7: S581–613. https://doi.org/10.1016/j.matlet.2012.02.059.

Bonetti, Lorenzo, Alice Caprioglio, Nina Bono, Gabriele Candiani, and Lina Altomare. 2023. "Mucoadhesive Chitosan–Methylcellulose Oral Patches for the Treatment of Local Mouth Bacterial Infections." *Biomaterials Science* 11 (8): 2699–710. https://doi.org/10.1039/D2BM01540D.

Borkowski, Leszek, Anna Sroka-Bartnicka, Piotr Drączkowski, Agnieszka Ptak, Emil Zięba, Anna Ślósarczyk, and Grażyna Ginalska. 2016. "The Comparison Study of Bioactivity between Composites Containing Synthetic Non-Substituted and Carbonate-Substituted Hydroxyapatite." *Materials Science and Engineering: C* 62: 260–67. https://doi.org/10.1016/j.msec.2016.01.056.

Božić, Katarina, Miroslav M Pavlović, Gavrilo Šekularac, Stefan Panić, and Marijana Pantović Pavlović. 2023. "Application Aspects of Joint Anaphoresis/Substrate Anodization in Production of Biocompatible Ceramic Coatings: Survey." *Journal of the Serbian Chemical Society* 88 (7-8 SE-Materials): 685–704. https://doi.org/10.2298/JSC230118034B.

Brangule, Agnese, and Karlis Agris Gross. 2015. "Importance of FTIR Spectra Deconvolution for the Analysis of Amorphous Calcium Phosphates." *IOP Conference Series: Materials Science and Engineering* 77 (1): 12027. https://doi.org/10.1088/1757-899X/77/1/012027.

Budrugeac, P. 2008. "Kinetics of the Complex Process of Thermo-Oxidative Degradation of Poly(Vinyl Alcohol)." *Journal of Thermal Analysis and Calorimetry* 92 (1): 291–96. https://doi.org/10.1007/s10973-007-8770-8.

Bustos-Ramírez, Karina, Ana L Martínez-Hernández, Gonzalo Martínez-Barrera, Miguel D Icaza, Víctor M Castaño, and Carlos Velasco-Santos. 2013. "Covalently Bonded Chitosan on Graphene Oxide via Redox Reaction." *Materials*. https://doi.org/10.3390/ma6030911.

Cabrejos-Azama, Jatsue, Mohammad Hamdan Alkhraisat, Carmen Rueda, Jesús Torres, Concepción Pintado, Luis Blanco, and Enrique López-Cabarcos. 2016. "Magnesium Substitution in Brushite Cements: Efficacy of a New Biomaterial Loaded with Vancomycin for the Treatment of Staphylococcus Aureus Infections." *Materials Science and Engineering: C* 61: 72–78. https://doi.org/10.1016/j.msec.2015.10.092.

Cacciotti, Ilaria. 2016. "Cationic and Anionic Substitutions in Hydroxyapatite." In *Handbook of Bioceramics and Biocomposites*, edited by Iulian Vasile Antoniac, 146–88. Cham: Springer International Publishing. https://doi.org/10.1007/978-3-319-12460-5_7.

Capanema, Nádia SV, Alexandra AP Mansur, Sandhra M Carvalho, Alexandra RP Silva, Virginia S Ciminelli, and Herman S Mansur. 2015. "Niobium-Doped Hydroxyapatite Bioceramics: Synthesis, Characterization and In Vitro Cytocompatibility." *Materials*. https://doi.org/10.3390/ma8074191.

Caroline Victoria, E, and FD Gnanam. 2002. "Synthesis and Characterisation of Biphasic Calcium Phosphate." *Trends in Biomaterials and Artificial Organs* 16: 12–14.

Charnley, J. 1960. "Anchorage of the Femoral Head Prosthesis to the Shaft of the Femur." *The Journal of Bone and Joint Surgery. British Volume* 42-B (February): 28–30. https://doi.org/10.1302/0301-620X.42B1.28.

Chaves, Thiago P, Felipe Hugo A Fernandes, Cleildo P Santana, Jocimar S Santos, Francinalva D Medeiros, Délcio C Felismino, Vanda L Santos, Raïssa Mayer R Catão, Henrique Douglas M Coutinho, and Ana Cláudia D Medeiros. 2016. "Evaluation of the Interaction between the Poincianella Pyramidalis (Tul.) LP Queiroz Extract and Antimicrobials Using Biological and Analytical Models." *PLoS One* 11 (5): e0155532.

Cheary, RW, and A Coelho. 1992. "A Fundamental Parameters Approach to X-Ray Line-Profile Fitting." *Journal of Applied Crystallography* 25 (2): 109–21. https://doi.org/10.1107/S0021889891010804.

Cheong, M, and I Zhitomirsky. 2008. "Electrodeposition of Alginic Acid and Composite Films." *Colloids and Surfaces A: Physicochemical and Engineering Aspects* 328 (1): 73–78. https://doi.org/10.1016/j.colsurfa.2008.06.019.

Chiara, Gardin, Ferroni Letizia, Favero Lorenzo, Stellini Edoardo, Stomaci Diego, Sivolella Stefano, Bressan Eriberto, and Zavan Barbara. 2012. "Nanostructured Biomaterials for Tissue Engineered Bone Tissue Reconstruction." *International Journal of Molecular Sciences*. https://doi.org/10.3390/ijms13010737.

Ciobanu, CS, SL Iconaru, I Pasuk, BS Vasile, AR Lupu, A Hermenean, A Dinischiotu, and D Predoi. 2013. "Structural Properties of Silver Doped Hydroxyapatite and Their Biocompatibility." *Materials Science and Engineering: C* 33 (3): 1395–402. https://doi.org/10.1016/j.msec.2012.12.042.

Clifford, A, and I Zhitomirsky. 2018. "Aqueous Electrophoretic Deposition of Drugs Using Bile Acids as Solubilizing, Charging and Film-Forming Agents." *Materials Letters* 227: 1–4. https://doi.org/10.1016/j.matlet.2018.05.026.

Corni, Ilaria, Mary P Ryan, and Aldo R Boccaccini. 2008. "Electrophoretic Deposition: From Traditional Ceramics to Nanotechnology." *Journal of the European Ceramic Society* 28 (7): 1353–67. https://doi.org/10.1016/j.jeurceramsoc.2007.12.011.

Cromme, Peter, Cordt Zollfrank, Lenka Müller, Frank A Müller, and Peter Greil. 2007. "Biomimetic Mineralisation of Apatites on Ca2+ Activated Cellulose Templates." *Materials Science and Engineering: C* 27 (1): 1–7. https://doi.org/10.1016/j.msec.2005.11.001.

Deen, I, and I Zhitomirsky. 2014. "Electrophoretic Deposition of Composite Halloysite Nanotube–Hydroxyapatite–Hyaluronic Acid Films." *Journal of Alloys and Compounds* 586: S531–34. https://doi.org/10.1016/j.jallcom.2013.01.088.

Depan, D, TC Pesacreta, and RDK Misra. 2014. "The Synergistic Effect of a Hybrid Graphene Oxide–Chitosan System and Biomimetic Mineralization on Osteoblast Functions." *Biomaterials Science* 2 (2): 264–74. https://doi.org/10.1039/C3BM60192G.

Djošić, Marija, Ana Janković, and Vesna Mišković-Stanković. 2021. "Electrophoretic Deposition of Biocompatible and Bioactive Hydroxyapatite-Based Coatings on Titanium." *Materials*. https://doi.org/10.3390/ma14185391.

Djošić, Marija, Ana Janković, Milena Stevanović, Jovica Stojanović, Maja Vukašinović-Sekulić, Vesna Kojić, and Vesna Mišković-Stanković. 2023. "Hydroxyapatite/Poly(Vinyl Alcohol)/Chitosan Coating with Gentamicin for Orthopedic Implants." *Materials Chemistry and Physics* 303: 127766. https://doi.org/10.1016/j.matchemphys.2023.127766.

Djošić, Marija S, VB Mišković-Stanković, S Milonjić, ZM Kačarević-Popović, N Bibić, and J Stojanović. 2008. "Electrochemical Synthesis and Characterization of Hydroxyapatite Powders." *Materials Chemistry and Physics* 111 (1): 137–42. https://doi.org/10.1016/j.matchemphys.2008.03.045.

Djošić, Marija S, Miodrag Mitrić, and Vesna B Mišković-Stankovic. 2015. "The Porosity and Roughness of Electrodeposited Calcium Phosphate Coatings in Simulated Body Fluid." *Journal of the Serbian Chemical Society* 80 (2): 237–51. https://doi.org/10.2298/JSC140626098D.

Dong, Zhihong, Yubao Li, and Qin Zou. 2009. "Degradation and Biocompatibility of Porous Nano-Hydroxyapatite/Polyurethane Composite Scaffold for Bone Tissue Engineering." *Applied Surface Science* 255 (12): 6087–91. https://doi.org/10.1016/j.apsusc.2009.01.083.

Đošić, Marija, Sanja Eraković, Ana Janković, Maja Vukašinović-Sekulić, Ivana Z Matić, Jovica Stojanović, Kyong Yop Rhee, Vesna Mišković-Stanković, and Soo-Jin Park. 2017. "In Vitro Investigation of Electrophoretically Deposited Bioactive Hydroxyapatite/Chitosan Coatings Reinforced by Graphene." *Journal of Industrial and Engineering Chemistry* 47: 336–47. https://doi.org/10.1016/j.jiec.2016.12.004.

Dupraz, A, TP Nguyen, M Richard, G Daculsi, and N Passuti. 1999. "Influence of a Cellulosic Ether Carrier on the Structure of Biphasic Calcium Phosphate Ceramic Particles in an Injectable Composite Material." *Biomaterials* 20 (7): 663–73. https://doi.org/10.1016/S0142-9612(98)00222-1.

Dwivedi, Charu, Himanshu Pandey, C Avinash Pandey, and W Pramod Ramteke. 2015. "Fabrication and Assessment of Gentamicin Loaded Electrospun Nanofibrous Scaffolds as a Quick Wound Healing Dressing Material." *Current Nanoscience*. https://doi.org/http://dx.doi.org/10.2174/1573413710666141003221954.

Dwivedi, Charu, Ishan Pandey, Himanshu Pandey, Sandip Patil, Shanti Bhushan Mishra, Avinash C Pandey, Paolo Zamboni, Pramod W Ramteke, and Ajay Vikram Singh. 2018. "In Vivo Diabetic Wound Healing with Nanofibrous Scaffolds Modified with Gentamicin and Recombinant Human Epidermal Growth Factor." *Journal of Biomedical Materials Research. Part A* 106 (3): 641–51. https://doi.org/10.1002/jbm.a.36268.

Eftekhari, Samin, Ihab El Sawi, Zahra Shaghayegh Bagheri, Ginette Turcotte, and Habiba Bougherara. 2014. "Fabrication and Characterization of Novel Biomimetic PLLA/Cellulose/Hydroxyapatite Nanocomposite for Bone Repair Applications." *Materials Science and Engineering: C* 39: 120–25. https://doi.org/10.1016/j.msec.2014.02.027.

El-Hendawy, Abdel-Nasser A. 2006. "Variation in the FTIR Spectra of a Biomass under Impregnation, Carbonization and Oxidation Conditions." *Journal of Analytical and Applied Pyrolysis* 75 (2): 159–66. https://doi.org/10.1016/j.jaap.2005.05.004.

El-Sayed, El Sayed M, Amina Omar, Medhat Ibrahim, and Wafa I Abdel-Fattah. 2009. "On the Structural Analysis and Electronic Properties of Chitosan/Hydroxyapatite Interaction." *Journal of Computational and Theoretical Nanoscience* 6 (7): 1663–69. https://doi.org/10.1166/jctn.2009.1228.

Eraković, Sanja, Ana Janković, Ivana Z Matić, Zorica D Juranić, Maja Vukašinović-Sekulić, Tatjana Stevanović, and Vesna Mišković-Stanković. 2013. "Investigation of Silver Impact on Hydroxyapatite/Lignin Coatings Electrodeposited on Titanium." *Materials Chemistry and Physics* 142 (2): 521–30. https://doi.org/10.1016/j.matchemphys.2013.07.047.

Erakovic, Sanja, Ana Jankovic, Gary CP Tsui, Chak-Yin Tang, Vesna Miskovic-Stankovic, and Tatjana Stevanovic. 2014. "Novel Bioactive Antimicrobial Lignin Containing Coatings on Titanium Obtained by Electrophoretic Deposition." *International Journal of Molecular Sciences*. https://doi.org/10.3390/ijms150712294.

Eraković, Sanja, Ana Janković, Djordje Veljović, Eriks Palcevskis, Miodrag Mitrić, Tatjana Stevanović, Djordje Janaćković, and Vesna Mišković-Stanković. 2013. "Corrosion Stability and Bioactivity in Simulated Body Fluid of Silver/Hydroxyapatite and Silver/Hydroxyapatite/Lignin Coatings on Titanium Obtained by Electrophoretic Deposition." *The Journal of Physical Chemistry B* 117 (6): 1633–43. https://doi.org/10.1021/jp305252a.

Eraković, Sanja, Djordje Veljović, Papa N Diouf, Tatjana Stevanović, Miodrag Mitrić, Djordje Janaćković, Ivana Z Matić, Zorica D Juranić, and Vesna Mišković-Stanković. 2012. "The Effect of Lignin on the Structure and Characteristics of Composite Coatings Electrodeposited on Titanium." *Progress in Organic Coatings* 75 (4): 275–83. https://doi.org/10.1016/j.porgcoat.2012.07.005.

Erakovic, Sanja, Djordje Veljovic, Papa Niokhor Diouf, Tatjana Stevanovic, Miodrag Mitric, Slobodan Milonjic, and Vesna B Miskovic-Stankovic. 2009. "Electrophoretic Deposition of Biocomposite Lignin/Hydroxyapatite Coatings on Titanium." *International Journal of Chemical Reactor Engineering* 7 (1): A62. https://doi.org/doi:10.2202/1542-6580.2088.

Fan, Zengjie, Jinqing Wang, Zhaofeng Wang, Zhangpeng Li, Yinong Qiu, Honggang Wang, Ye Xu, Lengyuan Niu, Peiwei Gong, and Shengrong Yang. 2013. "Casein Phosphopeptide-Biofunctionalized Graphene Biocomposite for Hydroxyapatite Biomimetic Mineralization." *The Journal of Physical Chemistry C* 117 (20): 10375–82. https://doi.org/10.1021/jp312163m.

Fidancevska, Emilija, Gordana Ruseska, Joerg Bossert, Yuan-Min Lin, and Aldo R Boccaccini. 2007. "Fabrication and Characterization of Porous Bioceramic Composites Based on Hydroxyapatite and Titania." *Materials Chemistry and Physics* 103 (1): 95–100. https://doi.org/10.1016/j.matchemphys.2007.01.015.

Filiaggi, MJ, RM Pilliar, and NA Coombs. 1993. "Post-Plasma-Spraying Heat Treatment of the HA Coating/Ti-6Al-4V Implant System." *Journal of Biomedical Materials Research* 27 (2): 191–98. https://doi.org/10.1002/jbm.820270208.

García, C, S Ceré, and A Durán. 2006. "Bioactive Coatings Deposited on Titanium Alloys." *Journal of Non-Crystalline Solids* 352 (32): 3488–95. https://doi.org/10.1016/j.jnoncrysol.2006.02.110.

Gebhardt, F, S Seuss, MC Turhan, H Hornberger, S Virtanen, and AR Boccaccini. 2012. "Characterization of Electrophoretic Chitosan Coatings on Stainless Steel." *Materials Letters* 66 (1): 302–4. https://doi.org/10.1016/j.matlet.2011.08.088.

Geetha, V, T Gomathi, and PN Sudha. 2015. "Preparation and Characterization of Graphene-Grafted- Chitosan / Hydroxyapatite Composite." *Journal of Chemical and Pharmaceutical Research* 7 (5): 871–76.

Geetha, M, AK Singh, R Asokamani, and AK Gogia. 2009. "Ti Based Biomaterials, the Ultimate Choice for Orthopaedic Implants – A Review." *Progress in Materials Science* 54 (3): 397–425. https://doi.org/10.1016/j.pmatsci.2008.06.004.

Geuli, Ori, Noah Metoki, Tal Zada, Meital Reches, Noam Eliaz, and Daniel Mandler. 2017. "Synthesis, Coating, and Drug-Release of Hydroxyapatite Nanoparticles Loaded with Antibiotics." *Journal of Materials Chemistry B* 5 (38): 7819–30. https://doi.org/10.1039/C7TB02105D.

Ghalme, Sachin G, Ankush Mankar, and Yogesh Bhalerao. 2016. "Biomaterials in Hip Joint Replacement." *International Journal of Materials Science and Engineering* 4 (2): 113–25. https://doi.org/10.17706/ijmse.2016.4.2.113-125.

Gibson, Iain R, and William Bonfield. 2002. "Novel Synthesis and Characterization of an AB-Type Carbonate-Substituted Hydroxyapatite." *Journal of Biomedical Materials Research* 59 (4): 697–708. https://doi.org/10.1002/jbm.10044.

Gluck, Themistocles. 2011. "The Classic: Report on the Positive Results Obtained by the Modern Surgical Experiment Regarding the Suture and Replacement of Defects of Superior Tissue, as Well as the Utilization of Re-Absorbable and Living Tamponade in Surgery." *Clinical Orthopaedics and Related Research®* 469 (6): 1528–35. https://doi.org/10.17706/ijmse.

Grohmann, Steffi, Manuela Menne, Diana Hesse, Sabine Bischoff, René Schiffner, Michael Diefenbeck, and Klaus Liefeith. 2019. "Biomimetic Multilayer Coatings Deliver Gentamicin and Reduce Implant-Related Osteomyelitis in Rats." *Biomedical Engineering / Biomedizinische Technik, Biomedical Engineering / Biomedizinische Technik* 64 (4): 383–95. https://doi.org/doi:10.1515/bmt-2018-0044.

Guthrie, James W, and Noel Fitzpatrick. 2019. "Single-Stage Revision of an Infected Total Hip Replacement Using Antibiotic-Impregnated Bioabsorbable Beads in a Canine Patient." *VCOT Open* 02 (01): e5–12. https://doi.org/10.1055/s-0038-1677523.

Hamdan, Nazirah, Deny Susanti Darnis, and Wan Khartini Wan Abdul Khodir. 2021. "In Vitro Evaluation of Crosslinked Polyvinyl Alcohol/Chitosan - Gentamicin Sulfate Electrospun Nanofibers." *Malaysian Journal of Chemistry* 23 (2): 1–10. https://doi.org/10.55373/mjchem.v23i2.992.

Han, Changjun, Yao Yao, Xian Cheng, Jiaxin Luo, Pu Luo, Qian Wang, Fang Yang, Qingsong Wei, and Zhen Zhang. 2017. "Electrophoretic Deposition of Gentamicin-Loaded Silk Fibroin Coatings on 3D-Printed Porous Cobalt–Chromium–Molybdenum Bone Substitutes to Prevent Orthopedic Implant Infections." *Biomacromolecules* 18 (11): 3776–87. https://doi.org/10.1021/acs.biomac.7b01091.

Harun, WSW, RIM Asri, J Alias, FH Zulkifli, K Kadirgama, SAC Ghani, and JHM Shariffuddin. 2018. "A Comprehensive Review of Hydroxyapatite-Based Coatings Adhesion on Metallic Biomaterials." *Ceramics International* 44 (2): 1250–68. https://doi.org/10.1016/j.ceramint.2017.10.162.

Hsu, CH, and F Mansfeld. 2001. "Technical Note: Concerning the Conversion of the Constant Phase Element Parameter Y0 into a Capacitance." *Corrosion* 57 (9): 747–48. https://doi.org/10.5006/1.3280607.

Hu, Wenbing, Cheng Peng, Weijie Luo, Min Lv, Xiaoming Li, Di Li Qing Huang, and Chunhai Fan. 2010. "Graphene-Based Antibacterial Paper." *ACS Nano* 4 (7): 4317–23. https://doi.org/10.1021/nn101097v.

Humayun, Ahmed, Yangyang Luo, and David K Mills. 2020. "Electrophoretic Deposition of Gentamicin-Loaded ZnHNTs-Chitosan on Titanium." *Coatings*. https://doi.org/10.3390/coatings10100944.

Ibrahim, Ahlam M, Zainab M Al-Rashidy, Nabil A Abdel Ghany, Hanaa Y Ahmed, Areg E Omar, and Mohammad M Farag. 2021. "Bioactive and Antibacterial Metal Implant Composite Coating Based on Ce-Doped Nanobioactive Glass and Chitosan by Electrophoretic Deposition Method." *Journal of Materials Research* 36 (9): 1899–913. https://doi.org/10.1557/s43578-021-00246-x.

Ishikawa, K, P Ducheyne, and S Radin. 1993. "Determination of the Ca/P Ratio in Calcium-Deficient Hydroxyapatite Using X-Ray Diffraction Analysis." *Journal of Materials Science: Materials in Medicine* 4 (2): 165–68. https://doi.org/10.1007/BF00120386.

Ivanova, TI, OV Frank-Kamenetskaya, AB Kol'tsov, and VL Ugolkov. 2001. "Crystal Structure of Calcium-Deficient Carbonated Hydroxyapatite. Thermal Decomposition." *Journal of Solid State Chemistry* 160 (2): 340–49. https://doi.org/10.1006/jssc.2000.9238.

Jaćimović, Nevena, Marija Đošić, Ana Janković, Svetlana Grujić, Ivana Matić Bujagić, Jovica Stojanović, Maja Vukašinović-Sekulić, Vesna Kojić, and Vesna Mišković-Stanković. 2023. "Biocomposite Poly(Vinyl Alcohol)-Based Coatings on Titanium Substrate." *Macedonian Journal of Chemistry and Chemical Engineering* 42(2):249–262. https://mjcce.org.mk/index.php/MJCCE/article/view/2775/1237.

Jahanmard, F, FM Dijkmans, A Majed, HC Vogely, BCH van der Wal, DAC Stapels, SM Ahmadi, T Vermonden, and S Amin Yavari. 2020. "Toward Antibacterial Coatings for Personalized Implants." *ACS Biomaterials Science & Engineering* 6 (10): 5486–92. https://doi.org/10.1021/acsbiomaterials.0c00683.

Jamuna-Thevi, K, SA Bakar, S Ibrahim, N Shahab, and MRM Toff. 2011. "Quantification of Silver Ion Release, in Vitro Cytotoxicity and Antibacterial Properties of Nanostuctured Ag Doped TiO2 Coatings on Stainless Steel Deposited by RF Magnetron Sputtering." *Vacuum* 86 (3): 235–41. https://doi.org/10.1016/j.vacuum.2011.06.011.

Janković, Ana, Sanja Eraković, Antonija Dindune, Djordje Veljović, Tatjana Stevanović, Djordje Janaćković, and Vesna Miskovic-Stankovic. 2012. "Electrochemical Impedance Spectroscopy of a Silver-Doped Hydroxyapatite Coating in Simulated Body Fluid Used as a Corrosive Agent." *Journal of the Serbian Chemical Society* 77 (11): 1609–23. https://doi.org/10.2298/JSC120712086J.

Janković, Ana, Sanja Eraković, Miodrag Mitrić, Ivana Z Matić, Zorica D Juranić, Gary CP Tsui, Chak-yin Tang, Vesna Mišković-Stanković, Kyong Yop Rhee, and Soo Jin Park. 2015. "Bioactive Hydroxyapatite/Graphene Composite Coating and Its Corrosion Stability in Simulated Body Fluid." *Journal of Alloys and Compounds* 624: 148–57. https://doi.org/10.1016/j.jallcom.2014.11.078.

Janković, Ana, Sanja Eraković, Maja Vukašinović-Sekulić, Vesna Mišković-Stanković, Soo Jin Park, and Kyong Yop Rhee. 2015. "Graphene-Based Antibacterial Composite Coatings Electrodeposited on Titanium for Biomedical Applications." *Progress in Organic Coatings* 83: 1–10. https://doi.org/10.1016/j.porgcoat.2015.01.019.

Kadurugamuwa, JL, AJ Clarke, and TJ Beveridge. 1993. "Surface Action of Gentamicin on Pseudomonas Aeruginosa." *Journal of Bacteriology* 175 (18): 5798–805. https://doi.org/10.1128/jb.175.18.5798-5805.1993.

Kalbacova, Marie, Antonin Broz, Jing Kong, and Martin Kalbac. 2010. "Graphene Substrates Promote Adherence of Human Osteoblasts and Mesenchymal Stromal Cells." *Carbon* 48 (15): 4323–29. https://doi.org/10.1016/j.carbon.2010.07.045.

Kamaly, Nazila, Basit Yameen, Jun Wu, and Omid C Farokhzad. 2016. "Degradable Controlled-Release Polymers and Polymeric Nanoparticles: Mechanisms of Controlling Drug Release." *Chemical Reviews* 116 (4): 2602–63. https://doi.org/10.1021/acs.chemrev.5b00346.

Kamieniak, Joanna, Peter J Kelly, Craig E Banks, and Aidan M Doyle. 2018. "Mechanical, PH and Thermal Stability of Mesoporous Hydroxyapatite." *Journal of Inorganic and Organometallic Polymers and Materials* 28 (1): 84–91. https://doi.org/10.1007/s10904-017-0652-3.

Kaya, C, I Singh, and AR Boccaccini. 2008. "Multi-Walled Carbon Nanotube-Reinforced Hydroxyapatite Layers on Ti6Al4V Medical Implants by Electrophoretic Deposition (EPD)." *Advanced Engineering Materials* 10 (1–2): 131–38. https://doi.org/10.1002/adem.200700241.

Kim, Hyun-Min, Teruyuki Himeno, Tadashi Kokubo, and Takashi Nakamura. 2005. "Process and Kinetics of Bonelike Apatite Formation on Sintered Hydroxyapatite in a Simulated Body Fluid." *Biomaterials* 26 (21): 4366–73. https://doi.org/10.1016/j.biomaterials.2004.11.022.

Korsmeyer, Richard W, Robert Gurny, Eric Doelker, Pierre Buri, and Nikolaos A Peppas. 1983. "Mechanisms of Solute Release from Porous Hydrophilic Polymers." *International Journal of Pharmaceutics* 15 (1): 25–35. https://doi.org/10.1016/0378-5173(83)90064-9.

Kuilla, Tapas, Sambhu Bhadra, Dahu Yao, Nam Hoon Kim, Saswata Bose, and Joong Hee Lee. 2010. "Recent Advances in Graphene Based Polymer Composites." *Progress in Polymer Science* 35 (11): 1350–75. https://doi.org/10.1016/j.progpolymsci.2010.07.005.

Kung, Kuan-Chen, Tzer-Min Lee, and Truan-Sheng Lui. 2010. "Bioactivity and Corrosion Properties of Novel Coatings Containing Strontium by Micro-Arc Oxidation." *Journal of Alloys and Compounds* 508 (2): 384–90. https://doi.org/10.1016/j.jallcom.2010.08.057.

Kwok, CT, PK Wong, FT Cheng, and HC Man. 2009. "Characterization and Corrosion Behavior of Hydroxyapatite Coatings on Ti6Al4V Fabricated by Electrophoretic Deposition." *Applied Surface Science* 255 (13): 6736–44. https://doi.org/10.1016/j.apsusc.2009.02.086.

Lafon, JP, E Champion, D Bernache-Assollant, R Gibert, and AM Danna. 2003. "Termal Decomposition of Carbonated Calcium Phosphate Apatites." *Journal of Thermal Analysis and Calorimetry* 72 (3): 1127–34. https://doi.org/10.1023/A:1025036214044.

Landi, E, A Tampieri, G Celotti, and S Sprio. 2000. "Densification Behaviour and Mechanisms of Synthetic Hydroxyapatites." *Journal of the European Ceramic Society* 20 (14): 2377–87. https://doi.org/10.1016/S0955-2219(00)00154-0.

Laska, Aleksandra, and Michał Bartmański. 2020. "Parameters of the Electrophoretic Deposition Process and Its Influence on the Morphology of Hydroxyapatite Coatings. Review." *Inżynieria Materiałowa* 41 (1): 18–23. https://doi.org/10.15199/28.2020.1.3.

Lee, In-Seop, Chung-Nam Whang, Kyung-Sik Oh, Jong-Chul Park, Kwon-Yong Lee, Gun-Hwan Lee, Sung-Min Chung, and Xiao-Dan Sun. 2006. "Formation of Silver Incorporated Calcium Phosphate Film for Medical Applications." *Nuclear Instruments and Methods in Physics Research Section B: Beam Interactions with Materials and Atoms* 242 (1): 45–47. https://doi.org/10.1016/j.nimb.2005.08.010.

Li, P, Z Huang, R Liu, and X Xiao. 2009. "Preparation of Porous Hydroxyapatite Coating with Glucose as Pore Producer." *Journal of the Chinese Ceramic Society* 37: 1864–68.

Lian, Peichao, Xuefeng Zhu, Shuzhao Liang, Zhong Li, Weishen Yang, and Haihui Wang. 2010. "Large Reversible Capacity of High Quality Graphene Sheets as an Anode Material for Lithium-Ion Batteries." *Electrochimica Acta* 55 (12): 3909–14. https://doi.org/10.1016/j.electacta.2010.02.025.

Liang, Jiajie, Yi Huang, Long Zhang, Yan Wang, Yanfeng Ma, Tianyin Guo, and Yongsheng Chen. 2009. "Molecular-Level Dispersion of Graphene into Poly(Vinyl Alcohol) and Effective Reinforcement of Their Nanocomposites." *Advanced Functional Materials* 19 (14): 2297–302. https://doi.org/10.1002/adfm.200801776.

Liu, Chang, Jing Zhang, E Yifeng, Jingli Yue, Lianshan Chen, and Donghui Li. 2014. "One-Pot Synthesis of Graphene–Chitosan Nanocomposite Modified Carbon Paste Electrode for Selective Determination of Dopamine." *Electronic Journal of Biotechnology* 17 (4): 183–88. https://doi.org/10.1016/j.ejbt.2014.04.013.

Liu, Hongyan, Pinxian Xi, Guoqiang Xie, Yanjun Shi, Fengping Hou, Liang Huang, Fengjuan Chen, Zhengzhi Zeng, Changwei Shao, and Jun Wang. 2012. "Simultaneous Reduction and Surface Functionalization of Graphene Oxide for Hydroxyapatite Mineralization." *The Journal of Physical Chemistry C* 116 (5): 3334–41. https://doi.org/10.1021/jp2102226.

Liu, Jian, Haixue Yan, Mike J Reece, and Kyle Jiang. 2012. "Toughening of Zirconia/Alumina Composites by the Addition of Graphene Platelets." *Journal of the European Ceramic Society* 32 (16): 4185–93. https://doi.org/10.1016/j.jeurceramsoc.2012.07.007.

Liu, Jinzhao, Jia Dong, Ting Zhang, and Qiang Peng. 2018. "Graphene-Based Nanomaterials and Their Potentials in Advanced Drug Delivery and Cancer Therapy." *Journal of Controlled Release* 286: 64–73. https://doi.org/10.1016/j.jconrel.2018.07.034.

Liu, Yang, Peihong Ji, Huilin Lv, Yong Qin, and Linhong Deng. 2017. "Gentamicin Modified Chitosan Film with Improved Antibacterial Property and Cell Biocompatibility." *International Journal of Biological Macromolecules* 98: 550–56. https://doi.org/10.1016/j.ijbiomac.2017.01.121.

Liu, Yi, Jing Huang, and Hua Li. 2013a. "Synthesis of Hydroxyapatite-Reduced Graphite Oxide Nanocomposites for Biomedical Applications: Oriented Nucleation and Epitaxial Growth of Hydroxyapatite." *Journal of Materials Chemistry B* 1 (13): 1826–34. https://doi.org/10.1039/c3tb00531c.

———. 2013b. "Synthesis of Hydroxyapatite–Reduced Graphite Oxide Nanocomposites for Biomedical Applications: Oriented Nucleation and Epitaxial Growth of Hydroxyapatite." *Journal of Materials Chemistry B* 1 (13): 1826–34. https://doi.org/10.1039/C3TB00531C.

Maachou, Hamida, Michel J Genet, Djamel Aliouche, Christine C Dupont-Gillain, and Paul G Rouxhet. 2013. "XPS Analysis of Chitosan–Hydroxyapatite Biomaterials: From Elements to Compounds." *Surface and Interface Analysis* 45 (7): 1088–97. https://doi.org/10.1002/sia.5229.

Macha, Innocent J, Sophie Cazalbou, Besim Ben-Nissan, Kate L Harvey, and Bruce Milthorpe. 2015. "Marine Structure Derived Calcium Phosphate–Polymer Biocomposites for Local Antibiotic Delivery." *Marine Drugs*. https://doi.org/10.3390/md13010666.

Madupalli, Honey, Barbara Pavan, and Mary MJ Tecklenburg. 2017. "Carbonate Substitution in the Mineral Component of Bone: Discriminating the Structural Changes, Simultaneously Imposed by Carbonate in A and B Sites of Apatite." *Journal of Solid State Chemistry* 255: 27–35. https://doi.org/10.1016/j.jssc.2017.07.025.

Mahmoodi, S, L Sorkhi, M Farrokhi-Rad, and T Shahrabi. 2013. "Electrophoretic Deposition of Hydroxyapatite–Chitosan Nanocomposite Coatings in Different Alcohols." *Surface and Coatings Technology* 216: 106–14. https://doi.org/10.1016/j.surfcoat.2012.11.032.

Manivasagam, Geetha, Durgalakshmi Dhinasekaran, and Asokamani Rajamanickam. 2010. "Biomedical Implants: Corrosion and Its Prevention - A Review." *Recent Patents on Corrosion Science* 2 (1): 40–54. https://doi.org/10.2174/1877610801002010040.

Mansur, Herman S, AAP Mansur, and SMCM Bicallho. 2005. "Lignin-Hydroxyapatite/Tricalcium Phosphate Biocomposites: SEM/EDX and FTIR Characterization." *Key Engineering Materials* 284–286: 745–48. https://doi.org/10.4028/www.scientific.net/KEM.284-286.745.

Martin, Holly J, Kirk H Schulz, Joel D Bumgardner, and Judith A Schneider. 2008. "Enhanced Bonding of Chitosan to Implant Quality Titanium via Four Treatment Combinations." *Thin Solid Films* 516 (18): 6277–86. https://doi.org/10.1016/j.tsf.2007.12.001.

Martinez, MM, A Pacheco, and VM Vargas. 2009. "Histological Evaluation of the Biocompatibility and Bioconduction of a Hydroxyapatite-Lignin Compound Inserted in Rabbits Shinbones." *Revista MVZ Córdoba* 14: 1624–32.

McManamon, Colm, Johann P de Silva, Paul Delaney, Michael A Morris, and Graham LW Cross. 2016. "Characteristics, Interactions and Coating Adherence of Heterogeneous Polymer/Drug Coatings for Biomedical Devices." *Materials Science and Engineering: C* 59: 102–8. https://doi.org/10.1016/j.msec.2015.09.103.

Meejoo, Siwaporn, Weerakanya Maneeprakorn, and Pongtip Winotai. 2006. "Phase and Thermal Stability of Nanocrystalline Hydroxyapatite Prepared via Microwave Heating." *Thermochimica Acta* 447 (1): 115–20. https://doi.org/10.1016/j.tca.2006.04.013.

Metsemakers, WJ, R Kuehl, TF Moriarty, RG Richards, MHJ Verhofstad, O Borens, S Kates, and M Morgenstern. 2018. "Infection after Fracture Fixation: Current Surgical and Microbiological Concepts." *Injury* 49 (3): 511–22. https://doi.org/10.1016/j.injury.2016.09.019.

Mišković-Stanković, Vesna B. 2014. "Electrophoretic Deposition of Ceramic Coatings on Metal Surfaces." In *Electrodeposition and Surface Finishing. Fundamentals and Applications*, edited by Stojan S Djokić, 133–216. New York, NY: Springer. https://doi.org/10.1007/978-1-4939-0289-7_3.

Mišković-Stanković, Vesna B, Sanja Eraković, Ana Janković, Maja Vukašinović-Sekulić, Miodrag Mitrić, Young Chan Jung, Soo Jin Park, and Kyong Yop Rhee. 2015. "Electrochemical Synthesis of Nanosized Hydroxyapatite/ Graphene Composite Powder." *Carbon Letters* 16 (4): 233–40. https://doi.org/10.5714/CL.2015.16.4.233.

Mokabber, T. 2020. *Electrochemically Deposited Antimicrobial Hydroxyapatite Coatings.* University of Groningen. https://doi.org/10.33612/diss.132596200.

Moseke, Claus, Uwe Gbureck, Patrick Elter, Peter Drechsler, Andreas Zoll, Roger Thull, and Andrea Ewald. 2011. "Hard Implant Coatings with Antimicrobial Properties." *Journal of Materials Science: Materials in Medicine* 22 (12): 2711–20. https://doi.org/10.1007/s10856-011-4457-6.

Mosmann, Tim. 1983. "Rapid Colorimetric Assay for Cellular Growth and Survival: Application to Proliferation and Cytotoxicity Assays." *Journal of Immunological Methods* 65 (1): 55–63. https://doi.org/10.1016/0022-1759(83)90303-4.

Mostafa, Nasser Y. 2005. "Characterization, Thermal Stability and Sintering of Hydroxyapatite Powders Prepared by Different Routes." *Materials Chemistry and Physics* 94 (2): 333–41. https://doi.org/10.1016/j.matchemphys.2005.05.011.

Mouriño, Viviana, Juan Pablo Cattalini, and Aldo R Boccaccini. 2012. "Metallic Ions as Therapeutic Agents in Tissue Engineering Scaffolds: An Overview of Their Biological Applications and Strategies for New Developments." *Journal of the Royal Society Interface* 9 (68): 401–19. https://doi.org/10.1098/rsif.2011.0611.

Müller, Lenka, and Frank A Müller. 2006. "Preparation of SBF with Different HCO3- Content and Its Influence on the Composition of Biomimetic Apatites." *Acta Biomaterialia* 2 (2): 181–89. https://doi.org/10.1016/j.actbio.2005.11.001.

Navarro, M, A Michiardi, O Castaño, and JA Planell. 2008. "Biomaterials in Orthopaedics." *Journal of The Royal Society Interface* 5 (27): 1137–58. https://doi.org/10.1098/rsif.2008.0151.

Neelgund, Gururaj M, Aderemi Oki, and Zhiping Luo. 2013. "In Situ Deposition of Hydroxyapatite on Graphene Nanosheets." *Materials Research Bulletin* 48 (2): 175–79. https://doi.org/10.1016/j.materresbull.2012.08.077.

Niinomi, M, and M Nakai. 2011. "Titanium-Based Biomaterials for Preventing Stress Shielding between Implant Devices and Bone." Edited by Tadashi Kokubo. *International Journal of Biomaterials* 2011: 836587. https://doi.org/10.1155/2011/836587.

Nikpour, MR, SM Rabiee, and M Jahanshahi. 2012. "Synthesis and Characterization of Hydroxyapatite/Chitosan Nanocomposite Materials for Medical Engineering Applications." *Composites Part B: Engineering* 43 (4): 1881–86. https://doi.org/10.1016/j.compositesb.2012.01.056.

Offermanns, Stefan, and Walter Rosenthal, eds. 2008. *Encyclopedia of Molecular Pharmacology*. Berlin, Heidelberg: Springer. https://doi.org/10.1007/978-3-540-38918-7.

Ohno, Mitsuharu, and Tsutomu Abe. 1991. "Rapid Colorimetric Assay for the Quantification of Leukemia Inhibitory Factor (LIF) and Interleukin-6 (IL-6)." *Journal of Immunological Methods* 145 (1): 199–203. https://doi.org/10.1016/0022-1759(91)90327-C.

Okada, Masahiro, and Takuya Matsumoto. 2015. "Synthesis and Modification of Apatite Nanoparticles for Use in Dental and Medical Applications." *Japanese Dental Science Review* 51 (4): 85–95. https://doi.org/10.1016/j.jdsr.2015.03.004.

Orazem, ME, and B Tribollet, eds. 2008. *Electrochemical Impedance Spectroscopy*. Hoboken and New York: John Wiley & Sons, Inc. https://doi.org/10.1002/9780470381588.

Ordikhani, F, M Ramezani Farani, M Dehghani, E Tamjid, and A Simchi. 2015. "Physicochemical and Biological Properties of Electrodeposited Graphene Oxide/Chitosan Films with Drug-Eluting Capacity." *Carbon* 84: 91–102. https://doi.org/10.1016/j.carbon.2014.11.052.

Orimo, Hideo. 2010. "The Mechanism of Mineralization and the Role of Alkaline Phosphatase in Health and Disease." *Journal of Nippon Medical School* 77 (1): 4–12. https://doi.org/10.1272/jnms.77.4.

Palcevskis, E, A Dindune, L Kuznecova, A Lipe, and Z Kanepe. 2005. "Granulated Composite Powders on Basis of Hydroxyapatite and Plasma-Processed Zirconia and Alumina Nanopowders." *Latvian Journal of Chemistry* 2: 128–38.

Pan, Xuejun, John F Kadla, Katsunobu Ehara, Neil Gilkes, and Jack N Saddler. 2006. "Organosolv Ethanol Lignin from Hybrid Poplar as a Radical Scavenger: Relationship between Lignin Structure, Extraction Conditions, and Antioxidant Activity." *Journal of Agricultural and Food Chemistry* 54 (16): 5806–13. https://doi.org/10.1021/jf0605392.

Pang, X, and I Zhitomirsky. 2008. "Electrodeposition of Hydroxyapatite–Silver–Chitosan Nanocomposite Coatings." *Surface and Coatings Technology* 202 (16): 3815–21. https://doi.org/10.1016/j.surfcoat.2008.01.022.

Pankey, GA, and LD Sabath. 2004. "Clinical Relevance of Bacteriostatic versus Bactericidal Mechanisms of Action in the Treatment of Gram-Positive Bacterial Infections." *Clinical Infectious Diseases* 38 (6): 864–70. https://doi.org/10.1086/381972.

Pantović Pavlović, Marijana R, Sanja G Eraković, Miroslav M Pavlović, Jasmina S Stevanović, Vladimir V Panić, and Nenad L Ignjatović. 2019. "Anaphoretical/Oxidative Approach to the in-Situ Synthesis of Adherent Hydroxyapatite/Titanium Oxide Composite Coatings on Titanium." *Surface and Coatings Technology* 358 (September 2018): 688–94. https://doi.org/10.1016/j.surfcoat.2018.12.003.

Pantović Pavlović, Marijana R, Nenad L Ignjatović, Vladimir V Panić, Ivana I Mirkov, Jelena B Kulaš, Anastasija Lj Malešević, and Miroslav M Pavlović. 2023. "Immunomodulatory Effects Mediated by Nano Amorphous Calcium Phosphate/Chitosan Oligosaccharide Lactate Coatings Decorated with Selenium on Titanium Implants." *Journal of Functional Biomaterials*. https://doi.org/10.3390/jfb14040227.

Pantović Pavlović, Marijana R, Miroslav M Pavlović, Sanja Eraković, Jasmina S Stevanović, Vladimir V Panić, and Nenad Ignjatović. 2020. "Simultaneous Anodization/Anaphoretic Electrodeposition Synthesis of Nano Calcium Phosphate/Titanium Oxide Composite Coatings Assisted with Chitosan Oligosaccharide Lactate." *Materials Letters* 261 (February): 127121. https://doi.org/10.1016/j.matlet.2019.127121.

Pantović Pavlović, Marijana R, Boris P Stanojević, Miroslav M Pavlović, Marija D Mihailović, Jasmina S Stevanović, Vladimir V Panić, and Nenad L Ignjatović. 2021. "Anodizing/Anaphoretic Electrodeposition of Nano-Calcium Phosphate/Chitosan Lactate Multifunctional Coatings on Titanium with Advanced Corrosion Resistance, Bioactivity, and Antibacterial Properties." *ACS Biomaterials Science & Engineering* 7 (7): 3088–102. https://doi.org/10.1021/acsbiomaterials.1c00035.

Parente, P, AJ Sanchez-Herencia, MJ Mesa-Galan, and B Ferrari. 2013. "Functionalizing Ti-Surfaces through the EPD of Hydroxyapatite/NanoY2O3." *The Journal of Physical Chemistry B* 117 (6): 1600–7. https://doi.org/10.1021/jp305176h.

Park, Ji-Ho, Doug-Youn Lee, Keun-Taek Oh, Yong-Keun Lee, Kwang-Mahn Kim, and Kyoung-Nam Kim. 2006. "Bioactivity of Calcium Phosphate Coatings Prepared by Electrodeposition in a Modified Simulated Body Fluid." *Materials Letters* 60 (21): 2573–77. https://doi.org/10.1016/j.matlet.2005.07.091.

Park, Yoosup, WOS Doherty, and Peter J Halley. 2008. "Developing Lignin-Based Resin Coatings and Composites." *Industrial Crops and Products* 27 (2): 163–67. https://doi.org/10.1016/j.indcrop.2007.07.021.

Patel, Kapil D, Ahmed El-Fiqi, Hye-Young Lee, Rajendra K Singh, Dong-Ae Kim, Hae-Hyoung Lee, and Hae-Won Kim. 2012. "Chitosan–Nanobioactive Glass Electrophoretic Coatings with Bone Regenerative and Drug Delivering Potential." *Journal of Materials Chemistry* 22 (47): 24945–56. https://doi.org/10.1039/C2JM33830K.

Patel, Kapil D, Rajendra K Singh, Eun-Jung Lee, Cheol-Min Han, Jong-Eun Won, Jonathan C Knowles, and Hae-Won Kim. 2014. "Tailoring Solubility and Drug Release from Electrophoretic Deposited Chitosan–Gelatin Films on Titanium." *Surface and Coatings Technology* 242: 232–36. https://doi.org/10.1016/j.surfcoat.2013.11.049.

Pecheva, Emilia V, Liliana D Pramatarova, Manfred F Maitz, Mihn T Pham, and Alexey V Kondyuirin. 2004. "Kinetics of Hydroxyapatite Deposition on Solid Substrates Modified by Sequential Implantation of Ca and P Ions: Part I. FTIR and Raman Spectroscopy Study." *Applied Surface Science* 235 (1): 176–81. https://doi.org/10.1016/j.apsusc.2004.05.174.

Peng, Fei, Eric Veilleux, Megan Schmidt, and Mei Wei. 2012. "Synthesis of Hydroxyapatite Nanoparticles with Tailorable Morphologies and Carbonate Substitutions Using a Wet Precipitation Method." *Journal of Nanoscience and Nanotechnology* 12 (3): 2774–82. https://doi.org/10.1166/jnn.2012.5714.

Permyakova, Elizaveta S, Anton M Manakhov, Philipp V Kiryukhantsev-Korneev, Alexander N Sheveyko, Kristina Y Gudz, Andrey M Kovalskii, Josef Polčak, et al. 2021. "Different Concepts for Creating Antibacterial yet Biocompatible Surfaces: Adding Bactericidal

Element, Grafting Therapeutic Agent through COOH Plasma Polymer and Their Combination." *Applied Surface Science* 556: 149751. https://doi.org/10.1016/j.apsusc.2021.149751.

Phillips, Hugh J. 1973. "Dye Exclusion Tests for Cell Viability." In *Tissue Culture Methods and Applications*, edited by Paul F Kruse and MK Patterson, 406–8. Cambridge, MA: Academic Press. https://doi.org/10.1016/B978-0-12-427150-0.50101-7.

Pishbin, Fatemehsadat, Viviana Mouriño, Sabrina Flor, Stefan Kreppel, Vehid Salih, Mary P Ryan, and Aldo R Boccaccini. 2014. "Electrophoretic Deposition of Gentamicin-Loaded Bioactive Glass/Chitosan Composite Coatings for Orthopaedic Implants." *ACS Applied Materials & Interfaces* 6 (11): 8796–806. https://doi.org/10.1021/am5014166.

Purcar, Violeta, Valentin Rădiţoiu, Cornelia Nichita, Adriana Bălan, Alina Rădiţoiu, Simona Căprărescu, Florentina Monica Raduly, et al. 2021. "Preparation and Characterization of Silica Nanoparticles and of Silica-Gentamicin Nanostructured Solution Obtained by Microwave-Assisted Synthesis." *Materials (Basel, Switzerland)* 14 (8): 2086. https://doi.org/10.3390/ma14082086.

Qiu, Kexin, Bo Chen, Wei Nie, Xiaojun Zhou, Wei Feng, Weizhong Wang, Liang Chen, Xiumei Mo, Youzhen Wei, and Chuanglong He. 2016. "Electrophoretic Deposition of Dexamethasone-Loaded Mesoporous Silica Nanoparticles onto Poly(l-Lactic Acid)/Poly(ε-Caprolactone) Composite Scaffold for Bone Tissue Engineering." *ACS Applied Materials & Interfaces* 8 (6): 4137–48. https://doi.org/10.1021/acsami.5b11879.

Radda'a, Namir S, Wolfgang H Goldmann, Rainer Detsch, Judith A Roether, Luis Cordero-Arias, Sannakaisa Virtanen, Tomasz Moskalewicz, and Aldo R Boccaccini. 2017. "Electrophoretic Deposition of Tetracycline Hydrochloride Loaded Halloysite Nanotubes Chitosan/Bioactive Glass Composite Coatings for Orthopedic Implants." *Surface and Coatings Technology* 327: 146–57. https://doi.org/10.1016/j.surfcoat.2017.07.048.

Ragu, A, K Senthilarasan, and P Sakthivel. 2015. "Synthesis and Characterization of Nano Hydroxyapatite with Polyoxymethylene Nanocomposites for Bone Growth Studies." *International Journal of Scientific Engineering and Research (IJSER)* 3 (7): 120–23.

Rahighi, Reza, Mohammad Panahi, Omid Akhavan, and Mojtaba Mansoorianfar. 2021. "Pressure-Engineered Electrophoretic Deposition for Gentamicin Loading within Osteoblast-Specific Cellulose Nanofiber Scaffolds." *Materials Chemistry and Physics* 272: 125018. https://doi.org/10.1016/j.matchemphys.2021.125018.

Rameshbabu, N, TS Sampath Kumar, TG Prabhakar, VS Sastry, KVGK Murty, and K Prasad Rao. 2007. "Antibacterial Nanosized Silver Substituted Hydroxyapatite: Synthesis and Characterization." *Journal of Biomedical Materials Research Part A* 80A (3): 581–91. https://doi.org/10.1002/jbm.a.30958.

Rapacz-Kmita, Alicja, EWA Stodolak-Zych, Magdalena Ziabka, Agnieszka Rozycka, and Magdalena Dudek. 2015. "Instrumental Characterization of the Smectite Clay–Gentamicin Hybrids." *Bulletin of Materials Science* 38 (4): 1069–78. https://doi.org/10.1007/s12034-015-0943-7.

Raschip, Irina Elena, Cornelia Vasile, Diana Ciolacu, and Georgeta Cazacu. 2007. "Semi-Interpenetrating Polymer Networks Containing Polysaccharides. I Xanthan/Lignin Networks." *High Performance Polymers* 19 (5–6): 603–20. https://doi.org/10.1177/0954008307081202.

Rath, Purna C, Laxmidhar Besra, Bimal P Singh, and Sarama Bhattacharjee. 2012. "Titania/Hydroxyapatite Bi-Layer Coating on Ti Metal by Electrophoretic Deposition: Characterization and Corrosion Studies." *Ceramics International* 38 (4): 3209–16. https://doi.org/10.1016/j.ceramint.2011.12.026.

Rathbone, Christopher R, Jessica D Cross, Kate V Brown, Clinton K Murray, and Joseph C Wenke. 2011. "Effect of Various Concentrations of Antibiotics on Osteogenic Cell Viability and Activity." *Journal of Orthopaedic Research* 29 (7): 1070–74. https://doi.org/10.1002/jor.21343.

Rehman, Muhammad Atiq Ur, and Syeda Ammara Batool. 2022. "Development of Sustainable Antibacterial Coatings Based on Electrophoretic Deposition of Multilayers: Gentamicin-Loaded Chitosan/Gelatin/Bioactive Glass Deposition on PEEK/Bioactive Glass Layer." *The International Journal of Advanced Manufacturing Technology* 120 (5): 3885–900. https://doi.org/10.1007/s00170-022-09024-3.

Ren, Fuzeng, Yonghui Ding, and Yang Leng. 2014. "Infrared Spectroscopic Characterization of Carbonated Apatite: A Combined Experimental and Computational Study." *Journal of Biomedical Materials Research Part A* 102 (2): 496–505. https://doi.org/10.1002/jbm.a.34720.

Riahi, Zohreh, Shahab Ahmadi Seyedkhani, and SK Sadrnezhaad. 2019. "Electrophoretic Encapsulation for Slow Release of Vancomycin from Perpendicular TiO2 Nanotubes Grown on Ti6Al4V Electrodes." *Materials Research Express* 6 (12): 125424. https://doi.org/10.1088/2053-1591/ab6c98.

Rincón-López, July A, Jennifer A Hermann-Muñoz, Astrid L Giraldo-Betancur, Andrea De Vizcaya-Ruiz, Juan M Alvarado-Orozco, and Juan Muñoz-Saldaña. 2018. "Synthesis, Characterization and In Vitro Study of Synthetic and Bovine-Derived Hydroxyapatite Ceramics: A Comparison." *Materials*. https://doi.org/10.3390/ma11030333.

Ritger, Philip L, and Nikolaos A Peppas. 1987. "A Simple Equation for Description of Solute Release I. Fickian and Non-Fickian Release from Non-Swellable Devices in the Form of Slabs, Spheres, Cylinders or Discs." *Journal of Controlled Release* 5 (1): 23–36. https://doi.org/10.1016/0168-3659(87)90034-4.

Roop Kumar, R, and M Wang. 2002. "Modulus and Hardness Evaluations of Sintered Bioceramic Powders and Functionally Graded Bioactive Composites by Nano-Indentation Technique." *Materials Science and Engineering: A* 338 (1): 230–36. https://doi.org/10.1016/S0921-5093(02)00080-1.

Sakthivel, P, A Ragu, and K Senthilarasan. 2015. "Synthesis and Characterization of Hydroxyapatite with Tamarind Kernel Powder (Bio-Polymer) for Biomedical Applications." *International Journal of Engineering, Science and Technology* 4: 631–35.

Sayyar, S, E Murray, S Gambhir, G Spinks, GG Wallace, and DL Officer. 2016. "Synthesis and Characterization of Covalently Linked Graphene/Chitosan Composites." *JOM* 68 (1): 384–90. https://doi.org/10.1007/s11837-015-1549-7.

Sekaran, Saravanan, Selvaraj Vimalraj, and Lakshmi Thangavelu. 2021. "The Physiological and Pathological Role of Tissue Nonspecific Alkaline Phosphatase beyond Mineralization." *Biomolecules* 11 (11): 1564. https://doi.org/10.3390/biom11111564.

Shakil, Shazi, Rosina Khan, Raffaele Zarrilli, and Asad U Khan. 2008. "Aminoglycosides versus Bacteria – A Description of the Action, Resistance Mechanism, and Nosocomial Battleground." *Journal of Biomedical Science* 15 (1): 5–14. https://doi.org/10.1007/s11373-007-9194-y.

Sharma, Geeta, and SW Gosavi. 2014. "Thermoluminescence Properties of Graphene–Nano ZnS Composite." *Journal of Luminescence* 145: 557–62. https://doi.org/10.1016/j.jlumin.2013.08.021.

Shi, YY, M Li, Q Liu, ZJ Jia, XC Xu, Y Cheng, and YF Zheng. 2016. "Electrophoretic Deposition of Graphene Oxide Reinforced Chitosan–Hydroxyapatite Nanocomposite Coatings on Ti Substrate." *Journal of Materials Science: Materials in Medicine* 27 (3): 48. https://doi.org/10.1007/s10856-015-5634-9.

Shuai, Cijun, Yi Nie, Chengde Gao, Haibo Lu, Huanlong Hu, Xuejun Wen, and Shuping Peng. 2012. "Poly (l-Lactide Acid) Improves Complete Nano-Hydroxyapatite Bone Scaffolds through the Microstructure Rearrangement." *Electronic Journal of Biotechnology* 15 (6): 1–13. https://doi.org/10.2225/vol15-issue6-fulltext-3.

Simchi, A, E Tamjid, F Pishbin, and AR Boccaccini. 2011. "Recent Progress in Inorganic and Composite Coatings with Bactericidal Capability for Orthopaedic Applications." *Nanomedicine: Nanotechnology, Biology and Medicine* 7 (1): 22–39. https://doi.org/10.1016/j.nano.2010.10.005.

Sjögren, Göran, Gaynour Sletten, and Jon E Dahl. 2000. "Cytotoxicity of Dental Alloys, Metals, and Ceramics Assessed by Millipore Filter, Agar Overlay, and MTT Tests." *The Journal of Prosthetic Dentistry* 84 (2): 229–36. https://doi.org/10.1067/mpr.2000.107227.

Smičiklas, I, S Dimović, I Plećaš, and M Mitrić. 2006. "Removal of Co2+ from Aqueous Solutions by Hydroxyapatite." *Water Research* 40 (12): 2267–74. https://doi.org/10.1016/j.watres.2006.04.031.

Song, YW, DY Shan, and EH Han. 2008. "Electrodeposition of Hydroxyapatite Coating on AZ91D Magnesium Alloy for Biomaterial Application." *Materials Letters* 62 (17): 3276–79. https://doi.org/10.1016/j.matlet.2008.02.048.

Stevanović, Milena, Marija Djošić, Ana Janković, Vesna Kojić, Jovica Stojanović, Svetlana Grujić, Ivana Matić Bujagić, Kyong Yop Rhee, and Vesna Mišković-Stanković. 2021. "The Chitosan-Based Bioactive Composite Coating on Titanium." *Journal of Materials Research and Technology* 15: 4461–74. https://doi.org/10.1016/j.jmrt.2021.10.072.

Stevanović, Milena, Marija Đošić, Ana Janković, Vesna Kojić, Maja Vukašinović-Sekulić, Jovica Stojanović, Jadranka Odović, Milkica Crevar Sakač, Kyong Yop Rhee, and Vesna Mišković-Stanković. 2018. "Gentamicin-Loaded Bioactive Hydroxyapatite/Chitosan Composite Coating Electrodeposited on Titanium." *ACS Biomaterials Science & Engineering* 4 (12): 3994–4007. https://doi.org/10.1021/acsbiomaterials.8b00859.

———. 2020. "Antibacterial Graphene-Based Hydroxyapatite/Chitosan Coating with Gentamicin for Potential Applications in Bone Tissue Engineering." *Journal of Biomedical Materials Research. Part A* 108 (11): 2175–89. https://doi.org/10.1002/jbm.a.36974.

Stevanović, Milena, Marija Djošić, Ana Janković, Katarina Nešović, Vesna Kojić, Jovica Stojanović, Svetlana Grujić, Ivana Matić Bujagić, Kyong Yop Rhee, and Vesna Mišković-Stanković. 2020. "Assessing the Bioactivity of Gentamicin-Preloaded Hydroxyapatite/Chitosan Composite Coating on Titanium Substrate." *ACS Omega* 5 (25): 15433–45. https://doi.org/10.1021/acsomega.0c01583.

Stoch, A, A Brożek, G Kmita, J Stoch, W Jastrzębski, and A Rakowska. 2001. "Electrophoretic Coating of Hydroxyapatite on Titanium Implants." *Journal of Molecular Structure* 596 (1): 191–200. https://doi.org/10.1016/S0022-2860(01)00716-5.

Stoch, A, W Jastrzębski, A Brożek, B Trybalska, M Cichocińska, and E Szarawara. 1999. "FTIR Monitoring of the Growth of the Carbonate Containing Apatite Layers from Simulated and Natural Body Fluids." *Journal of Molecular Structure* 511–512: 287–94. https://doi.org/10.1016/S0022-2860(99)00170-2.

Stravinskas, Mindaugas, Malin Nilsson, Peter Horstmann, Michael Mørk Petersen, Sarunas Tarasevicius, and Lars Lidgren. 2018. "Antibiotic Containing Bone Substitute in Major Hip Surgery: A Long Term Gentamicin Elution Study." *Journal of Bone and Joint Infection* 3 (2): 68–72. https://doi.org/10.7150/jbji.23901.

Sun, Ruixue, Musen Li, Yupeng Lu, and Aijuan Wang. 2006. "Immersion Behavior of Hydroxyapatite (HA) Powders before and after Sintering." *Materials Characterization* 56 (3): 250–54. https://doi.org/10.1016/j.matchar.2005.11.012.

Surudžić, Rade, Ana Janković, Nataša Bibić, Maja Vukašinović-Sekulić, Aleksandra Perić-Grujić, Vesna Mišković-Stanković, Soo Jin Park, and Kyong Yop Rhee. 2016. "Physico–Chemical and Mechanical Properties and Antibacterial Activity of Silver/Poly(Vinyl Alcohol)/Graphene Nanocomposites Obtained by Electrochemical Method." *Composites Part B: Engineering* 85: 102–12. https://doi.org/10.1016/j.compositesb.2015.09.029.

Swetha, Maddela, Kolli Sahithi, Ambigapathi Moorthi, Narasimhan Srinivasan, Kumarasamy Ramasamy, and Nagarajan Selvamurugan. 2010. "Biocomposites Containing Natural Polymers and Hydroxyapatite for Bone Tissue Engineering." *International Journal of Biological Macromolecules* 47 (1): 1–4. https://doi.org/10.1016/j.ijbiomac.2010.03.015.

Szatkowski, T, A Kolodziejczak-Radzimska, J Zdarta, K Szwarc-Rzepka, D Paukszta, M Wysokowski, H Ehrlich, and T Jesionowski. 2015. "Synthesis and Characterization of Hydroxyapatite." *Physicochemical Problems of Mineral Processing* 51 (2): 575–85. https://doi.org/10.1002/jbm.10280.

Tangy, Frédéric, Maryam Moukkadem, Eric Vindimian, Marie-Louise Capmau, and François Le Goffic. 1985. "Mechanism of Action of Gentamicin Components: Characteristics of Their Binding to Escherichia Coli Ribosomes." *European Journal of Biochemistry* 147 (2): 381–86. https://doi.org/10.1111/j.1432-1033.1985.tb08761.x.

Ugartondo, Vanessa, Montserrat Mitjans, and María Pilar Vinardell. 2008. "Comparative Antioxidant and Cytotoxic Effects of Lignins from Different Sources." *Bioresource Technology* 99 (14): 6683–87. https://doi.org/10.1016/j.biortech.2007.11.038.

Vafa, Ehsan, Mohammad Ebrahim Bahrololoom, Reza Bazargan-lari, and Ali Mohammad Amani. 2022. "Effect of Polyvinyl Alcohol Concentration on Biomedical Application of Chitosan/Bioactive Glass Composite Coated on AZ91D Magnesium Alloy." *Materials Chemistry and Physics* 291: 126650. https://doi.org/10.1016/j.matchemphys.2022.126650.

Veljović, Dj, B Jokić, R Petrović, E Palcevskis, A Dindune, IN Mihailescu, and Dj Janaćković. 2009. "Processing of Dense Nanostructured HAP Ceramics by Sintering and Hot Pressing." *Ceramics International* 35 (4): 1407–13. https://doi.org/10.1016/j.ceramint.2008.07.007.

Venkatesan, Jayachandran, and Se Kwon Kim. 2010. "Chitosan Composites for Bone Tissue Engineering - An Overview." *Marine Drugs* 8 (8): 2252–66. https://doi.org/10.3390/md8082252.

Viornery, Carine, Yann Chevolot, Didier Léonard, Björn-Owe Aronsson, Péter Péchy, Hans Jörg Mathieu, Pierre Descouts, and Michael Grätzel. 2002. "Surface Modification of Titanium with Phosphonic Acid To Improve Bone Bonding: Characterization by XPS and ToF-SIMS." *Langmuir* 18 (7): 2582–89. https://doi.org/10.1021/la010908i.

Vugt, Tom AG van, Jacobus J Arts, and Jan AP Geurts. 2019. "Antibiotic-Loaded Polymethylmethacrylate Beads and Spacers in Treatment of Orthopedic Infections and the Role of Biofilm Formation." *Frontiers in Microbiology*. https://www.frontiersin.org/articles/10.3389/fmicb.2019.01626.

Wang, CX, M Wang, and X Zhou. 2002. "Electrochemical Impedance Spectroscopy Study of the Nucleation and Growth of Apatite on Chemically Treated Titanium." *Langmuir* 18 (20): 7641–47. https://doi.org/10.1021/la011877u.

Wang, J, J de Boer, and K de Groot. 2004. "Preparation and Characterization of Electrodeposited Calcium Phosphate/Chitosan Coating on Ti6Al4V Plates." *Journal of Dental Research* 83 (4): 296–301. https://doi.org/10.1177/154405910408300405.

Watling, Kym M, Jeff F Parr, Llew Rintoul, Christopher L Brown, and Leigh A Sullivan. 2011. "Raman, Infrared and XPS Study of Bamboo Phytoliths after Chemical Digestion." *Spectrochimica Acta Part A: Molecular and Biomolecular Spectroscopy* 80 (1): 106–11. https://doi.org/10.1016/j.saa.2011.03.002.

Witte, Frank. 2010. "The History of Biodegradable Magnesium Implants: A Review." *Acta Biomaterialia* 6 (5): 1680–92. https://doi.org/10.1016/j.actbio.2010.02.028.

Wopenka, Brigitte, and Jill D Pasteris. 2005. "A Mineralogical Perspective on the Apatite in Bone." *Materials Science and Engineering: C* 25 (2): 131–43. https://doi.org/10.1016/j.msec.2005.01.008.

Wu, Cheng-Chei, Shun-Te Huang, Tian-Wen Tseng, Qun-Li Rao, and Hong-Ching Lin. 2010. "FT-IR and XRD Investigations on Sintered Fluoridated Hydroxyapatite Composites." *Journal of Molecular Structure* 979 (1): 72–76. https://doi.org/10.1016/j.molstruc.2010.06.003.

Xianmiao, Cheng, Li Yubao, Zuo Yi, Zhang Li, Li Jidong, and Wang Huanan. 2009. "Properties and in Vitro Biological Evaluation of Nano-Hydroxyapatite/Chitosan Membranes for Bone Guided Regeneration." *Materials Science and Engineering: C* 29 (1): 29–35. https://doi.org/10.1016/j.msec.2008.05.008.

Xie, Xingyi, Kaiwen Hu, Dongdong Fang, Lihong Shang, Simon D Tran, and Marta Cerruti. 2015. "Graphene and Hydroxyapatite Self-Assemble into Homogeneous, Free Standing Nanocomposite Hydrogels for Bone Tissue Engineering." *Nanoscale* 7 (17): 7992–8002. https://doi.org/10.1039/c5nr01107h.

Xu, YX, KM Kim, MA Hanna, and D Nag. 2005. "Chitosan–Starch Composite Film: Preparation and Characterization." *Industrial Crops and Products* 21 (2): 185–92. https://doi.org/10.1016/j.indcrop.2004.03.002.

Yang, WH, XF Xi, JF Li, and KY Cai. 2013. "Comparison of Crystal Structure Between Carbonated Hydroxyapatite and Natural Bone Apatite with Theoretical Calculation." *Asian Journal of Chemistry* 25 (7 SE-Articles): 3673–78. https://doi.org/10.14233/ajchem.2013.13709.

Yao, ZQ, Yu Ivanisenko, T Diemant, A Caron, A Chuvilin, JZ Jiang, RZ Valiev, M Qi, and H.-J. Fecht. 2010. "Synthesis and Properties of Hydroxyapatite-Containing Porous Titania Coating on Ultrafine-Grained Titanium by Micro-Arc Oxidation." *Acta Biomaterialia* 6 (7): 2816–25. https://doi.org/10.1016/j.actbio.2009.12.053.

Ye, Hezhou, Xing Yang Liu, and Hanping Hong. 2009a. "Characterization of Sintered Titanium/Hydroxyapatite Biocomposite Using FTIR Spectroscopy." *Journal of Materials Science: Materials in Medicine* 20 (4): 843–50. https://doi.org/10.1007/s10856-008-3647-3.

———. 2009b. "Cladding of Titanium/Hydroxyapatite Composites onto Ti6Al4V for Load-Bearing Implant Applications." *Materials Science and Engineering: C* 29 (6): 2036–44. https://doi.org/10.1016/j.msec.2009.03.021.

Yoshizawa, S, D Fourmy, and JD Puglisi. 1998. "Structural Origins of Gentamicin Antibiotic Action." *The EMBO Journal* 17 (22): 6437–48. https://doi.org/10.1093/emboj/17.22.6437.

Zawadzki, Jerzy, and Halina Kaczmarek. 2010. "Thermal Treatment of Chitosan in Various Conditions." *Carbohydrate Polymers* 80 (2): 394–400. https://doi.org/10.1016/j.carbpol.2009.11.037.

Zhang, Jie, Zhaohui Wen, Meng Zhao, Guozhong Li, and Changsong Dai. 2016. "Effect of the Addition CNTs on Performance of CaP/Chitosan/Coating Deposited on Magnesium Alloy by Electrophoretic Deposition." *Materials Science and Engineering: C* 58: 992–1000. https://doi.org/10.1016/j.msec.2015.09.050.

Zhang, Kai, Dieter Peschel, Johanna Helm, Thomas Groth, and Steffen Fischer. 2011. "FT Raman Investigation of Novel Chitosan Sulfates Exhibiting Osteogenic Capacity." *Carbohydrate Polymers* 83 (1): 60–65. https://doi.org/10.1016/j.carbpol.2010.07.021.

Zhang, Lv, Weiwei Liu, Chunguang Yue, Taihua Zhang, Pei Li, Zhanwen Xing, and Yao Chen. 2013. "A Tough Graphene Nanosheet/Hydroxyapatite Composite with Improved in Vitro Biocompatibility." *Carbon* 61: 105–15. https://doi.org/10.1016/j.carbon.2013.04.074.

Zhang, Qiyi, Jiyong Chen, Jiaming Feng, Yang Cao, Chunlin Deng, and Xingdong Zhang. 2003. "Dissolution and Mineralization Behaviors of HA Coatings." *Biomaterials* 24 (26): 4741–48. https://doi.org/10.1016/S0142-9612(03)00371-5.

Zhitomirsky, D, JA Roether, AR Boccaccini, and I Zhitomirsky. 2009. "Electrophoretic Deposition of Bioactive Glass/Polymer Composite Coatings with and without HA Nanoparticle Inclusions for Biomedical Applications." *Journal of Materials Processing Technology* 209 (4): 1853–60. https://doi.org/10.1016/j.jmatprotec.2008.04.034.

Zhitomirsky, I, and A Hashambhoy. 2007. "Chitosan-Mediated Electrosynthesis of Organic–Inorganic Nanocomposites." *Journal of Materials Processing Technology* 191 (1): 68–72. https://doi.org/10.1016/j.jmatprotec.2007.03.043.

Zielinski, Andrzej, and Michal Bartmanski. 2020. "Electrodeposited Biocoatings, Their Properties and Fabrication Technologies: A Review." *Coatings*. https://doi.org/10.3390/coatings10080782.

4 Modeling of Drug Release Processes

Fractional Derivative Models and Comparison with Standard Models

4.1 ELEMENTS OF FRACTIONAL CALCULUS

The term "fractional calculus" (FC) is used to denote the study of integrals and derivatives of real (non-integer) and complex integrals and derivatives of arbitrary order. It originated in 1695 almost at the same time as classical integer-order calculus. Today it represents the area of applied mathematics that is developing very fast with a large number of publications in both theoretical and applied areas. FC is used in many fields of science and engineering due to the possibility that it offers a mathematical modeling of memory and non-local effect. Therefore, it is used in visco-elasticity, heat conduction, pharmacokinetics, nanomaterials, economy, nuclear reactor dynamics, etc. For the development of FC and its application, see Podlubny 1999; Kilbas, Srivastava, and Trujillo 2006; Atanacković, Pilipović et al. 2014a, 2014b; Diethelm et al. 2022; Samko, Kilbas, and Marichev 1993; Hilfer 2019. For application of fractional calculus in pharmacokinetics, see the review article by Sopasakis et al. (Sopasakis et al. 2018).

Probably the best way to introduce the concept of integrals and derivatives of non-integer order is the so-called Cauchy formula for repeated integration of a function that reads,

$$ {}_0I_t^n f(t) = \frac{1}{(n-1)!}\int_0^t (t-\tau)^{n-1} f(\tau)\,d\tau, \; n \in \mathbb{N}, \tag{4.1} $$

for the causal function, i.e., function that are vanishing for $t < 0$. Recall the definition of the Gamma function (see Gorenflo et al. 2014)

$$ \Gamma(s) = \int_0^\infty \exp(-t)\, t^{s-1} dt, \, s \in \mathbb{C} \tag{4.2} $$

The integral in (4.2) is convergent for all $s \in \mathbb{C}, \Re s > 0$. Here $\Re\, s$ denotes the real part of s.

It is easy to show that the following relation holds,

DOI: 10.1201/9781032668895-4

$$\Gamma(s+1)=s\Gamma(s). \tag{4.3}$$

From (4.2), (4.3) we conclude that $\Gamma(1)=1$ and that for $s=n=1,2,3,\ldots$,we have,

$$\Gamma(n+1)=n\Gamma(n)=n! \tag{4.4}$$

Also, for $s=-n,\ (n=0,1,2,3,\ldots)$ the function (4.2) has simple poles. Let $[a,b]$ denote a finite interval on the real axis and let f be a continuous function defined on $[a,b]$. Using (4.1), we define, for any α real, or complex, the left Riemann-Liouville fractional integral as (Samko, Kilbas, and Marichev 1993)

$${}_aI_t^{\alpha}f(t)=\frac{1}{\Gamma(\alpha)}\int_a^t(t-\tau)^{\alpha-1}f(\tau)d\tau,\ \Re\alpha>0,\ t>a. \tag{4.5}$$

Also, the right Riemann-Liouville fractional integral is defined as

$${}_tI_b^{\alpha}f(t)=\frac{1}{\Gamma(\alpha)}\int_t^b(t-\tau)^{\alpha-1}f(\tau)d\tau,\ \Re\alpha>0,\ t<b. \tag{4.6}$$

The left Riemann-Liouville derivative of arbitrary order α is defined as

$${}_aD_t^{\alpha}f(t)=\frac{d^n}{dt^n}\,{}_aI_t^{n-\alpha}f(t)=\frac{d^n}{dt^n}\frac{1}{\Gamma(n-\alpha)}\int_a^t\frac{f(\tau)}{(t-\tau)^{\alpha-n+1}}d\tau,\ n-1\le\Re\alpha<n. \tag{4.7}$$

Similarly, the right Riemann-Liouville fractional derivative of order α is defined as

$${}_tD_b^{\alpha}f(t)=\left(-\frac{d}{dt}\right)^n{}_tI_b^{n-\alpha}f(t)=\left(-\frac{d}{dt}\right)^n\frac{1}{\Gamma(n-\alpha)}\int_t^b\frac{f(\tau)}{(\tau-t)^{\alpha-n+1}}d\tau,\ n-1\le\Re\alpha<n. \tag{4.8}$$

For $\alpha\in\mathbb{R}, 0\le\alpha<1$ we obtain

$${}_aD_t^{\alpha}f(t)=\frac{d}{dt}\frac{1}{\Gamma(1-\alpha)}\int_a^t\frac{f(\tau)}{(t-\tau)^{\alpha}}d\tau,\ 0\le\alpha<1 \tag{4.9}$$

and

$${}_tD_b^{\alpha}f(t)=-\frac{d}{dt}\frac{1}{\Gamma(1-\alpha)}\int_t^b\frac{f(\tau)}{(\tau-t)^{\alpha}}d\tau,\ 0\le\alpha<1. \tag{4.10}$$

Another definition of the fractional derivative is proposed by M. Caputo. The left Caputo fractional derivative is defined as (Samko, Kilbas, and Marichev 1993)

$$ {}_{a}^{C}D_{t}^{\alpha}f(t) = {}_{a}I_{t}^{n-\alpha}\frac{d^{n}}{dt^{n}}f(t) = \frac{1}{\Gamma(n-\alpha)}\int_{a}^{t}\frac{f^{(n)}(\tau)}{(t-\tau)^{\alpha-n+1}}d\tau, \ n-1 \le \Re\alpha < n \quad (4.11) $$

Similarly, the right Caputo fractional derivative is defined as

$$ {}_{t}D_{b}^{\alpha}f(t) = (-1)^{n}{}_{t}I_{b}^{n-\alpha}\left(\frac{d}{dt}\right)^{n}f(t) = (-1)^{n}\frac{1}{\Gamma(n-\alpha)}\int_{t}^{b}\frac{f^{(n)}(\tau)}{(\tau-t)^{\alpha-n+1}}d\tau, \ n-1 \le \Re\alpha < n. \quad (4.12) $$

Again, for $\alpha \in \mathbb{R}$, $0 \le \alpha < 1$ we have

$$ {}_{a}^{C}D_{t}^{\alpha}f(t) = \frac{1}{\Gamma(1-\alpha)}\int_{a}^{t}\frac{f^{(1)}(\tau)}{(\tau-t)^{\alpha}}d\tau, \ 0 \le \Re\alpha < 1, \quad (4.13) $$

and

$$ {}_{t}^{C}D_{b}^{\alpha}f(t) = -\frac{1}{\Gamma(1-\alpha)}\int_{t}^{b}\frac{f^{(1)}(\tau)}{(\tau-t)^{\alpha}}d\tau, \ 0 \le \Re\alpha < 1. $$

The Riemann-Liouville fractional derivative of a constant is not zero, while the Caputo fractional derivative of a constant is zero. To prove this, we consider the functions $(t-a)^{\beta-1}$ and $(b-t)^{\beta-1}$. Then,

$$ {}_{a}D_{t}^{\alpha}(t-a)^{\beta-1} = \frac{\Gamma(\beta)}{\Gamma(\beta-\alpha)}(t-a)^{\beta-\alpha-1}, \ {}_{t}D_{b}^{\alpha}(b-t)^{\beta-1} = \frac{\Gamma(\beta)}{\Gamma(\beta-\alpha)}(b-t)^{\beta-\alpha-1} \quad (4.14) $$

while

$$ {}_{a}^{C}D_{t}^{\alpha}(t-a)^{\beta-1} = \frac{\Gamma(\beta)}{\Gamma(\beta-\alpha)}(t-a)^{\beta-1}, \ {}_{t}^{C}D_{b}^{\alpha}(b-t)^{\beta-1} = \frac{\Gamma(\beta)}{\Gamma(\beta-\alpha)}(b-t)^{\beta-1}. \quad (4.15) $$

By setting $\beta = 1$ we obtain the fractional derivative of a *const.* = 1 from (4.14) in the following form

$$ {}_{a}D_{t}^{\alpha}(1) = \frac{1}{\Gamma(1-\alpha)}(t-a)^{-\alpha}, \ {}_{t}D_{b}^{\alpha}(1) = \frac{1}{\Gamma(1-\alpha)}(b-t)^{-\alpha}. $$

Directly, from (4.13), for any $f(t) = C = const.$, we obtain,

$$ {}_{a}^{C}D_{t}^{\alpha}C = 0, \ {}_{t}^{C}D_{b}^{\alpha}C = 0, $$

since $f^{(1)} = 0$. We present one more type of fractional derivative called Liouville fractional integral and Liouville fractional derivative. They are defined on $\mathbb{R}$ and have the following forms,

$$ {}_0D_+^\alpha f(t) = \left(\frac{d}{dt}\right)^n \frac{1}{\Gamma(n-\alpha)} \int_{-\infty}^{t} \frac{f(\tau)}{(t-\tau)^{\alpha-n+1}} d\tau, \quad n-1 \le \Re\alpha < n, $$

and

$$ {}_tD_\infty^\alpha f(t) = \left(-\frac{d}{dt}\right)^n \frac{1}{\Gamma(n-\alpha)} \int_{t}^{\infty} \frac{f(\tau)}{(\tau-t)^{\alpha-n+1}} d\tau, \quad n-1 \le \Re\alpha < n, $$

and are called the left and right Liouville derivative, respectively.

For useful formulas of fractional integrals and fractional derivatives of elementary functions, see Valério et al. 2013; Garrappa, Kaslik, and Popolizio 2019.

There is a connection between the Riemann-Liouville and Caputo fractional derivative in the form,

$$ {}_a^CD_t^\alpha f(t) = {}_aD_t^\alpha \left(f(t) - \sum_{k=0}^{n-1} \frac{f^{(k)}(a)}{k!}(t-a)^k \right)(t), \tag{4.16} $$

and

$$ {}_t^CD_b^\alpha f(t) = {}_tD_b^\alpha \left(f(t) - \sum_{k=0}^{n-1} \frac{f^{(k)}(b)}{k!}(b-t)^k \right)(t). \tag{4.17} $$

Also, from (4.16), (4.17) with the use of (4.14), (4.15) we obtain,

$$ {}_a^CD_t^\alpha f(t) = {}_aD_t^\alpha f(t) - \sum_{k=0}^{n-1} \frac{f^{(k)}(a)}{\Gamma(k-\alpha+1)}(t-a)^{k-\alpha}, $$

and

$$ {}_t^CD_b^\alpha f(t) = {}_tD_b^\alpha f(t) - \sum_{k=0}^{n-1} \frac{f^{(k)}(b)}{\Gamma(k-\alpha+1)}(b-t)^{k-\alpha}. $$

From (4.16) and (4.17) follows that for the case $\alpha \in \mathbb{R}, 0 \le \alpha < 1$ we have

$$ {}_aD_t^\alpha f(t) = {}_a^CD_t^\alpha f(t), \text{ if } f(a) = 0; \quad {}_tD_b^\alpha f(t) = {}_t^CD_b^\alpha f(t), \text{ if } f(b) = 0. $$

We now state two important properties of the fractional integrals (4.5), (4.6) and fractional derivatives (4.7), (4.8). Recall that we assume $\Re\alpha \ge 0$:

1.

$$ {}_aI_t^\alpha \, {}_aD_t^\alpha f(t) = f(t) - \sum_{j=1}^{n} \frac{f_{n-\alpha}^{(n-j)}(a)}{\Gamma(\alpha-j+1)}(t-a)^{\alpha-j}, \tag{4.18} $$

where $f_{n-\alpha}(t) = {}_aI_t^{n-\alpha} f(t)$ and $f_{n-\alpha}^{(n-j)} = \frac{d^{(n-j)}}{(dt)^{(n-j)}} {}_aI_t^{n-\alpha} f(t)$,

$$ {}_tI_b^{\alpha}\, {}_tD_b^{\alpha} g(t) = g(t) - \sum_{j=1}^{n} \frac{(-1)^{(n-j)} g_{n-\alpha}^{(n-j)}(b)}{\Gamma(\alpha - j + 1)} (b-t)^{\alpha-j}, \tag{4.19} $$

where $g_{n-\alpha}(t) = {}_tI_b^{n-\alpha} g(t)$.

2.

$$ {}_aD_t^{\alpha}\, {}_aI_t^{\alpha} f(t) = f(t); \quad {}_tD_b^{\alpha}\, {}_tI_b^{\alpha} f(t) = f(t). \tag{4.20} $$

Properties 1 and 2 are fundamental to solving fractional differential equations. They correspond to the relations in integer-order integrals and derivatives, known as the First and Second Fundamental Theorems of Calculus

$$ \frac{d}{dt} \int_a^t f(\tau)\, d\tau = f(t), \tag{4.21} $$

and

$$ \int_a^t f^{(1)}(\tau)\, d\tau = f(t) - f(a), \tag{4.22} $$

respectively.

The conditions that the functions involved in (4.18)–(4.20) must satisfy are given in specialized books, for example by Kilbas et al. (Kilbas, Srivastava, and Trujillo 2006, pp. 74–76. Finally note that geometrical interpretation of fractional integrals and derivatives is a rather complex problem. For review of the results in this area, see Hilfer 2019.

When fractional derivatives are used in physical systems, we are often faced with nonlinear differential equations that contain fractional derivatives. In certain cases, the problems of numerical solution of such equations may become easier to handle if such systems are transformed into the systems of differential equations with integer-order derivatives. One such procedure is proposed in Atanacković and Stanković 2004, and it is based on an expansion formula for fractional derivative. We state the main result of this procedure for the special case when $0 < \alpha < 1$ as:

$$ {}_0D_t^{\alpha} f(t) = \frac{f(t)}{t^{\alpha}} A(N,\alpha) - \sum_{p=1}^{N} C_{p-1}(\alpha) \frac{V_{p-1}(f)(t)}{t^{p+\alpha}} + Q_{N+1}(f)(t), \tag{4.23} $$

where,

$$ A(N,\alpha) = \frac{\Gamma(N+1+\alpha)}{\alpha\Gamma(1-\alpha)\Gamma(\alpha)\mathrm{N}!}, \quad C_{p-1}(\alpha) = \frac{\Gamma(N+1+\alpha)}{\alpha\Gamma(1-\alpha)\Gamma(\alpha)(\mathrm{p}-1)!}. $$

Here V_q denotes the $q-$th moment of a function *f*, i.e.,

$$V_q(f)(t)=\int_0^t \tau^q f(\tau)d\tau. \tag{4.24}$$

Also, the following estimates hold,

$$\left|Q_{N+1}(f(t))\right| \leq \frac{CM_t}{\text{``}(1-\pm)\text{``}(\pm)} \frac{t^{1-\alpha}}{N^{\alpha_1}},\ \alpha_1 \in (0,1-\alpha),\ M_t = \max_{\tau\in[0,t]}\left|f^{(1)}(\tau)\right|, C>0,$$

and

$$\lim_{N\to\infty}\left\|Q_{N+1}(f)\right\|_{C([0,T])}=0.$$

For details of the derivation and application of (4.23) see Atanackovic and Stankovic 2008; Atanacković, Janev et al. 2014. Application of (4.23) to a nonlinear two-compartmental model of pharmacokinetics will be shown in Subsection 4.3.

Fractional derivatives may be used to expand a function, satisfying certain regularity conditions, in the Taylor's type formulas.

In Odibat and Shawagfeh 2007, the following expansion is presented for the case when $0 \leq \alpha \leq 1$

$$f(t)=\sum_{j=0}^{N} \frac{{}_aD_t^{j\alpha} f(t_0)}{\Gamma(j\alpha+1)}(t-t_0)^{j\alpha}+R_m, R_m=\frac{{}_aD_t^{(N+1)\alpha} f(\tau)}{\Gamma((N+1)\alpha+1)}(t-t_0)^{(N+1)\alpha},$$

where $t_0 \leq \tau \leq t, t_0 \in [a,T]$, and ${}_aD_t^{j\alpha} f \in C[a,T]$, $j=0,1,\ldots,N+1$.

For solving differential equations with fractional derivatives later in this chapter we shall need the Laplace transform of the fractional integrals and derivatives. Recall that for the functions exponentially bounded, i.e., $|f(t)| \leq M\exp(At)$, $A>0$ the Laplace transform is defined,

$$\mathscr{L}[f(t)](s)=\hat{f}(s)=\int_0^\infty f(t)\exp(-st)dt, \tag{4.25}$$

where $s \in \mathbb{C}$. The inverse Laplace transform for $t \in \mathbb{R}_+$ is given by the following expression,

$$\mathscr{L}^{-1}\left[\hat{f}\right](t)=f(t)=\frac{1}{2\pi i}\int_{x_0-i\infty}^{x_0+i\infty} \exp(st)\hat{f}(s)ds, \tag{4.26}$$

where $i=\sqrt{-1}$ and $x_0 > A$. Here A is the abscissa of convergence. It can be easily shown that,

$$\mathscr{L}\left[f^{(1)}\right](s)=s\hat{f}(s)-f(0). \tag{4.27}$$

The left Riemann-Liouville fractional integral and derivative have the following transforms,

$$\mathscr{L}\left[{}_0I_t^{\alpha}f\right](s)=s^{-\alpha}\hat{f}(s);\quad \Re s>A,$$

$$\mathscr{L}\left[{}_0D_t^{\alpha}f\right](s)=s^{\alpha}\hat{f}(s)-\sum_{k=0}^{n-1}s^{n-k-1}D^k\left({}_0I_t^{n-\alpha}f\right)(0_+),\tag{4.28}$$

$$\Re s>A,\, n-1\le\alpha<n.$$

In the special case when $\alpha\in\mathbb{R}, 0\le\alpha<1$ we obtain

$$\mathscr{L}\left[{}_0D_t^{\alpha}f\right](s)=s^{\alpha}\hat{f}(s)-{}_0I_t^{1-\alpha}f)(0_+),\quad \Re s>A, 0\le\alpha<1\tag{4.29}$$

For the Caputo fractional derivative, the Laplace transform reads,

$$\mathscr{L}\left[{}_0^CD_t^{\alpha}f\right](s)=s^{\alpha}\hat{f}(s)-\sum_{k=0}^{n-1}s^{\alpha-k-1}D^k(f)(0),\quad \Re s>A, n-1\le\alpha<n\tag{4.30}$$

For $\alpha\in\mathbb{R}, 0\le\alpha<1$ the equation (4.30) becomes

$$\mathscr{L}\left[{}_0^CD_t^{\alpha}f\right](s)=s^{\alpha}\hat{f}(s)-s^{\alpha-1}f(0),\quad \Re s>A, 0\le\alpha<1.\tag{4.31}$$

We present two useful formulas for inverse Laplace transform of functions important in fractional calculus:

$$\mathscr{L}^{-1}\left[\frac{s^{\alpha-\beta}}{s^{\alpha}\mp a}\right](t)=t^{\beta-1}E_{\alpha,\beta}\left(\pm at^{\alpha}\right),\quad \mathscr{L}^{-1}\left[\frac{1}{s^{\beta}}\right](t)=\frac{t^{\beta-1}}{\Gamma(\beta)}.$$

There are many generalizations of a definition of fractional integrals and derivatives. These generalizations are sometimes not mathematically well motivated. The problem is that, first, the following fundamental question must be answered: when can a linear operator be called fractional derivative? For a review of this question, see Ortigueira and Tenreiro Machado 2015 and Hilfer and Luchko 2019, and references given there.

Recently a new type of fractional derivatives named the general fractional derivatives (GFD) has been intensively studied. It is defined such that that the basic properties of integer-order derivatives are preserved while the properties of Riemann-Liouville and Caputo derivatives are extended. We stress that the basic requirement preserved in the definition of GFC is that it is a non-local convolution type operator, in time or space, depending on the independent variable and that conditions (4.21), (4.22) are satisfied. Thus, the general fractional calculus is a branch of mathematical analysis the deals with linear operators of the convolution type that are generalizations of integrals and derivatives of integer-order. These operators satisfy the fundamental theorems of the calculus (4.21), (4.22), see Tarasov 2019, 2021, 2022. More details on the topic are presented in Samko and Cardoso 2003; A. N. Kochubei 2011; Luchko 2021a, 2021c, 2021b; Hanyga 2020; Yang 2019; Yang, Gao, and Ju 2020.

The starting point of the general fractional calculus is the definition of a general fractional integral $I_{(M)}^{t}$ and general fractional derivative $D_{(K)}^{t}$ as

$$I_{(M)}^{t}[\tau]f(\tau)=\int_0^t M(t-\tau)f(\tau)d\tau,\quad D_{(K)}^{t}[\tau]f(\tau)=\frac{d}{dt}\int_0^t K(t-\tau)f(\tau)d\tau, \tag{4.32}$$

where the kernels, M and K satisfy certain condition. Those conditions are imposed in order that (4.21) and (4.22) hold. The general fractional derivative of the Caputo type with the kernel K is defined as

$$^{C}D_{(K)}^{t}f(\tau)=\int_0^t K(t-\tau)f^{(1)}(\tau)d\tau, \tag{4.33}$$

We state two conditions that the kernels K and M in (4.32) must satisfy:

1. $$M(t),K(t)\in C_{-1,0}(0,\infty),$$

2. $$\int_0^t M(t-\tau)K(\tau)d\tau=1, \tag{4.34}$$

where,

$$C_{a,b}(0,\infty)=\{f(t):f(t)=t^{p}Y(t),\ t>0,\ a<p<b,\ Y(t)\in C[0,\infty)\} \tag{4.35}$$

If the kernels satisfy $(4.34)_2$ they constitute the so-called Sonin pair. It can be shown that the condition $(4.34)_2$ in the Laplace domain, is equivalent to

$$s\hat{K}(s)\hat{M}(s)=1.$$

Note that the Riemann-Liouville kernels,

$$M(t)=\frac{t^{\alpha-1}}{\Gamma(\alpha)},\quad K(t)=\frac{t^{-\alpha}}{\Gamma(1-\alpha)},$$

satisfy (4.34), (4.35) and that, in this case (4.32) become Rieman-Liouville fractional integral and derivative whereas (4.33) becomes the Caputo fractional derivative.

There are many kernels that satisfy (4.34), (4.35) as shown in Tarasov 2021; Hanyga 2020; Samko and Cardoso 2003. We present several of them:

1. In Hanyga 2020 the following kernels are proposed

$$M(t)=\left[\frac{t^{-\beta}}{\Gamma(1-\beta)}+\frac{t^{\alpha-\beta}}{\Gamma(\alpha-\beta+1)}\right]H(t),$$

$$K(t)=\left[t^{\beta-1}E_{\alpha,\beta}\left(-t^{\alpha}\right)\right]H(t), t\in(0,\infty), \beta\geq 0, 0\leq\beta,$$

here H is the Heaviside step function and

$$E_{\alpha,\beta}(t)=\sum_{k=0}^{\infty}\frac{t^k}{\Gamma(k\alpha+\beta)},\quad \alpha>0, \beta\geq 0,$$

is a two-parameter Mittag-Lefler function (Gorenflo et al. 2014).

2. In Samko and Cardoso 2003 the following kernels are proposed

$$M(s)=\lambda^{\alpha}+\frac{\alpha}{\Gamma(1-\alpha)}\int_t^{\infty}\frac{\exp(-\lambda u)}{u^{1+\alpha}}du,\quad K(t)=\frac{t^{\alpha-1}}{\Gamma(\alpha)}\exp(-\lambda t), \tag{4.36}$$

where $\lambda\geq 0$. The GFD of the Caputo type that we use in this work is given, by (4.33) with the kernel $(4.36)_2$ so that,

$${}_0^C D_t^{\alpha,\lambda} f(t)={}^C D_{(K)}^t[f]=\frac{1}{\Gamma(1-\alpha)}\int_0^t\frac{\exp(-\lambda\tau)}{\tau^{\alpha}}f^{(1)}(t-\tau)d\tau. \tag{4.37}$$

The proof the M and K used in (4.36) satisfy $(4,34)_2$ is given in Samko and Cardoso 2003.

3. Another proposal from Samko and Cardoso 2003 is,

$$M(t)=1-\frac{\lambda}{\Gamma(\alpha)}t^{\alpha-1};\quad K(t)=\lambda t^{\alpha}E_{1-\alpha,1-\alpha}\left(\lambda t^{1-\alpha}\right) \tag{4.38}$$

where $\lambda>0$ and $E_{1-\alpha,1-\alpha}$ is a two-parameter Mittag-Lefler function (Gorenflo et al. 2014).

For other choices of the functions M and K see Tarasov 2022 and the references given there.

The kernel $(4.36)_2$ is called *Truncated power-law kernel*, and is used in Sandev et al. 2015, 2017 for the study of anomalous diffusion and in Molina-Garcia et al. 2018 for friction kernel for a model of lipid motion in lipid bilayer system. Also, it is used in Miskovic-Stankovic, Janev, and Atanackovic 2023 and in Miskovic-Stankovic and Atanackovic 2023.

From (4.37) we can define the distributed order fractional derivatives. Subsection 4.4.3 will provide an example of this type of fractional derivative.

We stress that in the analysis that follows we shall use the GFD with the kernel (4.37). The theory of fractional calculus with more general kernels is presented in Luchko 2023, where, also, the generalized convolution Taylor formulas and the generalized convolution Taylor series is presented.

4.2 CLASSICAL COMPARTMENTAL MODELS

Here we recall some formulas from the compartmental method in pharmacokinetics. The detailed analysis can be found in Rescigno 2003. The compartmental models were used in physics for the description of radioactive decay and in pharmacokinetics to describe the time evolution of drugs. It has been found that the number of radioactive atoms decaying is proportional to the number of radioactive atoms present in the material. This idea was generalized and led to the following model, consisting of N compartments. We shall here use compartments connected in series only, as shown in Figure 4.1

The system of differential equations describing the mass of certain element Q_i, drag for example in the $i-$th compartment, $i=1,\ldots,N$ is,

$$
\begin{aligned}
\frac{dQ_1}{dt} &= -k_{12}\left(\frac{Q_1}{V_1}-\frac{Q_2}{V_2}\right)+f_{11}-f_{10}, \\
\frac{dQ_2}{dt} &= k_{12}\left(\frac{Q_1}{V_1}-\frac{Q_2}{V_2}\right)-f_{20}, \\
&\ldots\ldots\ldots\ldots\ldots\ldots\ldots\ldots, \\
\frac{dQ_i}{dt} &= k_{i-1,i}\left(\frac{Q_{i-1}}{V_{i-1}}-\frac{Q_i}{V_i}\right)-f_{i0}, \\
\frac{dQ_n}{dt} &= k_{n-1,n}\left(\frac{Q_{n-1}}{V_{n-1}}-\frac{Q_n}{V_n}\right)-f_{n0}.
\end{aligned}
\tag{4.39}
$$

In (4.39) we used Q_i to denote the amount of material, such as drag, in the $i-$th compartment, V_i denotes the volume of the $i-$th compartment, k_{ij} are constants

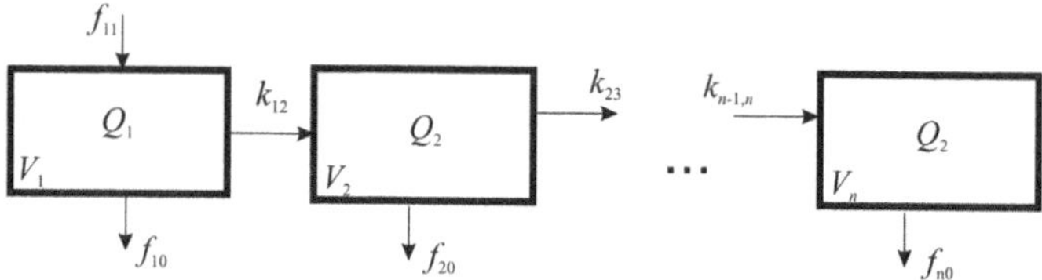

FIGURE 4.1 Simplified multi-compartmental system

that control mass transfer between compartments and are connected with diffusion coefficients, f_{11} denotes the amount of material introduced in the first compartment and f_{i0} denotes the loss of material in the $i-$th compartment. In writing (4.39) we assumed system's, dynamics, i.e., the mass transfer between compartments, obeys Fick's kinetics. The initial conditions for (4.39) are prescribed as

$$Q_i(0) = Q_{0i} \tag{4.40}$$

The solution of the system (4.39) with initial conditions (4.40) is, usually, obtained by using the Laplace transform methods.

The fractional calculus was introduced into the compartmental analysis in Dokoumetzidis and Macheras 2009. It was also used in Popović et al. 2010; Dokoumetzidis, Magin, and Macheras 2010a, 2010b; Verotta 2010; Sopasakis et al. 2018. In Pereira 2010 the concepts of fractal and fractional are connected by showing that the macroscopic flux of mass, across a fractal interface is described by the generalized diffusion equation, i.e., fractional diffusion. For two-compartmental systems, with fractional dynamics of Fick's type with Caputo type fractional derivatives, see (4.13); we propose the following generalization of the system (4.39)

$$a\frac{1}{V_1}\,{}_0^C D_t^{\alpha_1} Q_1(t) = -k_{12}\left(\frac{Q_1}{V_1} - \frac{Q_2}{V_2}\right) + f_{11} - f_{10},$$

$$b\frac{1}{V_2}\,{}_0^C D_t^{\alpha_2} Q_2(t) = K\left(\frac{Q_1}{V_1} - \frac{Q_2}{V_2}\right) - f_{20}, \tag{4.41}$$

where $0 < \alpha_1 \leq 1, 0 < \alpha_2 \leq 1$. The constants a and b, have dimensions $T^{\alpha_1 - 1}$ and $T^{\alpha_2 - 1}$, respectively, where T is the time unit. The constant k_{12} and K may be equal, as in the case when $\alpha_1 = \alpha_2, a = b$ or K may be a function specially determined. Which of these two cases is occurring in (4.41) depends on the type of system that we model. We shall discuss this question later in this Section. The initial conditions we assume in the form,

$$Q_1(0) = Q_{01}; \quad Q_2(0) = 0. \tag{4.42}$$

We shall solve (4.41), (4.42) in the next Subsection and discuss the mass conservation for the special case when,

$$f_{11} = f_{10} = f_{20} = 0; V_1 = V_2. \tag{4.43}$$

Note that the generalization of integer-order systems describing a specific physical phenomenon requires some principles to be observed. Those principles are discussed in Tarasov 2019.

We comment on the form of (4.41). If $V_1 = V_2$ the system (4.41) represents the dynamical equations for the pharmacokinetics expressed in terms of concentrations (see (4.47) below). However, we often want the results in terms of masses $Q_i, i = 1,2$, or amounts (see Rescigno 2003, pp. 31–32), and we want to determine diffusion coefficient D form the value of k_{12}. Recall the definition of diffusion coefficient D: mass of the substance that diffuses through a unit surface in a unit time at a concentration gradient of unity. In this case, we modify the system (4.41) to a Fick-type equation by introducing a gradient of the concentration on the right-hand side of (4.41) and we omit the volumes of the compartments $V_i, i = 1,2$ on the left-hand side, so that

$$ {}_0^C D_t^{\alpha_1} Q_1(t) = -k_{12} \text{ grad } c + f_{11} - f_{10}, $$

$$ {}_0^C D_t^{\alpha_2} Q_2(t) = K \text{ grad } c - f_{20} \tag{4.44} $$

The definition of concentration gradient $\text{grad}\, c$ from $\left(\frac{Q_1}{V_1} - \frac{Q_2}{V_2}\right)$ will be explained later (see (4.96). The system (4.42), (4.44) is based on Fick-type diffusion, which states that the driving force for mass exchange is difference in concentration in compartments of the substance that is exchanged. The radioactive decay type of kinetics, of successive transformation (see Rescigno 2003, p. 27) may be, obtained from (4.39) if we consider $V_i = V, i = 1,\ldots,N$ and neglect the term $\frac{Q_2}{V_2}$ in the first compartment, neglect the production terms and write the "the driving terms" $\left(\frac{Q_{i-1}}{V_{i-1}} - \frac{Q_i}{V_i}\right)$ in a different form, so that we obtain

$$ \begin{aligned} \frac{dQ_1}{dt} &= -k_{12}\frac{Q_1}{V_1}, \\ \frac{dQ_2}{dt} &= k_{12}\frac{Q_1}{V_1} - k_{21}\frac{Q_2}{V_2}, \\ &\cdots\cdots\cdots\cdots, \\ \frac{dQ_n}{dt} &= k_{n-1,n}\frac{Q_{n-1}}{V_{n-1}} - k_n\frac{Q_n}{V_n}. \end{aligned} \tag{4.45} $$

Formally the fractional derivative version of (4.45) for two-compartmental system, with $k_{21} = 0$ becomes,

$$ {}_0^C D_t^{\alpha_1} Q_1(t) = -k_{12}\frac{Q_1}{V_1}, $$

$$ {}_0^C D_t^{\alpha_2} Q_2(t) = K\frac{Q_1}{V_1} - K_{20}\frac{Q_2}{V_2}. \tag{4.46} $$

The mass conservation implies that the constant K is equal to k_{12} if $\alpha_1 = \alpha_2$. Next, we shall discuss the relation between K and k_{12}.

4.3 COMPARTMENTAL MODELS WITH FRACTIONAL DERIVATIVES

The comparison between the integer-order models and fractional derivative models may not be easy and straightforward. We demonstrate this by solving the system (4.40) – (4.41) with $a = b$ which we write as

$$\begin{aligned} {}_0^C D_t^{\alpha_1} c_1(t) &= -k_{12}(c_1 - c_2), \\ {}_0^C D_t^{\alpha_2} c_2(t) &= k_{12}(c_1 - c_2), \end{aligned} \tag{4.47}$$

where $c_i, i = 1,2$ are concentrations, i.e., $c_1 = \frac{Q_1}{V_1}, c_2 = \frac{Q_2}{V_2}$ and where we shall use (4.42). Also we assume that $0 < \alpha_1, \alpha_2 < 1$ so that we need only $c_1(0)$ and $c_2(0)$. Note that in the system (4.47) we do not have property that the total mass is conserved i.e., that the amount of material that leaves compartment **1** in the time interval dt is equal to the amount of material that enters the compartment **2** in the same time interval, unless $\alpha_1 = \alpha_2$, see discussion about this point in Dokoumetzidis, Magin, and Macheras 2010a. We shall show that this is a consequence of the fact that, as in integer-order model, we took the same constant k_{12} in both equations of the system (4.47).

Using (4,42) the initial conditions corresponding to (4.47) are

$$c_1(0) = c_{01}; \quad c_2(0) = 0. \tag{4.48}$$

By applying the Laplace transform to (4.47) and by using (4.31) we obtain

$$s^{\alpha_1}\hat{c}_1(s) - s^{\alpha_1 - 1}c_{10} = -k_{12}(\hat{c}_1(s) - \hat{c}_2(s)),$$

$$s^{\alpha_2}\hat{c}_2(s) = k_{12}(\hat{c}_1(s) - \hat{c}_2(s)). \tag{4.49}$$

From (4.49) we have

$$s^{\alpha_1}\left(\left[\hat{c}_1(s) + s^{\alpha_2 - \alpha_1}\hat{c}_2(s)\right] - \frac{c_{10}}{s}\right) = 0, \tag{4.50}$$

so that by using the uniqueness for the inverse Laplace transform (Doetsch 1974), it follows

$$\mathscr{L}^{-1}\left[\left(\left[\hat{c}_1(s) + s^{\alpha_2 - \alpha_1}\hat{c}_2(s)\right] - \frac{c_{10}}{s}\right)\right](t) = 0,$$

or

$$c_1(t) + {}_0^C D_t^{\alpha_1-\alpha_2} c_2(t) = c_{10} H(t), \tag{4.51}$$

where H is the Heaviside step function and we used the index law for Caputo fractional derivatives. Expression (4.51) represents the *conservation law* for the system of equations (4.47) in the sense that it is a relation between concentrations $c_1(t)$ and $c_2(t)$ and fractional derivative ${}_0^C D_t^{\alpha_1-\alpha_2} c_2(t)$ of concentration c_2. For the definition and properties of conservation laws for fractional system of differential equations, see Atanacković et al. 2009 and references given there.

In expanded form (4.51) reads

$$c_1(t) + \frac{1}{\Gamma(1-\alpha_2+\alpha_1)} \int_0^t \frac{\exp(-\lambda\tau)}{\tau^{\alpha_2-\alpha_1}} c_2^{(1)}(t-\tau)\, d\tau = c_{10} H(t).$$

For the special case when $\alpha_1 = \alpha_2$ it becomes the conservation of *mass* relation

$$c_1(t) + c_2(t) = c_{10},\ t \geq 0.$$

Since $c_1 = \frac{Q_1}{V_1}, c_2 = \frac{Q_2}{V_2}, V_1 = V_2$ we have

$$Q_1(t) + Q_2(t) = Q_1(0).$$

If we want to model a system with mass conservation in the sense that the mass that leaves compartment **1** equals to the mass that enters compartment **2**, and we assume that $\alpha_1 \neq \alpha_2$ we must modify the system (4.47) as follows. We write it as

$$\begin{aligned} {}_0^C D_t^{\alpha_1} c_1(t) &= -k_{12}(c_1 - c_2), \\ {}_0^C D_t^{\alpha_2} c_2(t) &= K(c_1)(c_1 - c_2), \end{aligned} \tag{4.52}$$

where K is an operator to be determined, acting on c_1. We multiply $(4.52)_1$ by

$$\frac{{}_0^C D_t^{\alpha_2} c_1(t)}{{}_0^C D_t^{\alpha_1} c_1(t)},$$

so that, instead of (4.52) we have

$${}_0^C D_t^{\alpha_2} c_1(t) = -k_{12}(c_1 - c_2) \frac{{}_0^C D_t^{\alpha_2} c_1(t)}{{}_0^C D_t^{\alpha_1} c_1(t)},$$

$${}_0^C D_t^{\alpha_2} c_2(t) = K(c_1)(c_1 - c_2). \tag{4.53}$$

Since the order of fractional derivatives on the left-hand side of (4.53) is the same (α_2) the condition of mass conservation reads

$$k_{12}\frac{{}_0^C D_t^{\alpha_2} c_1(t)}{{}_0^C D_t^{\alpha_1} c_1(t)} = K(c_1). \tag{4.54}$$

This is easily seen if we add equations in (4.53) and use (4.54) to obtain,

$${}_0^C D_t^{\alpha_2}[c_1(t)+[c_1(t)]=0,$$

so that

$$[c_1(t)+[c_1(t)]=const.,$$

since Caputo fractional derivative of a constant is zero. Now from $(4.52)_1$ and (4.54) we conclude that (4.52) may be written as

$${}_0^C D_t^{\alpha_1} c_1(t) = -k_{12}(c_1 - c_2),$$

$${}_0^C D_t^{\alpha_2} c_2(t) = k_{12}\frac{{}_0^C D_t^{\alpha_2} c_1(t)}{{}_0^C D_t^{\alpha_1} c_1(t)}(c_1 - c_2).$$

By using the first equation in the previous system in the second one, we obtain,

$${}_0^C D_t^{\alpha_1} c_1(t) = -k_{12}(c_1 - c_2)$$

$${}_0^C D_t^{\alpha_2} c_2(t) = -{}_0^C D_t^{\alpha_2} c_1(t) \tag{4.55}$$

The solution to $(4.55)_2$ is easily obtained as $c_1(t)+c_2(t)=c_{10}$ so that (4.55) reduces to

$${}_0^C D_t^{\alpha_1} c_1(t) = -k_{12}(2c_1(t) - c_{10})$$

$$c_2(t) = c_{10} - c_1(t) \tag{4.56}$$

Finally, we write $(4.56)_1$ as

$${}_0^C D_t^{\alpha_1} c_1(t) + 2k_{12}c_1(t) = k_{12}c_{10}.$$

Let $C_1(t) = c_1(t) - \frac{c_{10}}{2}$ so that,

$${}_0^C D_t^{\alpha_1} C_1(t) + 2k_{12}C_1(t) = 0,$$

with

$$C_1(0) = \frac{c_{10}}{2}.$$

The solution $C_1(\mathrm{t})$, is, given as $C_1(t) = \frac{c_{10}}{2} E_\alpha\left(-2k_{12}t^\alpha\right)$, see Kilbas, Srivastava, and Trujillo 2006, p. 313, so that,

$$c_1(t) = \frac{c_{10}}{2}\left[1 + E_\alpha\left(-2k_{12}t^\alpha\right)\right], \tag{4.57}$$

where $E_\alpha(x)$ is the Mittag-Leffler function of order α, (Gorenflo et al. 2014). Note that,

$$\lim_{t\to\infty} c_1(t) = \frac{c_{10}}{2}, \lim_{t\to\infty} c_2(t) = \frac{c_{10}}{2}.$$

We conclude by stressing that the "fractionalization" of (4.39) in the form (4.52) leads to different systems with different solutions. Therefore, not only the order of the derivatives, but also other parameters in the system may sometimes require changes during the fractionalization in which integer-order derivatives are replaced with the non-integer ones. In our case, k_{12} is replaced in the second equation with $K(c_1)$ given with (4.54).

Similar analysis can be carried out for the radioactive decay type of kinetics given in (4.46) that we write as

$$ {}_0^C D_t^{\alpha_1} c_1(t) = -k_{12}c_1(t),$$

$$ {}_0^C D_t^{\alpha_2} c_2(t) = Kc_1(t) - K_{20}c_2(t). \tag{4.58}$$

Multiplying (4.58) by

$$\frac{{}_0^C D_t^{\alpha_2} c_1(t)}{{}_0^C D_t^{\alpha_1} c_1(t)}$$

we obtain,

$$ {}_0^C D_t^{\alpha_2} c_1(t) = -k_{12}\frac{{}_0^C D_t^{\alpha_2} c_1(t)}{{}_0^C D_t^{\alpha_1} c_1(t)} c_1(t),$$

$$ {}_0^C D_t^{\alpha_2} c_2(t) = Kc_1(t) - K_{20}c_2(t),$$

so that

$$K = k_{12}\frac{{}_0^C D_t^{\alpha_2} c_1(t)}{{}_0^C D_t^{\alpha_1} c_1(t)}.$$

System (4.57) becomes,

$$ {}_0^C D_t^{\alpha_1} c_1(t) = -k_{12} c_1(t), $$

$$ {}_0^C D_t^{\alpha_2} c_2(t) = k_{12} \frac{{}_0^C D_t^{\alpha_2} c_1(t)}{{}_0^C D_t^{\alpha_1} c_1(t)} c_1(t) - K_{20} c_2(t). \tag{4.59} $$

By using $(4.59)_1$ in $(4.59)_2$ we finally obtain

$$ {}_0^C D_t^{\alpha_1} c_1(t) = -k_{12} c_1(t), $$

$$ {}_0^C D_t^{\alpha_2} c_2(t) = -{}_0^C D_t^{\alpha_2} c_1(t), \tag{4.60} $$

as the system that must be solved.

There is an interesting approach to fractionalization of (4.39) that is proposed by Dokoumetzidis, Magin and Macheras (Dokoumetzidis, Magin, and Macheras 2010a) slightly different from the method presented so far. In their seminal paper (Dokoumetzidis, Magin, and Macheras 2010b) the procedure is proposed that generalizes the classical compartmental system (4.39) for the radioactive decay type of systems. We present their results for two-compartmental system. The authors assumed that compartment **1**, which they refer to as *central*, represents general circulation and well perfused tissues, while compartment **2**, *peripheral*, represents deeper tissues. The transfer from the central compartment to the peripheral compartment is assumed to follow classical kinetics, while a flux from the peripheral to the central compartment is assumed to follow fractional kinetics, which accounts for tissue trapping. Thus, they considered the following system of differential equations,

$$ \frac{dc_1}{dt} = -(k_{12} + f_{10}) c_1 + k_{21} {}_0^C D_t^{1-\alpha} c_2(t), $$

$$ \frac{dc_2}{dt} = k_{12} c_1 - k_{21} {}_0^C D_t^{1-\alpha} c_2(t). \tag{4.61} $$

The system (4.61) with specified initial conditions is solved in Dokoumetzidis, Magin, and Macheras 2010b. The term $k_{21} {}_0^C D_t^{1-\alpha} c_2(t)$ represents the amount of material (drug, for example) that returns from compartment **2** (peripheral compartment) to compartment **1** (central compartment). This process is assumed to exhibit memory effects and is described by fractional derivative of order $1-\alpha$. After the application of the Laplace transform, the solution to (4.61) with initial conditions

$$ c_1(0) = c_{10}, c_2(0) = 0, $$

is (Dokoumetzidis, Magin, and Macheras 2010b),

$$c_1(t) = \mathscr{L}^{-1}\left[\frac{c_{10}(s^\alpha + k_{21})}{(s + k_{12} + f_{10})(s^\alpha + k_{21}) - k_{12}k_{21}}\right](t),$$

$$c_2(t) = \mathscr{L}^{-1}\left[\frac{c_{10}k_{12}s^{\alpha-1}}{(s + k_{12} + f_{10})(s^\alpha + k_{21}) - k_{12}k_{21}}\right](t). \tag{4.62}$$

A possible generalization of (4.61) is the case when the transport of drug from compartment **1** to compartment **2** and from compartment **2** to compartment **1** has different kinetics. In this case, we would have

$$\frac{dc_1}{dt} = -(k_{12} + f_{10})c_1 + k_{21}\,{}_0^C D_t^{1-\alpha} c_2(t)$$

$$\frac{dc_2}{dt} = k_{12}c_1 - K_{21}(c_2)\,{}_0^C D_t^{1-\beta} c_2(t) \tag{4.63}$$

with $\alpha \neq \beta$. It is clear that to maintain mass balance between compartments **1** and **2** we must determine K_{21} by the procedure used treating (4.52). Therefore, by calculating the amount of mass entering compartment **2** from compartment **1** in the time interval dt and equating it with the amount of mass leaving compartment **2** and entering compartment **1** in the same time interval, we obtain,

$$k_{21}\,{}_0^C D_t^{1-\alpha} c_2(t)\,dt = K_{21}(c_2)\,{}_0^C D_t^{1-\beta} c_2(t)\,dt,$$

so that

$$K_{21}(c_2) = k_{21}\frac{{}_0^C D_t^{1-\alpha} c_2(t)}{{}_0^C D_t^{1-\beta} c_2(t)}. \tag{4.64}$$

Therefore, (4.63) becomes,

$$\frac{dc_1}{dt} = -(k_{12} + f_{10})c_1 + k_{21}\,{}_0^C D_t^{1-\alpha} c_2(t),$$

$$\frac{dc_2}{dt} = k_{12}c_1 - k_{21}(c_2)\,{}_0^C D_t^{1-\alpha} c_2(t). \tag{4.65}$$

We conclude from (4.65) that if mass balance is to be preserved in (4.63) we must have $\alpha = \beta$ and $K_{21} = k_{12}$.

The analysis presented here implies that the coefficients in the model are constrained/limited by the condition that the mass leaving the compartment **1** is equal to the mass entering the compartment **2**. In the case where the orders of differential equations describing the kinetics of the compartments are not equal, the restrictions must be determined, for example, as is done in (4.54). However, for some systems, some mass may be lost at the compartmental boundaries. In such cases, it could be of interest to consider the cases where the total mass of the system is not conserved.

We present the results for the generalized model (4.47) described by the following system of equations,

$$\begin{aligned} {}_0^C D_t^{\alpha_1} c_1(t) &= -k_{12}(c_1 - c_2), \\ {}_0^C D_t^{\alpha_2} c_2(t) &= k_{12}(c_1 - c_2) - k_{20} c_2(t), \end{aligned} \tag{4.66}$$

subject to the initial conditions

$$c_1(0) = c_{10}, c_2(0) = c_{20}. \tag{4.67}$$

Since $\alpha_1 \neq \alpha_2$ and the coefficient k_{12} in the second equation was left unchanged in (4.66), we can conclude that the total mass is not conserved. If we wish to impose the condition that the total mass is conserved, we could consider the following system, see (4.54)

$${}_0^C D_t^{\alpha_1} c_1(t) = -k_{12}(c_1 - c_2)$$

$$,$$

$${}_0^C D_t^{\alpha_2} c_2(t) = -{}_0^C D_t^{\alpha_2} c_1(t) - k_{20} c_2(t),$$

subject to (4.67). This system has the conservation of mass in the sense that the mass leaving the first compartment is equal to the mass entering the second compartment although the total mass is not preserved due to the term, $k_{20} c_2(t)$ in $(4.66)_2$.

We shall solve the system (4.66), (4.67) since its solution has interesting properties. Applying the Laplace transform, we obtain

$$\begin{aligned} s^{\alpha_1} \hat{c}_1(s) - s^{\alpha_1 - 1} c_{10} &= -k_{12}(\hat{c}_1(s) - \hat{c}_2(s)), \\ s^{\alpha_2} \hat{c}_2(s) - s^{\alpha_2 - 1} c_{20} &= k_{12}(\hat{c}_1(s) - \hat{c}_2(s)) - k_{20} \hat{c}_2(s). \end{aligned} \tag{4.68}$$

By solving (4.68) for $\hat{c}_1(s)$ and $\hat{c}_2(s)$, we arrive at

$$\begin{aligned} \hat{c}_1(s) &= \frac{c_{10} s^{\alpha_1 - 1}}{s^{\alpha_1} + k_{12}} + \frac{k_{12} c_{20} s^{\alpha_2 - 1}}{(s^{\alpha_1} + k_{12})(s^{\alpha_2} + k_{12} + k_{20})} + \frac{k_{12} c_{10} s^{\alpha_1 - 1}}{(s^{\alpha_2} + k_{12} + k_{20})(s^{\alpha_1} + k_{12})}, \\ \hat{c}_2(s) &= \frac{c_{20} s^{\alpha_2 - 1}}{s^{\alpha_2} + k_{12} + k_{20}} + \frac{k_{12} c_{10} s^{\alpha_1 - 1}}{(s^{\alpha_2} + k_{12} + k_{20})(s^{\alpha_1} + k_{12})}. \end{aligned} \tag{4.69}$$

Note that denominators in (4.69) do not have zeros with positive real part, since $k_{12} > 0$ and $k_{20} > 0$. Consequently, we may express inversion of (4.69) as (Doetsch 1974)

$$c_1(t) = \lim_{p\to\infty} \frac{1}{2\pi} \int_{x_0-ip}^{x_0+ip} \exp((x_0+ip)t[\frac{c_{10}s^{\alpha_1-1}}{s^{\alpha_1}+k_{12}}$$

$$+\frac{k_{12}c_{20}s^{\alpha_2-1}}{(s^{\alpha_1}+k_{12})(s^{\alpha_2}+k_{12}+k_{20})}$$

$$+\frac{k_{12}c_{10}s^{\alpha_1-1}}{(s^{\alpha_2}+k_{12}+k_{20})(s^{\alpha_1}+k_{12})}]dp \quad (4.70)$$

$$c_2(t) = \lim_{p\to\infty} \frac{1}{2\pi} \int_{x_0-ip}^{x_0+ip} \exp((x_0+ip)t[\frac{c_{20}s^{\alpha_2-1}}{s^{\alpha_2}+k_{12}+k_{20}}$$

$$+\frac{k_{12}c_{10}s^{\alpha_1-1}}{(s^{\alpha_2}+k_{12}+k_{20})(s^{\alpha_1}+k_{12})}]dp$$

where $x_0 > 0$ is arbitrary.

For the system (4.66), we can formulate a conservation law in the following form. By adding the system's equations, we obtain,

$${}_0^C D_t^{\alpha_1}[c_1(t) + {}_0^C D_t^{\alpha_2-\alpha_1} c_2(t)] = -k_{20}c_2(t),$$

where we used the index law for fractional derivatives. By setting $k_{20} = 0,$ we obtain the conservation law, instead of mass conservation, as

$$[c_1(t) + {}_0^C D_t^{\alpha_2-\alpha_1} c_2(t) = const.$$

In the special case $\alpha_1 = \alpha_2$ this becomes the conservation of mass equation $c_1(t)+c_2(t)=c_{10}$. From (4.69) we obtain the concentrations estimated by using the final value theorems, see (Cohen 2007). With the appropriate assumptions about the functions involved, we have that if the limiting values exist, $\lim_{t\to 0} c_i(t) = c_i(0), \lim_{t\to\infty} c_i(t) = c_i(\infty), i = 1,2$ they satisfy,

$$\lim_{s\to\infty} s\hat{c_1}(s) = c_1(0) = \lim_{s\to\infty} \frac{c_{10}s^{\alpha_1}}{s^{\alpha_1}+k_{12}} + \frac{k_{12}c_{20}s^{\alpha_2}}{(s^{\alpha_1}+k_{12})(s^{\alpha_2}+k_{12}+k_{20})}$$

$$+\frac{k_{12}c_{10}s^{\alpha_1}}{(s^{\alpha_2}+k_{12}+k_{20})(s^{\alpha_1}+k_{12})} = c_{10}$$

$$\lim_{s\to 0} s\hat{c}_1(s) = c_1(\infty) = \lim_{s\to 0} \frac{c_{10}s^{\alpha_1}}{s^{\alpha_1}+k_{12}} + \frac{k_{12}c_{20}s^{\alpha_2}}{\left(s^{\alpha_1}+k_{12}\right)\left(s^{\alpha_2}+k_{12}+k_{20}\right)}$$

$$+\frac{k_{12}c_{10}s^{\alpha_1}}{\left(s^{\alpha_2}+k_{12}+k_{20}\right)\left(s^{\alpha_1}+k_{12}\right)} = 0 \quad (4.71)$$

$$\lim_{s\to\infty} s\hat{c}_2(s) = c_2(0) = \lim_{s\to\infty} \frac{c_{20}s^{\alpha_2}}{s^{\alpha_2}+k_{12}+k_{20}} + \frac{k_{12}c_{10}s^{\alpha_1}}{\left(s^{\alpha_2}+k_{12}+k_{20}\right)\left(s^{\alpha_1}+k_{12}\right)}$$

$$= c_{20} = 0$$

$$\lim_{s\to 0} s\hat{c}_2(s) = c_2(\infty) = \lim_{s\to 0} \frac{c_{20}s^{\alpha_2}}{s^{\alpha_2}+k_{12}+k_{20}} + \frac{k_{12}c_{10}s^{\alpha_1}}{\left(s^{\alpha_2}+k_{12}+k_{20}\right)\left(s^{\alpha_1}+k_{12}\right)}$$

$$= 0$$

We can conclude from (4.71) that for $k_{20} > 0$, the limiting values for the system (4.66) are equal to zero.

We now present an example of a nonlinear compartmental system for which a solution can be obtained by applying expansion formula (4.23). Consider the following two-compartmental model of the form,

$$\tau_1^{\alpha_1-1}\, {}_0^C D_t^{\alpha_1} Q_1(t) = -k_{12} f(Q_1(t),$$

$$\tau_2^{\alpha_2-1}\, {}_0^C D_t^{\alpha_2} Q_2(t) = Kf\left(Q_1(t),t\right) - k_{02}Q_2(t) \quad (4.72)$$

with the initial conditions

$$Q_1(0) = Q_{01}, Q_2(0) = 0 \quad (4.73)$$

Here $f\left(q_1(t),t\right)$ is given nonlinear function. In the analysis that follows we assume that $\alpha_1 = \alpha_2$ and $\tau_1 = \tau_2 = \tau$ so that $K = k_{12}$. Given the aforementioned assumption the system's nonlinear version may be written as

$$\begin{aligned} {}_0D_t^{\alpha} q_1(t) &= -K_{12} f\left(q_1(t),t\right) + f_{11} - f_{10},\ t\in[0,T], \\ {}_0D_t^{\alpha} q_2(t) &= K_{12} f\left(q_1(t),t\right) - K_{02} q_2(t),\ t\in[0,T], \end{aligned} \quad (4.74)$$

subject to (4.72).

We follow the procedure proposed in Atanackovic and Stankovic 2008 and apply the ${}_0D_t^{1-\alpha}(\cdot)$ derivative on both sides of equation (4.73). Then, in the special case $f_{11} = f_{10} = 0$ we have

$$q_1^{(1)}(t) = -{}_0D_t^{1-\alpha}[K_{12}f(q_1(t),t)]$$
$$q_2^{(1)}(t) = {}_0D_t^{1-\alpha}[K_{12}f(q_1(t),t)] - {}_0D_t^{1-\alpha}[K_{02}q_2(t)],\ t \in [0,T] \tag{4.75}$$

By using the expansion formula (4.23), we write

$${}_0D_t^{1-\alpha}\left[K_{12}f(q_1(t),t)\right]$$
$$= K_{12}\left[\frac{f(q_1(t),t)}{t^{1-\alpha}}A(N,1-\alpha)\right.$$
$$\left. -\sum_{p=1}^{N} C_{p-1}(1-\alpha)\frac{W_{p-1}(f(q_1(t),t))(t)}{t^{p+1-\alpha}}\right]$$

Now the system (4.75) becomes,

$$q_1^{(1)}(t) = -K_{12}\left[\frac{f(q_1(t),t)}{t^{1-\alpha}}A(N,1-\alpha)\right.$$
$$\left. -\sum_{p=1}^{N} C_{p-1}(1-\alpha)\frac{W_{p-1}(f(q_1(t),t))(t)}{t^{p+1-\alpha}}\right]$$
$$q_2^{(1)}(t) = K_{12}\left[\frac{f(q_1(t),t)}{t^{1-\alpha}}A(N,1-\alpha) - \sum_{p=1}^{N} C_{p-1}(1-\alpha)\frac{W_{p-1}(f(q_1(t),t))(t)}{t^{p+1-\alpha}}\right]$$
$$-K_{02}\left[\frac{q_2(t)}{t^{1-\alpha}}A(N,1-\alpha) - \sum_{p=1}^{N} C_{p-1}(1-\alpha)\frac{\bar{W}_{p-1}(q_2)(t)}{t^{p+1-\alpha}}\right]. \tag{4.76}$$

The moments of the function $f(q_1(t),t)$ are denoted by W_{p-1} and the moments of the function q_2 are denoted by $\bar{W}_{p-1}$. We adjoin the following system of the first order differential equations for moments to the system (4.75)

$$W_{p-1}^{(1)}(t) = t^{p-1}f(q_1(t),t), \quad \bar{W}_{p-1}^{(1)}(t) = t^{p-1}q_2(t), p = 1,\ldots,N \tag{4.77}$$

with the initial conditions

$$q_1(0) = q_{10}, q_2(0) = 0, \quad W_{p-1}(0) = \bar{W}_{p-1}(0) = 0. \tag{4.78}$$

The system (4.76) – (4.78) is the system of $p+2$ first order differential equations with specified initial values. Also

$$A(N,1-\alpha)=\frac{\Gamma(N+2-\alpha)}{\alpha\Gamma(\alpha)\Gamma(1-\alpha)N!},C_{p-1}(1-\alpha)=\frac{\Gamma(N+2-\alpha)}{\alpha\Gamma(\alpha)\Gamma(1-\alpha)(p-1)!}.$$

Similar procedure can be applied to the case where the derivatives on the left-hand side of (4.74) have a different order.

4.4 GENERAL FRACTIONAL DERIVATIVES IN PHARMACOKINETICS

In this Subsection we formulate differential equations for two-compartmental system general fractional derivatives to describe the dynamics of the system. We shall analyze the special general fractional derivative given by (4.37); in other words, we use,

$$ {}_0^C D_t^{\alpha,\lambda} f(t)=\frac{1}{\Gamma(1-\alpha)}\int_0^t \frac{\exp(-\lambda\tau)}{\tau^{\alpha}} f^{(1)}(t-\tau)\,d\tau \tag{4.79}$$

Miskovic-Stankovic, Janev, and Atanackovic (Miskovic-Stankovic, Janev, and Atanackovic 2023) propose the generalization for two-compartmental model (4.39), which reads,

$$\frac{1}{V_1}\left[a\,{}_0^C D_t^{\alpha_1,\lambda_1}+b\,{}_0^C D_t^{\beta_2,\lambda_2}\right]Q_1(t)=-k\left(\frac{Q_1(t)}{V_1}-\frac{Q_2(t)}{V_2}\right)+f_1(t)$$

$$\frac{1}{V_2}\left[a\,{}_0^C D_t^{\alpha_1,\lambda_1}+b\,{}_0^C D_t^{\beta_2,\lambda_2}\right]Q_2(t)=k\left(\frac{Q_1(t)}{V_1}-\frac{Q_2(t)}{V_2}\right) \tag{4.80}$$

where, again, $Q_i, V_i, i=1,2$ denote the mass of drug and volume of the compartment i, respectively, and the derivatives $a\,{}_0^C D_t^{\alpha,\lambda_1}(\cdot)$ and ${}_0^C D_t^{\alpha,\lambda_2}(\cdot)$ are given by (4.79). The parameters a and b have dimensions $T^{\alpha-1}$ and $T^{\beta-1}$, respectively, where T is the characteristic time of the compartments, in [s] or in our experiments in [days]. Basically, we are replacing the first derivatives $\frac{d}{dt}(\cdot)$ in (4.39) with a linear combination of two general fractional derivatives of different orders,

$$a\,{}_0^C D_t^{\alpha_1,\lambda_1}(\cdot)+b\,{}_0^C D_t^{\beta_2,\lambda_2}(\cdot).$$

Note that for $\lambda_i=0, i=1,2, \alpha=1, \beta=1, V_1=V_2$ the system (4.80) reduces to (4.39).

We now discuss a possible generalization of (4.80) when $V_1=V_2$ and on the left-hand side we have different combinations of GFD. With concentrations as dependent variables, (4.80) becomes

$$\left[a_1 {}_0^C D_t^{\alpha_1,\lambda_1} c_1(t) + b_1 {}_0^C D_t^{\beta_1,\lambda_1} c_1(t)\right] = -k\left(c_1(t) - c_2(t)\right)$$
$$\left[a_2 {}_0^C D_t^{\alpha_2,\lambda_2} c_2(t) + b_2 {}_0^C D_t^{\beta_2,\lambda_2} c_2(t)\right] = K\left(c_1(t) - c_2(t)\right) + f_{20}(t) \tag{4.81}$$

If we multiply the first equation in (4.81) by

$$\frac{\left[a_2 {}_0^C D_t^{\alpha_2,\lambda_2} c_1(t) + b_2 {}_0^C D_t^{\beta_2,\lambda_2} c_1(t)\right]}{\left[a_1 {}_0^C D_t^{\alpha_1,\lambda_1} c_1(t) + b_1 {}_0^C D_t^{\beta_1,\lambda_1} c_1(t)\right]},$$

we conclude that for (4.81) the conservation of mass, i.e., the amount that leaves compartment **1** equals the amount that enters compartment **2** leads to the value of K given as

$$K = k\frac{\left[a_2 {}_0^C D_t^{\alpha_2,\lambda_2} c_1(t) + b_2 {}_0^C D_t^{\beta_2,\lambda_2} c_1(t)\right]}{\left[a_1 {}_0^C D_t^{\alpha_1,\lambda_1} c_1(t) + b_1 {}_0^C D_t^{\beta_1,\lambda_1} c_1(t)\right]},$$

so that (4.81) becomes,

$$\left[a_1 {}^C D^{\alpha_1,\lambda_1} c_1(t) + b_1 {}^C D^{\beta_1,\lambda_1} c_1(t)\right] = -k\left(c_1(t) - c_2(t)\right)$$
$$\left[a_2 {}^C D^{\alpha_2,\lambda_2} c_2(t) + b_2 {}^C D^{\beta_2,\lambda_2} c_2(t)\right]$$
$$= k\frac{\left[a_2 {}^C D^{\alpha_2,\lambda_2} c_2(t) + b_2 {}^C D^{\beta_2,\lambda_2} c_2(t)\right]}{\left[a_1 {}^C D^{\alpha_1,\lambda_1} c_1(t) + b_1 {}^C D^{\beta_1,\lambda_1} c_1(t)\right]}\left(c_1(t) - c_2(t)\right) \tag{4.82}$$
$$+ f_{20}(t)$$

subject to

$$c_1(0) = c_{10}, c_2(0) = c_{20}.$$

The system (4.82) is expressed as

$$\left[a_1 {}_0^C D_t^{\alpha_1,\lambda_1} c_1(t) + b_1 {}_0^C D_t^{\beta_1,\lambda_1} c_1(t)\right] = -k\left(c_1(t) - c_2(t)\right),$$
$$\left[a_2 {}^C D^{\alpha_2,\lambda_2} c_2(t) + b_2 {}^C D^{\beta_2,\lambda_2} c_2(t)\right] \tag{4.83}$$
$$= \left[a_1 {}^C D^{\alpha_1,\lambda_1} c_1(t) + b_1 {}^C D^{\beta_1,\lambda_1} c_1(t)\right] + f_{20}(t),$$

By adding more terms on the left-hand side of (4.81) we may, heuristically, define a *distributed* order general fractional derivative as

$${}_0^C \bar{D}_t^{\alpha,\lambda} f(t) = \int_0^1 \varphi\left(\alpha(\alpha), \lambda(\alpha)\right) {}_0^C D_t^{\alpha,\lambda(\alpha)} f(t)\, d\alpha \tag{4.84}$$

In (4.84) the function $\varphi(\alpha(\alpha),\lambda(\alpha))$, $\alpha\in[0,1]$ denotes a weighting function. The functions $\varphi(\alpha(\alpha),\lambda(\alpha))$, $\alpha(\alpha)$ and $\lambda(\alpha)$ are assumed to be known. The homogeneity of dimension in (4.84) implies that φ must have dimension $=[\dim \mathrm{t}]^{\alpha}$ i.e., $\dim\varphi(\alpha(\alpha),\lambda(\alpha))=[\dim \mathrm{t}]^{\alpha}$. The simplest form of such function, that we shall use in (4.84) is $\varphi(\alpha(\alpha),\lambda(\alpha)=\lambda=const.)=\psi(\alpha,\lambda)a^{\alpha}$ where $\dim a=\dim \mathrm{t}$. Also, we assume that $\lambda\geq 0$ and $\psi(\alpha,\lambda),\alpha\in[0,1]$ is a dimensionless function. In the analysis that follows we assume $\psi(\alpha,\lambda)=1$. Then (4.84) becomes

$$ {}_{0}^{C}\bar{D}_{t}^{\alpha,\lambda}f(t)=\int_{0}^{1}a^{\alpha}\,{}_{0}^{C}D_{t}^{\alpha,\lambda}f(t)\,d\alpha \tag{4.85}$$

The compartmental system with the derivatives of the type (4.85) and its generalization will be analyzed in Subsection 4.4.3.

4.4.1 Gentamicin Release From Poly(Vinyl Alcohol)/Gentamicin Hydrogel

This issue was treated in Miskovic-Stankovic, Janev, and Atanackovic 2023, while the experiments are presented in Section 2.2.2.4. We shall use (4.80), which is a model with two general fractional derivatives (GFD) on the left-hand side. The system (4.41), i.e., a Fick-type equation with GFD becomes

$$\begin{aligned} a\,{}_{0}^{C}D_{t}^{\alpha,\lambda_a}Q_1(t)+b\,{}_{0}^{C}D_{t}^{\alpha,\lambda_b}Q_1(t)&=-k_{12}\left(\frac{Q_1}{V_1}-\frac{Q_2}{V_2}\right)\\ a\,{}_{0}^{C}D_{t}^{\alpha,\lambda_a}Q_2(t)+b\,{}_{0}^{C}D_{t}^{\alpha,\lambda_b}Q_2(t)&=k_{12}\left(\frac{Q_1}{V_1}-\frac{Q_2}{V_2}\right)\end{aligned}\tag{4.86}$$

or

$$\begin{aligned} &a\frac{1}{\Gamma(1-\alpha)}\int_0^t\frac{\exp(-\lambda_a\tau)}{\tau^{\alpha}}Q_1^{(1)}(t-\tau)\,d\tau\\ &\quad+b\frac{1}{\Gamma(1-\alpha)}\int_0^t\frac{\exp(-\lambda_b\tau)}{\tau^{\alpha}}Q_1^{(1)}(t-\tau)\,d\tau=-k\left(\frac{Q_1(t)}{V_1}-\frac{Q_2(t)}{V_2}\right)\\ &a\frac{1}{\Gamma(1-\alpha)}\int_0^t\frac{\exp(-\lambda_a\tau)}{\tau^{\alpha}}Q_2^{(1)}(t-\tau)\,d\tau\\ &\quad+b\frac{1}{\Gamma(1-\alpha)}\int_0^t\frac{\exp(-\lambda_b\tau)}{\tau^{\alpha}}Q_2^{(1)}(t-\tau)\,d\tau=k\left(\frac{Q_1(t)}{V_1}-\frac{Q_2(t)}{V_2}\right)\end{aligned}\tag{4.87}$$

The initial conditions corresponding to (4.87) are

$$Q_1(0)=Q_0, Q_2(0)=0. \tag{4.88}$$

Further, note that for the case when $V_2 \to \infty$ the system (4.86) becomes,

$$\begin{aligned}
&a\frac{1}{\Gamma(1-\alpha)}\int_0^t \frac{\exp(-\lambda_a\tau)}{\tau^\alpha}Q_1^{(1)}(t-\tau)d\tau \\
&\quad +b\frac{1}{\Gamma(1-\alpha)}\int_0^t \frac{\exp(-\lambda_b\tau)}{\tau^\alpha}Q_1^{(1)}(t-\tau)d\tau=-k\frac{Q_1(t)}{V_1}+f_1(t) \\
&a\frac{1}{\Gamma(1-\alpha)}\int_0^t \frac{\exp(-\lambda_a\tau)}{\tau^\alpha}Q_2^{(1)}(t-\tau)d\tau \\
&\quad +b\frac{1}{\Gamma(1-\alpha)}\int_0^t \frac{\exp(-\lambda_b\tau)}{\tau^\alpha}Q_2^{(1)}(t-\tau)d\tau=k\frac{Q_1(t)}{V_1}
\end{aligned} \tag{4.89}$$

System (4.89) represents the generalized two-compartmental model with general fractional derivative for radioactive decay.

Solution of the system (4.87), (4.88)

We use the Laplace transform method in solving (4.87), (4.88). The Laplace transform of general fractional derivative (4.37) is

$$\begin{aligned}
\mathscr{L}\left[{}_0^C D_t^{\alpha,\lambda} f(t)\right](s)&=\mathscr{L}\left[\frac{1}{\Gamma(1-\alpha)}\int_0^t \frac{\exp(-\lambda\tau)}{\tau^\alpha}f^{(1)}(t-\tau)d\tau\right](s) \\
&=\frac{s}{(s+\lambda_1)^{1-\alpha}}\left[\hat{f}(s)-sf(0)\right]
\end{aligned}$$

Therefore, the Laplace transform of (4.87) is

$$\begin{aligned}
&\left[a\frac{s}{(s+\lambda_1)^{1-\alpha}}+b\frac{s}{(s+\lambda_1)^{1-\beta}}\right]\hat{Q}_1(s)=-k\left[\frac{\hat{Q}_1(s)}{V_1}-\frac{\hat{Q}_2(s)}{V_2}\right] \\
&\qquad +\left[a\frac{s}{(s+\lambda_1)^{1-\alpha}}+b\frac{s}{(s+\lambda_1)^{1-\beta}}\right]Q_1(0) \\
&\left[a\frac{s}{(s+\lambda_1)^{1-\alpha}}+b\frac{s}{(s+\lambda_1)^{1-\beta}}\right]\hat{Q}_2(s)=k\left[\frac{\hat{Q}_1(s)}{V_1}-\frac{\hat{Q}_2(s)}{V_2}\right]
\end{aligned} \tag{4.90}$$

Note that (4.90) leads to

$$\hat{Q}_1(s)+\hat{Q}_2(s)=\frac{Q_1(0)}{s},$$

so that by taking the inverse Laplace transform,

$$Q_1(t)+Q_2(t)=Q_1(0), t\geq 0,$$

we obtain the conservation of mass law. Also, the following limiting values are obtained,

$$\lim_{s\to\infty} s\hat{Q}_1(s)=Q_1(0), \lim_{s\to 0} s\hat{Q}_1(s)=Q_1(\infty)=Q_1(0)\frac{V_1}{V_1+V_2}.$$

$$\lim_{s\to 0} s\hat{Q}_2(s)=Q_2(\infty)=Q_1(0)\frac{V_1}{V_1+V_2}.$$

The parameters in the model $\alpha,\beta,\lambda_1,\lambda_2,a,b$ will be determined by measuring values of $Q_2(t)$ at various time instants, $t_j, j=1,2....6$.

In the analysis that follows we shall use the dimensionless quantities defined as

$$q_1(t)=\frac{Q_1(t)}{Q_1(0)},\quad q_2(t)=\frac{Q_2(t)}{Q_1(0)} \tag{4.91}$$

to represent the results graphically.

We present the results of numerical inversion of (4.90). By solving (4.90) for $\hat{Q}_1(s)$ and $\hat{Q}_2(s)$ we obtain

$$\hat{Q}_1(s)=Q_1(0)\frac{1}{s}-\left[\frac{k}{V_1}\frac{1}{s\left[a\frac{s}{(s+\lambda_1)^{1-\alpha}}+b\frac{s}{(s+\lambda_2)^{1-\beta}}+k\left(\frac{1}{V_1}+\frac{1}{V_2}\right)\right]}\right], \tag{4.92}$$

$$\hat{Q}_2(s)=Q_1(0)\frac{k}{V_1}\frac{1}{s\left[a\frac{s}{(s+\lambda_1)^{1-\alpha}}+b\frac{s}{(s+\lambda_2)^{1-\beta}}+k\left(\frac{1}{V_1}+\frac{1}{V_2}\right)\right]}.$$

Using the argument principle, it can be easily shown that the function,

$$s\left[a\frac{s}{(s+\lambda_1)^{1-\alpha}}+b\frac{s}{(s+\lambda_2)^{1-\beta}}+k\left(\frac{1}{V_1}+\frac{1}{V_2}\right)\right],$$

has no zeros with positive real part. Therefore

$$Q_2(t) = \lim_{P\to\infty} Q_1(0)\frac{k}{V_1}\frac{1}{\pi}\int_{x_0-iP}^{x_0+iP} \frac{exp(x_0+ip)t}{(x_0+ip)\left[a\frac{(x_0+ip)}{(x_0+ip+\lambda_1)^{1-\alpha}}+b\frac{(x_0+ip)}{(x_0+ip+\lambda_2)^{1-\beta}}+k\left(\frac{1}{V_1}+\frac{1}{V_2}\right)\right]}dp \tag{4.93}$$

Here $x_0 > 0$ is arbitrary and we used the following property $\hat{Q}_2(s) = -\hat{Q}_2(-s)$. Also, in the numerical inversion of (4.93) the parameter P is set to be $P = 120$. Note that $Q_1(t)$ is determined from,

$$Q_1(t) = Q_1(0) - Q_2(t).$$

The parameters in the model are determined so that the squared difference between measured and calculated values of Q_2 at five measured points is minimal. Thus, by using (4.90) we defined,

$$Z(\alpha,\beta,\lambda_1,\lambda_2,k,a,b) = \sum_{j=1}^{5}\left(q_2(t_j) - q_{2measured}(t_j)\right)^2, \tag{4.94}$$

where $q_2(t_j)$ denotes the values determined from (4.92) and $q_{2measured}(t_j)$ are measured at time instant t_j. By using (4.91), the measured values are presented in Table 4.1.

The parameters in the model $\alpha^*,\beta^*,\lambda_1^*,\lambda_2^*,k^*,a^*,b^*$ are determined from the condition (4.93) as

TABLE 4.1
The Measured Values of q_2 and Corresponding Values of q_1 (Reprinted from Miskovic-Stankovic, Janev, and Atanackovic 2023 with Permission from Springer Nature)

t [days]	$q_1 = 1 - q_{2measured}(t_j)$	$q_{2measured}(t_j)$
0	1	0
1	0.582	0.418
2	0.402	0.598
4	0.389	0.611
7	0.3884	0.6115
14	0.3880	0.612

$$\min_{(\alpha,\beta,\lambda_1,\lambda_2,k,a,b)} Z\left(\alpha,\beta,\lambda_1,\lambda_2,k,a,b\right)=Z\left(\alpha^*,\beta^*,\lambda_1^*,\lambda_2^*,k^*,a^*,b^*\right). \tag{4.95}$$

We considered the following restrictions during the minimization process,

$$0<\alpha\leq 1,0\left\langle \beta\leq 1,\lambda_1\geq 0,\lambda_2\geq 0,k\right\rangle 0,a\geq 0,b\geq 0.$$

In experiments, described in Section 2.2.2.4, the following values where used: V_1 = 254.5 mm^3, V_2 = 1000 mm^3 and the diffusion area is A= 2.40 cm^2. From (4.95) we determined the following values of parameters

$$\alpha=0,\beta=0.99913,\ \lambda_1=8.7\times 10^{-7}\text{day}^{-1},\ \lambda_2=6.75\,\text{day}^{-1}$$

$$k=0.0199\frac{\text{cm}^4}{\text{day}},\ a=0.0284\,\text{day}^{-1.0},\ b=0.104\,\text{day}^{-0.000286},$$

where we omitted stars for the optimal values. The value of Z for parameters given by (4.95) is $Z\left(\alpha^*,\beta^*,\lambda_1^*,\lambda_2^*,k^*,a^*,b^*\right)=1.591\times 10^{-3}$. The values of the constants given by (4.95) agree with the results presented in Miskovic-Stankovic, Janev, and Atanackovic 2023 where $1-\alpha$ and $1-\beta$ are denoted by α and β. From the value of $k=0.0199\frac{cm^4}{day}$ we now determine the diffusion coefficient D. Since D is the coefficient of proportionality in Fick's law, we have to define a gradient of concentration in model (4.86). Let Δ be a length of the transition region, i.e., the region in which concentration changes from the value c_1 in compartment **1** to the value c_2 in compartment **2**. The gradient of concentration is defined as

$$\text{grad}\,c=\frac{\frac{Q_1}{V_1}-\frac{Q_2}{V_2}}{\Delta}. \tag{4.96}$$

Then we write (4.86) as

$$a\frac{1}{V_1}\,{}_0^C D_t^{\alpha,\lambda_a}Q_1\left(t\right)+b\frac{1}{V_1}\,{}_0^C D_t^{\alpha,\lambda_b}Q_1\left(t\right)=-k_{12}\Delta\frac{\left(\frac{Q_1}{V_1}-\frac{Q_2}{V_2}\right)}{\Delta}=-k_{12}\delta\text{grad}\,c,$$

$$a\frac{1}{V_2}\,{}_0^C D_t^{\alpha,\lambda_a}Q_2\left(t\right)+b\frac{1}{V_2}\,{}_0^C D_t^{\alpha,\lambda_b}Q_2\left(t\right)=k_{12}\Delta\frac{\left(\frac{Q_1}{V_1}-\frac{Q_2}{V_2}\right)}{\Delta}=k_{12}\delta\text{grad}\,c,$$

Now by dividing $k_{12}\Delta$ by the area of the exchange A, we obtain

$$D=\frac{\Delta\delta}{A}.$$

Since the shape of the hydrogel is cylindrical with a diameter of 9 mm and a height (thickness) of 4 mm, the area of the diffusion was calculated to be $A = 2.4\ \text{cm}^2$. The value of δ has no effect on the minimization (4.95). The diffusion coefficient determined in this manner is $D = 0.0333$ cm²/day or $D = 9.64\text{x}10^{-8}$ cm²/s, which is consistent with the literature data for gentamicin release from different polymer matrices ranging from $7.2\text{x}10^{-5}$ to $1.6\text{x}10^{-9}$ cm²/s[1] (Simovic et al. 2010; Thakur, Wanchoo, and Singh 2011; Croitoru et al. 2020; Bajpai, Shah, and Bajpai 2017; Della Porta et al. 2016). In addition, the value of diffusion coefficient, D, calculated from the GFD model, agrees well with the value of the diffusion coefficient calculated for the same PVA/Gent hydrogel using the modified ETA model,

$$D = 7.16 \times 10^{-8} \text{cm}^2 \text{s}^{-1} \left(\textit{Section } 2.2.2.4 \right)$$

Figures 4.2a and 4.2b show the agreement between experimental values of q_1 and q_2 with the values calculated according to (4.93) with the use of (4.91).

The collected data (GFD model) are compared to several theoretical models to clarify the diffusion parameters. We shall compare our data with the Makoid-Banakar, Korsmeyer-Peppas, and Kopcha models described by equations (4.97), (4.98), and (4.99), respectively.

$$\frac{C_t}{C_0} = \text{k}_{\text{MB}} \cdot t^{\text{n}} \cdot \exp\left(-\text{c} \cdot t\right) \tag{4.97}$$

$$\frac{C_t}{C_0} = \text{k}_{\text{KP}} \cdot t^{\text{n}} \tag{4.98}$$

$$\frac{C_t}{C_0} = \text{A} \cdot t^{1/2} + \text{B} \cdot t \tag{4.99}$$

Physical quantities and constants in (4.97)–(4.99) have the following meanings: c_t –the concentration of gentamicin released from hydrogel over time; c_0–the initial concentration of gentamicin inside the hydrogel; k_{MB}– Makoid-Banakar constant; c – Makoid-Banakar parameter (related to dissolution limitations as the function approaches maximum value); k_{KP} – Korsmeyer-Peppas constant; n – coefficient that describes transport mechanism ($\text{n} < 0.5$ – Fickian diffusion, $\text{n} > 0.5$ – non-Fickian/ anomalous diffusion, $\text{n} = 1$ – Case II transport; A and B – Kopcha's constants, which depend on the dominant transport phenomenon during release.

The calculated parameters and the fit quality evaluated using minimization of square residual, Z, for different models are listed in Table 4.2.

The models are presented along with experimental data in Figures 4.3a, 4.3b, and 4.3c for the Makoid-Banakar, Korsmeyer-Peppas, and Kopcha models and compared with GFD model (4.86), respectively. It should be noted that $q_2(t)$ in (4.86) is proportional to the concentration c_t, while $q_1(0)$ is proportional to the concentration, c_0.

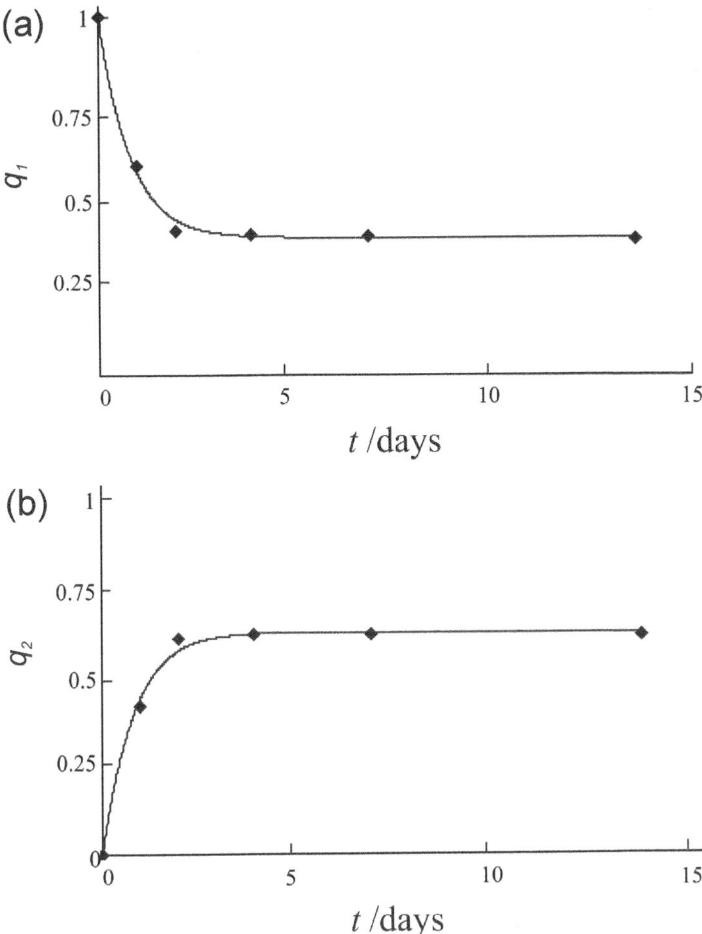

FIGURE 4.2 Change of relative mass in compartments: (a) decrease in amount of gentamicin remained in PVA/Gent hydrogel, q_1, with time, ♦experimental points, – GFD model, (b) increase in relative mass of released gentamicin from PVA/Gent hydrogel, q_2, with time, ♦experimental points, – GFD model (reprinted from Miskovic-Stankovic, Janev, and Atanackovic 2023 with permission from Springer Nature)

From Figure 4.3 and the values of square residuals, Z, presented in Table 4.2 it may be concluded that the GFD model (4.92) fits the experimental data better than the other models.

4.4.2 Gentamicin Release From Poly(Vinyl Alcohol)/Chitosan/Gentamicin Hydrogel

The experiments of gentamicin release from poly(vinyl alcohol)/chitosan/gentamicin hydrogel (PVA/CHI/Gent) are described in Section 2.2.2.4. The relative mass of the

TABLE 4.2
Fitting Parameters for Different Models of Gentamicin Release from PVA/Gent Hydrogel

Model GFD								
α	β	λ_1 day^{-1}	λ_2 day^{-1}	k (cm^4/day)	D (cm^{2}s^{-1})	a day$^{-1.0}$	b day$^{-0.000286}$	Z
0	0.99913	8.7×10^{-7}	6.75	0.0199	9.64×10^{-8}	0.028	0.103	0.0016
Krosmeyer-Peppas model								
k_{KP} (s^{-n})	n							Z
0.494	0.103							0.01358857
Makoid-Banakar model								
k_{MB} (s^{-n})	n	c						Z
0.493	0.189	0.0198						0.00819
Kopcha model								
A ($s^{-1/2}$)	B (s^{-1})							Z
0.228	-5×10^{-7}							0.194

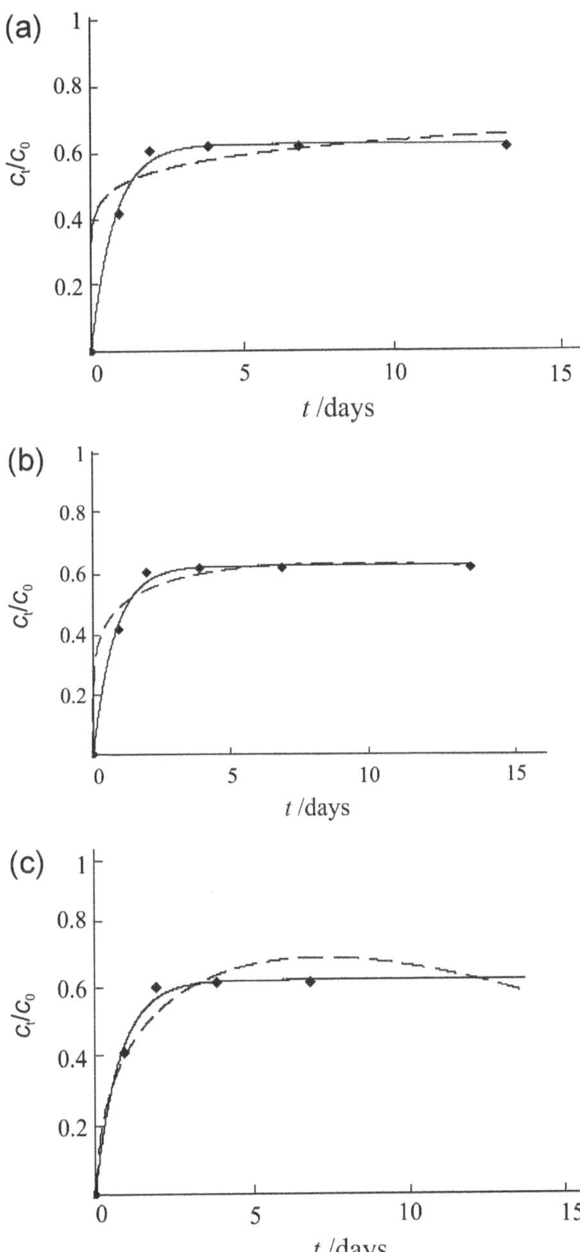

FIGURE 4.3 Comparison of (a) Korsmeyer-Peppas (dash line) and GFD models (solid line), (b) Makoid-Banakar (dash line) and GFD models (solid line), (c) Kopcha (dash line) and GFD models (solid line), for PVA/Gent hydrogel,, ♦experimental points

TABLE 4.3
The Measured Values of q_2 and Corresponding Values of q_1 (Reprinted from Miskovic-Stankovic and Atanackovic 2023 with Permission from MDPI)

t [days]	$q_1 = 1 - q_{2measured}(t_j)$	$q_{2measured}(t_j)$
0	1	0
1	0.72389	0.27611
2	0.330933	0.69067
4	0.2612	0.73880
7	0.25229	0.74771
14	0.25164	0.74836

gentamicin in hydrogel, q_1, and the relative mass of released gentamicin in deionized water surrounding hydrogel, q_2, are defined in (4.91) and presented in Table 4.3.

We determined the parameters in model (4.86), denoted as $\left(\alpha^*, \beta^*, \lambda_1^*, \lambda_2^*, a^*, b^*, k^*\right)$ from the condition (4.94). Thus, the optimal values $\left(\alpha^*, \beta^*, \lambda_1^*, \lambda_2^*, a^*, b^*, k^*\right)$ satisfy

$$\min_{(\alpha,\beta,\lambda_1,\lambda_2,a,b,k)} Z(\alpha,\beta,\lambda_1,\lambda_2,a,b,k) = Z\left(\alpha^*,\beta^*,\lambda_1^*,\lambda_2^*,a^*,b^*,k^*\right).$$

Again, in the minimization process we considered restrictions,

$$0 < \alpha \leq 1, 0 < \beta \leq 1, \lambda_1 \geq 0, \lambda_2 \geq 0, a \geq 0, b \geq 0, k \geq 0.$$

Experiments were performed with $V_1 = 254.5$ mm^3, $V_2 = 1000$ mm^3 and the area over which diffusion takes place A=2.40 cm^2. Condition (4.94) with Z given by (4.93) lead to

$$\alpha = 0.0, \beta = 0.9994, \lambda_1 = 8.7\times10^{-7}\text{day}^{-1},\ \lambda_2 = 6.63\ \text{day}^{-1}, a = 5.8\times10^{-3}\ \text{day}^{1},$$

$$b = 0.02501\ \text{day}^{-0.0006}, \qquad k\Delta = 0.0339\ \text{cm}^4/\text{day}$$

The corresponding diffusion coefficient, D, is calculated as follows. The shape of the hydrogel is cylinder with diameter 9 mm and height (thickness) 4 mm. The area of the diffusion is calculated to be A=2.4 cm^2. Therefore, diffusion coefficient is,

$$D = \frac{k}{A} = 2.50\times10^{-8}\ \text{cm}^2\text{s}^{-1}$$

The value of the coefficient of diffusion, D, calculated from the GFD model agrees well with the value of the diffusion coefficient calculated for the same PVA/CHI/Gent hydrogel using the modified ETA model, $D = 4.29\times10^{-8}\text{cm}^2\text{s}^{-1}$ (Section 2.2.2.4).

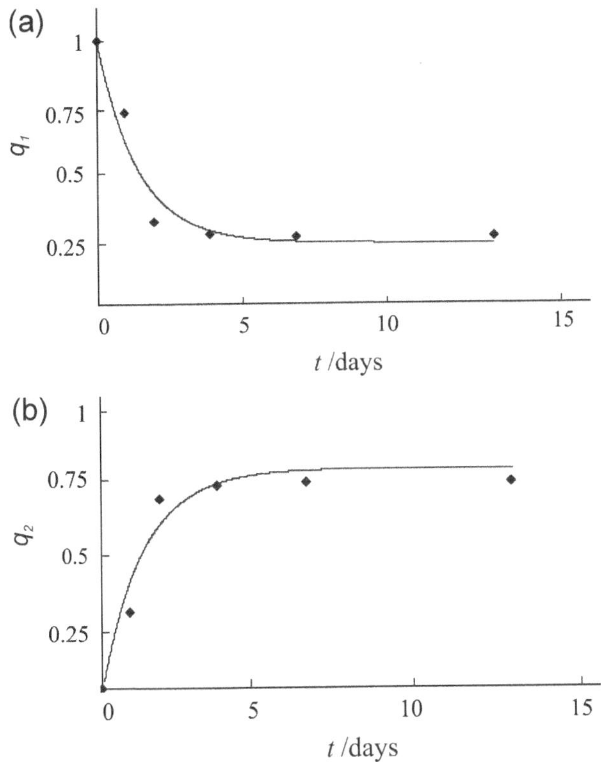

FIGURE 4.4 Change of relative mass in compartments: (a) decrease in amount of gentamicin remained in PVA/CHI/Gent hydrogel, q_1, with time, ◆ experimental points, – GFD model, (b) increase in relative mass of released gentamicin from PVA/CHI/Gent hydrogel, q_2, with time, ◆experimental points – GFD model (reprinted from Miskovic-Stankovic and Atanackovic 2023 with permission from MDPI)

Figures 4.4a and 4.4b depict the agreement between experimental values of q_1 and q_2 and the values calculated according to (4.93).

The parameters of GFD model (4.93) obtained from the condition (4.94), the Makoid-Banakar, Korsmeyer-Peppas, and Kopcha models described by (4.97)–(4.99), respectively, as well as the fit quality evaluated using minimization of square residual, Z, are listed in the Table 4.4.

The models are presented along with experimental profiles in Figures 4.5a, 4.5b, and 4.5c for Makoid-Banakar, Korsmeyer-Peppas, and Kopcha models compared with GFD model (4.93), respectively. It should be noted that $q_2(t)$ in our (4.93) is proportional to the concentration c_t, while $q_1(0)$ is proportional to the concentration, c_0.

It can be observed that equation (4.93) provided the lowest value of Z, i.e., the notably better correlation with the experimental data with respect to the other models. The Korsmeyer-Peppas and the Makoid-Banakar models did not differ

TABLE 4.4
Fitting Parameters for Different Models of Gentamicin Release from PVA/CHI/Gent Hydrogel

Model GFD								
α	β	λ_1 day^{-1}	λ_2 day^{-1}	k (cm^4/day)	D (cm^2s^{-1})	a $day^{-1.0}$	b $day^{-0.0006}$	Z
0	0.9994	$8.7x10^{-7}$	6.63	0.0339	$2.504x10^{-8}$	0.0058	0.026	0.0256
Krosmeyer-Peppas Model								
k_{KP} (s^{-n})	n							Z
0.474	0.214							0.0773
Makoid-Banakar Model								
k_{MB} (s^{-n})	n	c						Z
0.42	0.629	0.080						0.0367
Kopcha Model								
A $(s^{-1/2})$	B (s^{-1})							Z
0.473	0.21							0.2045

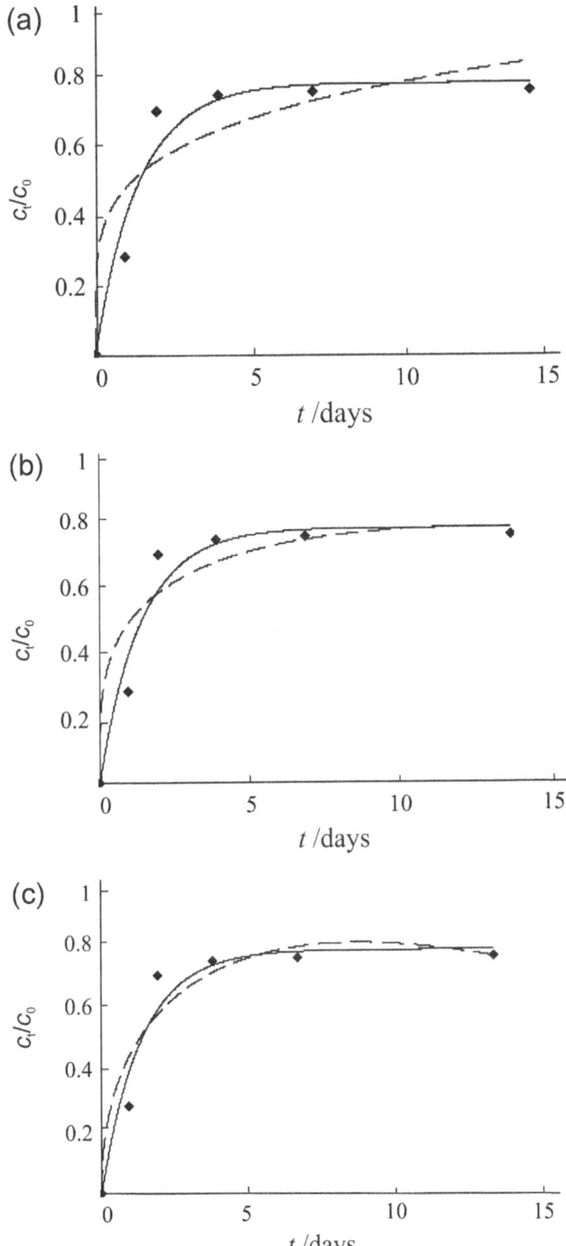

FIGURE 4.5 Comparison of (a) Korsmeyer-Peppas (dash line) and GFD models (solid line), (b) Makoid-Banakar (dash line) and GFD models (solid line), (c) Kopcha (dash line) and GFD models (solid line) for PVA/CHI/Gent hydrogel,◆ experimental points.

significantly, which was not surprising, as the Korsmeyer-Peppas model (4.98) can be consider as an approximation of the Makoid-Banakar model (4.97), in the case when $c \to 0$. From Table 4.4, it is obvious that the c parameter from the Makoid-Banakar model had small value, while parameter n, and k_{KP} and k_{MB} constants had similar values, indicating that the Makoid-Banakar and Korsmeyer-Peppas models were similar for gentamicin-loaded hydrogel. The time exponent n is an indication of the dominant diffusion mechanism, and, as its values were less than 0.5 (Table 4.4), it can be concluded that the release of gentamicin from hydrogel obeys the Fickian diffusion behavior and was governed mainly by the concentration gradient of released gentamicin. This was also proved by the Kopcha model as the absolute values of the parameter A were higher compared to |B|, indicating that the predominant driving force for the release is the diffusion and not the polymer matrix relaxation.

The general conclusion is that novel GFD model exhibited the best fitting with experimental data in comparison with the Korsmeyer-Peppas, Makoid-Banakar, and Kopcha models based on the minimal value of square residual Z. In addition, the diffusion coefficient of gentamicin was determined for entire period of the release in respect to ETA model that considers the initial release period. Finally, the diffusion coefficient of gentamicin release from PVA/CHI/Gent hydrogel (2.50×10^{-8} cm^2 s^{-1}) is lower than the diffusion coefficient of gentamicin for PVA/Gent hydrogel (9.64×10^{-8} cm^2 s^{-1}) due to more cross-linked hydrogel matrix as a consequence of the greater number of established hydrogen bonds on chitosan.

4.4.3 Gentamicin Release From Hydroxyapatite/Poly(Vinyl Alcohol)/Chitosan/Gentamicin Coating on Titanium Substrate. Distributed Order Fractional Models

We define a new model for the release of gentamicin from hydroxyapatite/poly(vinyl alcohol)/chitosan/gentamicin (HAP/PVA/CS/Gent) coating on titanium substrate. We start with (4.85)

$${}_0^C\bar{D}_t^{\alpha,\lambda} f(t) = \int_0^1 a^{\alpha}\, {}_0^C D_t^{\alpha} f(t)\, d\alpha.$$

where $a = const$. We shall use this equation to define kinetics of a two-compartmental model of pharmacokinetics. Recall that the classical two-compartmental model of pharmacokinetics, with different volumes of compartments is described as

$$\begin{aligned} \frac{dQ_1}{dt} &= -k\left(\frac{Q_1(t)}{V_1} - \frac{Q_2(t)}{V_2}\right) + f_1(t), \\ \frac{dQ_2}{dt} &= k\left(\frac{Q_1(t)}{V_1} - \frac{Q_2(t)}{V_2}\right) + f_2(t), \end{aligned} \tag{4.100}$$

We propose the generalization of this system of equations in which we replace first derivatives on the left-hand side by linear combination of general fractional derivative of order β given by (4.79) and distributed order general fractional derivative (4.85). Then for a Fick-type equation, i.e., (4.100) we obtain,

$$
\begin{aligned}
& b^{\beta}\,{}_0^C D_t^{\beta,\Lambda} Q_1(t) + {}_0^C \bar{D}_t^{\alpha,\lambda} Q_1(t) = -k\left(\frac{Q_1(t)}{V_1} - \frac{Q_2(t)}{V_2}\right) + f_1(t) \\
& b^{\beta}\,{}_0^C D_t^{\beta,\Lambda} Q_2(t) + {}_0^C \bar{D}_t^{\alpha,\lambda} Q_2(t) = k\left(\frac{Q_1(t)}{V_1} - \frac{Q_2(t)}{V_2}\right) + f_2(t)
\end{aligned}
\tag{4.101}
$$

where, again, $Q_i, V_i, i = 1,2$ denote the drug mass and volume of the compartment i, respectively. We also assume that a and b have the dimension of time.

Note that the expressions the left-hand side of (4.101) may be expressed in the form (4.84) with weighting functions taken as

$$
\varphi(\alpha(\alpha),\lambda(\alpha)) = \varphi_1\left(\delta(\alpha-\beta)b^{\alpha}, \Lambda = const.\right) + \varphi_2\left(a^{\alpha}, \lambda = const.\right),
$$

where δ denotes the Dirac distribution.

The system (4.101) is written in an expanded form as

$$
\begin{aligned}
& b^{\beta} a \frac{1}{\Gamma(1-\beta)} \int_0^t \frac{\exp(-\rangle\,\tau)}{\tau^{\beta}} Q_1^{(1)}(t-\tau)\,d\tau \\
& + \int_0^1 a^{\alpha}\left[\frac{1}{\Gamma(1-\alpha)} \int_0^t \frac{\exp(-\lambda\tau)}{\tau^{\alpha}} Q_1^{(1)}(t-\tau)\,d\tau\right] d\alpha \\
& = -k\Delta \frac{\left(\frac{Q_1(t)}{V_1} - \frac{Q_2(t)}{V_2}\right)}{\Delta} + f_1(t) \\
& b^{\beta} a \frac{1}{\Gamma(1-\beta)} \int_0^t \frac{\exp(-\Lambda\tau)}{\tau^{\beta}} Q_2^{(1)}(t-\tau)\,d\tau \\
& + \int_0^1 a^{\alpha}\left[\frac{1}{\Gamma(1-\alpha)} \int_0^t \frac{\exp(-\lambda\tau)}{\tau^{\alpha}} Q_2^{(1)}(t-\tau)\,d\tau\right] d\alpha \\
& = k\Delta \frac{\left(\frac{Q_1(t)}{V_1} - \frac{Q_2(t)}{V_2}\right)}{\Delta} + f_2(t)
\end{aligned}
\tag{4.102}
$$

To (4.102) we assign the following initial conditions that are used in our experiments

$$Q_1(0) = Q_0, \quad Q_2(0) = 0 \tag{4.103}$$

System (4.102) represents the two-compartmental model with general fractional derivative that we use in the analysis that follows.

Solution of the system (4.102), (4.103)

We use the Laplace transform method in solving (4.102), (4.103). Since

$$\mathscr{L}\left[{}_0^C D_t^{\alpha,\lambda} Q_i(t)\right](s) = \mathscr{L}\left[\frac{1}{\Gamma(1-\alpha)}\int_0^t \frac{\exp(-\lambda\tau)}{\tau^\alpha} Q_i^{(1)}(t-\tau)\,d\tau\right](s)$$

$$= \frac{s}{(s+\lambda_1)^{1-\alpha}}\left[s\hat{Q}_i(s) - Q_i(0)\right],\ i = 1,2,$$

by applying the Laplace transform to (4.85) we obtain

$$\mathscr{L}\left[{}_0^C \bar{D}_t^{\alpha,\lambda} Q_1(t)\right](s)$$

$$= \int_0^1 a^\alpha \left[\frac{s}{(s+\lambda)^{1-\alpha}}\hat{Q}_1(s) - \frac{1}{(s+\lambda)^{1-\alpha}} Q_1(0)\right] d\alpha$$

$$= a\int_0^1 \left[\frac{s}{\left[a(s+\lambda)\right]^{1-\alpha}}\hat{Q}_1(s) - \frac{1}{\left[a(s+\lambda)\right]^{1-\alpha}} Q_1(0)\right] d\alpha.$$

Let

$$K(s) = \int_0^1 \frac{d\alpha}{\left[a(s+\lambda)\right]^{1-\alpha}} = \frac{1-\left[a(s+\lambda)\right]^{-1}}{\ln\left[a(s+\lambda)\right]} = \frac{a(s+\lambda)-1}{a(s+\lambda)\ln\left[a(s+\lambda)\right]}, \tag{4.104}$$

so that

$$\mathscr{L}\left[{}_0^C \bar{D}_t^{\alpha,\lambda} Q_1(t)\right](s) = aK(s)\left(s\hat{Q}_1(s) - Q_1(0)\right) \tag{4.105}$$

We now apply the Laplace transform to (4.102), (4.103) and obtain,

$$\begin{aligned}
&\left[\frac{b}{\left[b(s+\Lambda)\right]^{1-\beta}} + aK(s)\right]\left[s\hat{Q}_1(s) - Q_1(0)\right] = -k\left(\frac{\hat{Q}_1(s)}{V_1} - \frac{\hat{Q}_2(s)}{V_2}\right) + \hat{f}_1(s),\\
&\left[\frac{b}{\left[b(s+\Lambda)\right]^{1-\beta}} + aK(s)\right] s\hat{Q}_2(s) = k\left(\frac{\hat{Q}_1(s)}{V_1} - \frac{\hat{Q}_2(s)}{V_2}\right) + \hat{f}_2(s).
\end{aligned} \tag{4.106}$$

By solving (4.106) we obtain the Laplace transform of Q_1 and Q_2 as

$$\hat{Q}_2(s) = \frac{1}{V_1} \frac{k\left(Q_1(0) + \dfrac{\hat{f}_1(s) + \hat{f}_2(s)}{\dfrac{b}{\left[b(s+\Lambda)\right]^{1-\beta}} + aK(s)} \right)}{s\left[\dfrac{bs}{\left[b(s+\Lambda)\right]^{1-\beta}} + asK(s) + k\left(\dfrac{1}{V_1} + \dfrac{1}{V_2} \right) \right]}, \quad (4.107)$$

and

$$\hat{Q}_1(s) = \frac{Q_1(0)}{s} - \frac{\hat{f}_1(s) + \hat{f}_2(s)}{s\left[\dfrac{b}{\left[b(s+\Lambda)\right]^{1-\beta}} + aK(s) \right]} - \frac{1}{V_1} \frac{k\left(Q_1(0) + \dfrac{\hat{f}_1(s) + \hat{f}_2(s)}{aK(s)} \right)}{s\left[\dfrac{bs}{\left[b(s+\Lambda)\right]^{1-\beta}} + asK(s) + k\left(\dfrac{1}{V_1} + \dfrac{1}{V_2} \right) \right]}. \quad (4.108)$$

Note that from (4.106) we obtain the following conservation of mass law,

$$Q_1(t) + Q_2(t) = Q_1(0) + {}^{-1}\left[\frac{\hat{f}_1(s) + \hat{f}_2(s)}{aK(s)} \right].$$

In the special case when $f_1(t) = f_2(t) = 0$, i.e., there is no addition/loss of the mass in the compartments, we have, as expected,

$$Q_1(t) + Q_2(t) = Q_1(0).$$

By using initial and final value theorems, for the case $f_1(t) = f_2(t) = 0$ the following estimates are obtained from (4.107), (4.108)

$$\lim_{s\to\infty} s\hat{Q}_1(s) = Q_1(0), \lim_{s\to 0} s\hat{Q}_1(s) = Q_1(\infty) = Q_1(0)\frac{V_1}{V_1+V_2}$$

$$\lim_{s\to 0} s\hat{Q}_2(s) = Q_2(\infty) = Q_1(0)\frac{V_2}{V_1+V_2} \quad (4.109)$$

Therefore, the limiting concentrations in each compartment $c_i = \frac{Q_i}{V_i}, i = 1,2$ are equal,

$$c_1(\infty) = c_2(\infty) = \frac{Q_1(\infty)}{V_1} = \frac{Q_2(\infty)}{V_2} = \frac{Q_1(0)}{V_1 + V_2},$$

in accordance with Fick's model of diffusion.

We present the results of numerical inversion of (4.107). Since in our experiments we have $f_1(t) = f_2(t) = 0$ the equation (4.107) reduces to

$$\hat{Q}_2(s) = \frac{1}{V_1} \frac{kQ_1(0)}{s\left[\frac{bs}{\left[b(s+\Lambda)\right]^{1-\beta}} + asK(s) + k\left(\frac{1}{V_1} + \frac{1}{V_2}\right)\right]},$$

so that

$$Q_2(t) = Q_1(0)\frac{k}{V_1}\frac{1}{2\pi}$$

$$\times \int_{x_0 - i\infty}^{x_0 + i\infty} \frac{\exp(x_0 + ip)t}{(x_0 + ip)\left[\frac{b(x_0 + ip)}{\left[b(x_0 + ip + \lambda_1)\right]^{1-\beta}} + a(x_0 + ip)K((x_0 + ip)) + k\left(\frac{1}{V_1} + \frac{1}{V_2}\right)\right]} dp \tag{4.110}$$

where x_0 chosen so that all zeros in the denominator of (4.107) are with the real part less than x_0. In the equation (4.110) it is necessary that $x_0 > 0$.

To improve the numerical minimization square residual, we introduce here the following dimensionless quantities, slightly different from that in (4.90) and in Miskovic-Stankovic and Atanackovic 2023

$$q_1(t) = \frac{Q_1(t)}{Q_1(0)},\ q_2(t) = \frac{Q_2(t)}{Q_1(0)},\ v_1 = \frac{V_1}{V_1},\ v_2 = \frac{V_2}{V_1},\ \bar{k} = \frac{k\Delta A}{V_1},$$

where Δ is characteristic length, see (4.96) and A denotes the area of the through which diffusion takes place and in our experiments was $A = 1$ cm². Note that $\Delta A / V_1$ represents the characteristic length of the system and $\dim k = \dim \bar{k} = \mathrm{s}$. The diffusion coefficient *D*, from the coefficient $\bar{k}$ is determined as $D = \frac{\bar{k}}{A}$. Multiplying (4.110) with $\frac{A}{Q_1(0)}$ we obtain,

$$q_2(t) = \bar{k}\frac{1}{2\pi}$$

$$\times \int_{x_0 - i\infty}^{x_0 + i\infty} \frac{\exp(x_0 + ip)t}{(x_0 + ip)\left[\frac{b(x_0 + ip)}{\left[b(x_0 + ip + \lambda_1)\right]^{1-\beta}} + a(x_0 + ip)K((x_0 + ip)) + \bar{k}\left(1 + \frac{V_1}{V_2}\right)\right]} dp, \tag{4.111}$$

where we used $A = 1\text{cm}^2$. Parameters in the model $,\bar{k},\lambda,b,\beta,\Lambda$, as in the previous examples, are determined by the least square method, i.e., the sum squared residuals Z between measured and calculated values of q_2 at five measured points, is minimized, that is,

$$Z(a,\bar{k},\lambda,b,\beta,\Lambda) = \sum_{j=1}^{5} (q_2(t_j) - q_{2measured}(t_j))^2.$$

Table 4.5 presents the measured values of $q_2(t)$ and calculated values of $q_1(t)$ from the mass conservation relation.

The parameters in the model $\left(a^*,\bar{k}^*,\lambda^*,b^*,\beta^*,\Lambda^*\right)$ are determined from the condition,

$$\min_{(a,k,\lambda,b,\beta,\Lambda)} Z(a,\bar{k},\lambda,b,\beta,\Lambda) = Z\left(a^*,\bar{k}^*,\lambda^*,b^*,\beta^*,\Lambda^*\right) \tag{4.112}$$

In the minimization process we considered restrictions

$$a > 0, b > 0, \bar{k} > 0,$$

TABLE 4.5
The Measured Values of q_2 and Corresponding Values of q_1 (Reprinted from Miskovic-Stankovic and Atanackovic 2023 with Permission from MDPI)

Time t [days]	$q_1 = 1 - q_{2measured}(t_j)$	$q_{2measured}(t_j)$
0	1	0
1	0.78	0.22
2	0.70	0.30
7	0.68	0.32
14	0.69	0.31
21	0.69	0.31

since a and b represent relaxation times and k relates to diffusion coefficient. Also, $\lambda \geq 0, \Lambda \geq 0$,
since this is required by the definition of general fractional derivative. Finally, we are dealing with Fick's diffusion, the function $Q_2(t), t \geq 0$ must be monotonically increasing. Since fractional derivative (4.101) for $\beta > 1$ has oscillatory behavior, we must have,

$$0 \leq \beta \leq 1.$$

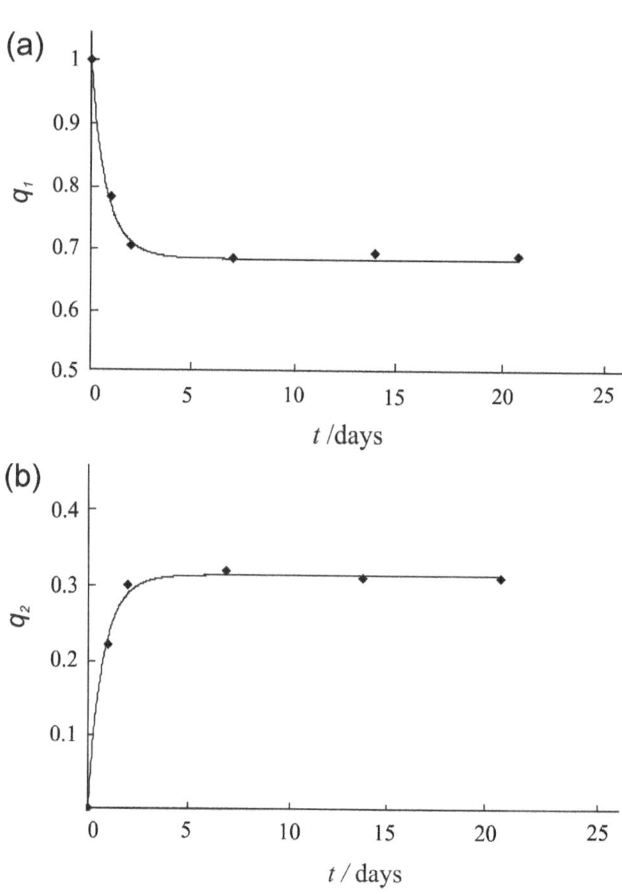

FIGURE 4.6 Change of relative mass in compartments: (a) decrease in amount of gentamicin remained in HAP/PVA/CS/Gent coating, q_1, with time, ◆ experimental points, – GFD model, (b) increase in relative mass of released gentamicin from HAP/PVA/CS/Gent coating, q_2, with time, ◆ experimental points – GFD model (reprinted from Miskovic-Stankovic and Atanackovic 2023 with permission from MDPI)

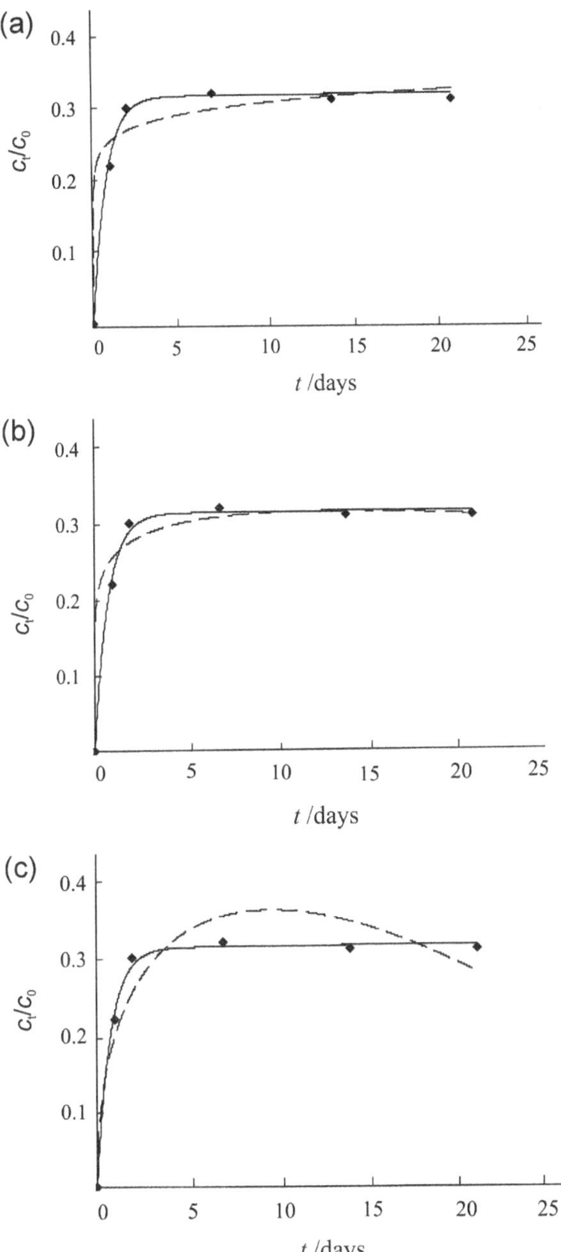

FIGURE 4.7 Comparison of (a) Korsmeyer-Peppas (dash line) and GFD models (solid line), (b) Makoid-Banakar (dash line) and GFD models (solid line), (c) Kopcha (dash line) and GFD models (solid line), for HAP/PVA/CS/Gent coating, ♦experimental points.

TABLE 4.6
Fitting Parameters for Different Models of Gentamicin Release from HAP/PVA/CS/Gent Coating

(4.111) Model							
A	**b**	**λ**	**Λ**	$\bar{k}$ **(cm^4/day)**	***D*** **(cm^2 s^{-1})**	**β**	***Z***
7.73×10^{-5}	0.158	8.476×10^{-4}	0.170	6.44×10^{-2}	7.455×10^{-7}	1	0.000263
Krosmeyer-Peppas Model							
k_{KP} (s^{-n})	**n**						
0.254	0.0808						0.00289
Makoid-Banakar Model							
k_{MB} (s^{-n})	**n**	**c**					
0.256	0.1288	0.00941					0.00194
A (s$^{-1/2}$)	**B (s^{-1})**						
0.233	-0.037						0.00606

Experiments described in Section 3.2.5.5 were performed with $V_1 = 254.5\ \text{mm}^3$, $V_2 = 1000\ \text{mm}^3$ and A=1 cm^2 , the area over which diffusion takes place. The condition $D = \frac{\bar{k}}{A}$ and (4.111) lead to

$$a = 7.7 \times 10^{-5}\text{day}, \quad \bar{k} = 6.44 \times 10^{-2}\text{day}, \quad \lambda = 8.47 \times 10^{-4}\text{day}^{-1}, \quad b = 0.158\ \text{day},$$

$$\beta = 1, \quad \Lambda = 0.170\ \text{day}^{-1}, \quad D = 7.45 \times 10^{-7} \frac{\text{cm}^2}{\text{s}}.$$

Figures 4.7a and 4.7b represent numerical results obtained from (4.111) with parameters determined from (4.112), showing excellent agreement between experimental (points) and calculated (line) values.

GFD model (4.102), i.e., (4.111) is compared with models (4.97)–(4.99) of Korsmeyer-Peppas, Makoid-Banakar, and Kopcha in Figures 4.7a–4.7c, respectively.

The calculated parameters and the fit quality evaluated using minimization of square residual, Z, for different models are listed in Table 4.6.

From the Figure 4.7 and the values of square residuals, Z, presented in Table 4.6 it may be concluded that the GFD model (4.110) fits experimental data better than the other models.

We conclude this section with remarks concerning the minimization of (4.112.). The numerical minimization may lead to different values for parameters $a, \bar{k}, \lambda, b, \beta, \Lambda$. To obtain a physically relevant solution, we must impose a restriction on the minimization procedure based on the physical laws that we describe. We are specifically using the Fick's diffusion. Therefore, the "driving force" of the mass exchange is the difference in concentrations. In equation $(4.102)_2$ the right-hand side is positive and therefore the left-hand side must be positive. From the definition of (4.13) we may conclude that $Q_2^{(1)}(t) \geq 0$. This implies, in turn, that $0 \leq \beta \leq 1$. This condition was observed in obtaining Figures 4.7a and 4.7b. However, if we let $1 \leq \beta \leq 2$ and minimize (4.112) we obtain a non-monotonic curves through the same experimental points. These curves approximate the measured points better; however, this solution is irrelevant since it predicts a mass flow with negative concentration gradient.

The general conclusion is that novel GFD model exhibited the best fitting with experimental data in comparison with the Korsmeyer-Peppas, Makoid-Banakar, and Kopcha models, based on the minimal value of square residual Z.

REFERENCES

Atanacković, Teodor M, Marko Janev, Sanja Konjik, Stevan Pilipović, and Dušan Zorica. 2014. "Expansion Formula for Fractional Derivatives in Variational Problems." *Journal of Mathematical Analysis and Applications* 409 (2): 911–24. https://doi.org/10.1016/j.jmaa.2013.07.071.

Atanacković, Teodor M, Sanja Konjik, Stevan Pilipović, and Srboljub Simić. 2009. "Variational Problems with Fractional Derivatives: Invariance Conditions and Nöther's Theorem." *Nonlinear Analysis, Theory, Methods and Applications* 71 (5–6): 1504–17. https://doi.org/10.1016/j.na.2008.12.043.

Atanacković, Teodor M, Stevan Pilipović, Bogoljub Stanković, and Dušan Zorica. 2014a. *Fractional Calculus with Applications in Mechanics: Vibrations and Diffusion Processes*. New York: John Wiley & Sons, Inc. https://doi.org/10.1002/9781118577530.

———. 2014b. *Fractional Calculus With Applications in Mechanics: Wave Propagation, Impact and Variational Principles*. New York: John Wiley & Sons, Inc. https://doi.org/10.1002/9781118909065.

Atanacković, Teodor M, and B Stanković. 2004. "An Expansion Formula for Fractional Derivatives and Its Application." *Fractional Calculus and Applied Analysis* 7 (3): 365–78.

———. 2008. "On a Numerical Scheme for Solving Differential Equations of Fractional Order." *Mechanics Research Communications* 35 (7): 429–38. https://doi.org/10.1016/j.mechrescom.2008.05.003.

Bajpai, SK, FF Shah, and M Bajpai. 2017. "Dynamic Release of Gentamicin Sulfate (GS) from Alginate Dialdehyde (AD)-Crosslinked Casein (CAS) Films for Antimicrobial Applications." *Designed Monomers and Polymers* 20 (1): 18–32. https://doi.org/10.1080/15685551.2016.1231037.

Cohen, Alan M. 2007. *Numerical Methods for Laplace Transform Inversion*. Edited by Claude Brezinski. New York: Springer Science Business Media. https://doi.org/10.1007/978-0-387-68855-8.

Croitoru, Catalin, Ionut Claudiu Roata, Alexandru Pascu, and Elena Manuela Stanciu. 2020. "Diffusion and Controlled Release in Physically Crosslinked Poly (Vinyl Alcohol)/Iota-Carrageenan Hydrogel Blends." *Polymers* 12 (7): 1–25. https://doi.org/10.3390/polym12071544.

Diethelm, K, V Kiryakova, Y Luchko, JA Tenreiro Machado, and VE Tarasov. 2022. "Trends, Directions for Further Research, and Some Open Problems of Fractional Calculus." *Nonlinear Dynamics* 107 (4): 3245–70. https://doi.org/10.1007/s11071-021-07158-9.

Doetsch, Gustav. 1974. *Introduction to the Theory and Application of the Laplace Transformation*. Berlin, Heidelberg and New York: Springer-Verlag. https://doi.org/10.1007/978-3-642-65690-3.

Dokoumetzidis, Aristides, and Panos Macheras. 2009. "Fractional Kinetics in Drug Absorption and Disposition Processes." *Journal of Pharmacokinetics and Pharmacodynamics* 36 (2): 165–78. https://doi.org/10.1007/s10928-009-9116-x.

Dokoumetzidis, Aristides, Richard Magin, and Panos Macheras. 2010a. "Fractional Kinetics in Multi-Compartmental Systems." *Journal of Pharmacokinetics and Pharmacodynamics* 37 (5): 507–24. https://doi.org/10.1007/s10928-010-9170-4.

———. 2010b. "A Commentary on Fractionalization of Multi-Compartmental Models." *Journal of Pharmacokinetics and Pharmacodynamics* 37 (2): 203–7. https://doi.org/10.1007/s10928-010-9153-5.

Garrappa, Roberto, Eva Kaslik, and Marina Popolizio. 2019. "Evaluation of Fractional Integrals and Derivatives of Elementary Functions: Overview and Tutorial." *Mathematics*. https://doi.org/10.3390/math7050407.

Gorenflo, Rudolf, Anatoly A Kilbas, Francesco Mainardi, and Sergei V Rogosin. 2014. *Mittag-Leffler Functions, Related Topics and Applications*. Springer Monographs in Mathematics. Berlin, Heidelberg: Springer. https://doi.org/10.1007/978-3-662-43930-2.

Hanyga, Andrzej. 2020. "A Comment on a Controversial Issue: A Generalized Fractional Derivative Cannot Have a Regular Kernel." *Fractional Calculus and Applied Analysis* 23 (1): 211–23. https://doi.org/doi:10.1515/fca-2020-0008.

Hilfer, Rudolf. 2019. "Mathematical and Physical Interpretations of Fractional Derivatives and Integrals. Volume 1: Basic Theory." In *Handbook of Fractional Calculus with Applications*, edited by Anatoly Kochubei and Yuri Luchko, 47–85. Berlin: de Gruyter. https://doi.org/10.1515/9783110571622.

Hilfer, Rudolf, and Yuri Luchko. 2019. "Desiderata for Fractional Derivatives and Integrals." *Mathematics*. https://doi.org/10.3390/math7020149.

Kilbas, Anatoly A, Hari M Srivastava, and Juan J Trujillo, eds. 2006. *Theory and Applications of Fractional Differential Equations*. Amsterdam: Elsevier.

Kochubei, AN. 2011. "General Fractional Calculus, Evolution Equations, and Renewal Processes." *Integral Equations and Operator Theory* 71 (4): 583–600. https://doi.org/10.1007/s00020-011-1918-8.

Luchko, Yuri. 2021a. "General Fractional Integrals and Derivatives of Arbitrary Order." *Symmetry*. https://doi.org/10.3390/sym13050755.

———. 2021b. "General Fractional Integrals and Derivatives with the Sonine Kernels." *Mathematics*. https://doi.org/10.3390/math9060594.

———. 2021c. "Operational Calculus for the General Fractional Derivative and Its Applications." *Fractional Calculus and Applied Analysis* 24 (2): 338–75. https://doi.org/10.1515/fca-2021-0016.

———. 2023. "On the 1st-Level General Fractional Derivatives of Arbitrary Order." *Fractal and Fractional*. https://doi.org/10.3390/fractalfract7020183.

Miskovic-Stankovic, Vesna, and Teodor M Atanackovic. 2023. "On a System of Equations with General Fractional Derivatives Arising in Diffusion Theory." *Fractal and Fractional*. https://doi.org/10.3390/fractalfract7070518.

Miskovic-Stankovic, Vesna, Marko Janev, and Teodor M Atanackovic. 2023. "Two Compartmental Fractional Derivative Model with General Fractional Derivative." *Journal of Pharmacokinetics and Pharmacodynamics* 50 (2): 79–87. https://doi.org/10.1007/s10928-022-09834-8.

Molina-Garcia, Daniel, Trifce Sandev, Hadiseh Safdari, Gianni Pagnini, Aleksei Chechkin, and Ralf Metzler. 2018. "Crossover from Anomalous to Normal Diffusion: Truncated Power-Law Noise Correlations and Applications to Dynamics in Lipid Bilayers." *New Journal of Physics* 20: 103027. https://doi.org/10.1088/1367-2630/aae4b2.

Odibat, Zaid M., and Nabil T Shawagfeh. 2007. "Generalized Taylor's Formula." *Applied Mathematics and Computation* 186 (1): 286–93. https://doi.org/10.1016/j.amc.2006.07.102.

Ortigueira, Manuel D, and JA Tenreiro Machado. 2015. "What Is a Fractional Derivative?" *Journal of Computational Physics* 293: 4–13. https://doi.org/10.1016/j.jcp.2014.07.019.

Podlubny, I. 1999. *Fractional Differential Equations*. San Diego: Academic Press.

Popović, Jovan K, Milica T Atanacković, Ana S Pilipović, Milan R Rapaić, Stevan Pilipović, and Teodor M Atanacković. 2010. "A New Approach to the Compartmental Analysis in Pharmacokinetics: Fractional Time Evolution of Diclofenac." *Journal of Pharmacokinetics and Pharmacodynamics* 37 (2): 119–34. https://doi.org/10.1007/s10928-009-9147-3.

Porta, Giovanna Della, Roberta Campardelli, Vincenzo Cricchio, Francesco Oliva, Nicola Maffulli, and Ernesto Reverchon. 2016. "Injectable PLGA/Hydroxyapatite/Chitosan Microcapsules Produced by Supercritical Emulsion Extraction Technology: An In Vitro Study on Teriparatide/Gentamicin Controlled Release." *Journal of Pharmaceutical Sciences* 105 (7): 2164–72. https://doi.org/10.1016/j.xphs.2016.05.002.

Rescigno, Aldo. 2003. *Foundations of Pharmacokinetics*. New York: Kluwer Academic/Plenum Publishers.

Samko, Stefan G, and Rogério P Cardoso. 2003. "Integral Equations of the First Kind of Sonine Type." *International Journal of Mathematics and Mathematical Sciences* 2003 (57): 3609–32. https://doi.org/10.1155/S0161171203211455.

Samko, Stefan G, Anatoly A Kilbas, and OI Marichev. 1993. "Fractional Integrals and Derivatives: Theory and Applications." https://api.semanticscholar.org/CorpusID:118631078.

Sandev, Trifce, Aleksei Chechkin, Holger Kantz, and Ralf Metzler. 2015. "Diffusion and Fokker-Planck-Smoluchowski Equations with Generalized Memory Kernel." *Fractional Calculus and Applied Analysis* 18 (4): 1006–38. https://doi.org/10.1515/fca-2015-0059.

Sandev, Trifce, Igor M Sokolov, Ralf Metzler, and Aleksei Chechkin. 2017. "Beyond Monofractional Kinetics." *Chaos, Solitons & Fractals* 102: 210–17. https://doi.org/10.1016/j.chaos.2017.05.001.

Simovic, Ljiljana, Petar Skundric, Ivana Pajic-Lijakovic, Katarina Ristic, Adela Medovic, and Goran Tasić. 2010. "Mathematical Model of Gentamicin Sulfate Release from a Bioactive Textile Material as a Transdermal System under in Vitro Conditions." *Journal of Applied Polymer Science* 117 (3): 1424–30. https://doi.org/10.1002/app.31964.

Sopasakis, Pantelis, Haralambos Sarimveis, Panos Macheras, and Aristides Dokoumetzidis. 2018. "Fractional Calculus in Pharmacokinetics." *Journal of Pharmacokinetics and Pharmacodynamics* 45 (1): 107–25. https://doi.org/10.1007/s10928-017-9547-8.

Tarasov, Vasily E. 2019. "Rules for Fractional-Dynamic Generalizations: Difficulties of Constructing Fractional Dynamic Models." *Mathematics*. https://doi.org/10.3390/math7060554.

———. 2021. "General Fractional Dynamics." *Mathematics*. https://doi.org/10.3390/math9131464.

———. 2022. "General Non-Local Continuum Mechanics: Derivation of Balance Equations." *Mathematics*. https://doi.org/10.3390/math10091427.

Thakur, A, RK Wanchoo, and P Singh. 2011. "Hydrogels of Poly(Acrylamide-Co-Acrylic Acid): In-Vitro Study on Release of Gentamicin Sulfate." *Chemical and Biochemical Engineering Quarterly* 25 (4): 471–82.

Verotta, D. 2010. "Fractional Compartmental Models and Multi-Term Mittag–Leffler Response Functions." *Journal of Pharmacokinetics and Pharmacodynamics* 37 (2): 209–15. https://doi.org/10.1007/s10928-010-9155-3.

Valério, D, JJ Trujillo, M Rivero, JAT Machado, and D Baleanu. 2013. "Fractional Calculus: A Survey of Useful Formulas." *The European Physical Journal Special Topics* 222 (8): 1827–46. https://doi.org/10.1140/epjst/e2013-01967-y.

Yang, Xiao-Jun. 2019. *General Fractional Derivatives Theory, Methods and Applications*, 1st ed. Boca Raton, FL: CRC Press Taylor & Francis Group.

Yang, Xiao-Jun, Feng Gao, and Yang Ju. 2020. *General Fractional Derivatives with Applications in Viscoelasticity*. London: Academic Press.

Index

For Product Safety Concerns and Information please contact our EU representative GPSR@taylorandfrancis.com Taylor & Francis Verlag GmbH, Kaufingerstraße 24, 80331 München, Germany

Batch number: 10397790

Printed by Printforce, the Netherlands